Neurology for the Non-Neurologist

Editor

TRACEY A. MILLIGAN

MEDICAL CLINICS
OF NORTH AMERICA

www.medical.theclinics.com

Consulting Editor
BIMAL H. ASHAR

March 2019 • Volume 103 • Number 2

ELSEVIER

1600 John F. Kennedy Boulevard ● Suite 1800 ● Philadelphia, Pennsylvania, 19103-2899

http://www.theclinics.com

MEDICAL CLINICS OF NORTH AMERICA Volume 103, Number 2
March 2019 ISSN 0025-7125, ISBN-13: 978-0-323-65471-5

Editor: Jessica McCool
Developmental Editor: Kristen Helm

Medical Clinics of North America (ISSN 0025-7125) is published bimonthly by Elsevier Inc., 360 Park Avenue South, New York, NY 10010-1710. Months of publication are January, March, May, July, September, and November. Business and editorial offices: 1600 John F. Kennedy Boulevard, Suite 1800, Philadelphia, PA 19103-2899. Periodicals postage paid at New York, NY, and additional mailing offices. Subscription prices are USD $284.00 per year (US individuals), $611.00 per year (US institutions), $100.00 per year (US Students), $353.00 per year (Canadian individuals), $794.00 per year (Canadian institutions), $200.00 per year (Canadian and foreign students), $406.00 per year (foreign individuals), and $794.00 per year (foreign institutions). To receive student/resident rate, orders must be accompanied by name of affiliated institution, date of term, and the signature of program/residency coordinator on institution letterhead. Orders will be billed at individual rate until proof of status is received. Foreign air speed delivery is included in all Clinics' subscription prices. All prices are subject to change without notice. **POSTMASTER:** Send address changes to *Medical Clinics of North America*, Elsevier Health Sciences Division, Subscription Customer Service, 3251 Riverport Lane, Maryland Heights, MO 63043. **Customer Service: Telephone: 1-800-654-2452** (U.S. and Canada); **1-314-447-8871** (outside U.S. and Canada). **Fax: 314-447-8029. E-mail: journalscustomerserviceusa@elsevier.com** (for print support); **journalsonlinesupport-usa@elsevier.com** (for online support).

Reprints. For copies of 100 or more of articles in this publication, please contact the Commercial Reprints Department, Elsevier Inc., 360 Park Avenue South, New York, NY 10010-1710. Tel.: 212-633-3874; Fax: 212-633-3820; E-mail: reprints@elsevier.com.

Medical Clinics of North America is also published in Spanish by McGraw-Hill Interamericana Editores S. A., P.O. Box 5-237, 06500 Mexico, D.F., Mexico.

Medical Clinics of North America is covered in *MEDLINE/PubMed (Index Medicus), Current Contents, ASCA, Excerpta Medica, Science Citation Index,* and *ISI/BIOMED.*

PROGRAM OBJECTIVE
The goal of the *Medical Clinics of North America* is to keep practicing physicians up to date with current clinical practice by providing timely articles reviewing the state of the art in patient care.

TARGET AUDIENCE
All practicing physicians and other healthcare professionals.

LEARNING OBJECTIVES
Upon completion of this activity, participants will be able to:
1. Review the etiology, signs, and symptoms of common entrapment neuropathies of the upper and lower extremities and strategies for selecting treatment modalities.
2. Discuss identification, diagnosis, and management of concussion.
3. Recognize diagnostic challenges and preventive treatment options for migraine and treatment of tension-type headache

ACCREDITATION
The Elsevier Office of Continuing Medical Education (EOCME) is accredited by the Accreditation Council for Continuing Medical Education (ACCME) to provide continuing medical education for physicians.

The EOCME designates this enduring material for a maximum of 15 *AMA PRA Category 1 Credit*(s)™. Physicians should claim only the credit commensurate with the extent of their participation in the activity.

All other healthcare professionals requesting continuing education credit for this enduring material will be issued a certificate of participation.

DISCLOSURE OF CONFLICTS OF INTEREST
The EOCME assesses conflict of interest with its instructors, faculty, planners, and other individuals who are in a position to control the content of CME activities. All relevant conflicts of interest that are identified are thoroughly vetted by EOCME for fair balance, scientific objectivity, and patient care recommendations. EOCME is committed to providing its learners with CME activities that promote improvements or quality in healthcare and not a specific proprietary business or a commercial interest.

The planning committee, staff, authors and editors listed below have identified no financial relationships or relationships to products or devices they or their spouse/life partner have with commercial interest related to the content of this CME activity:
Bimal H. Ashar, MD, MBA, FACP; Kelsey Barrell, MD; Shamik Bhattacharyya, MD, MS; Michael P. Bowley, MD, PhD; Rebecca Burch, MD; Fan Z. Caprio, MD; Christopher T. Doughty, MD; Kristin M. Galetta, MD; Kristen Helm; William T. Jackson, MD; Emily L. Johnson, MD; Alison Kemp; Jessica McCool; Tracey A. Milligan, MD, MS, FAAN; Stephen G. Reich, MD; Paul B. Rizzoli, MD; Michael Ronthal, MbBCh; Joseph M. Savitt, MD, PhD; A. Gordon Smith, MD; Farzaneh A. Sorond, MD, PhD; Jeyanthi Surendrakumar; Angeliki Vgontzas, MD; Gregory T. Whitman, MD.

The planning committee, staff, authors and editors listed below have identified financial relationships or relationships to products or devices they or their spouse/life partner have with commercial interest related to the content of this CME activity:
Alireza Atri, MD, PhD: is a consultant/advisor for Allergan, Eisia Co., Ltd, and Grifols, S.A., Suven Life Sciences Limited, and Synexus Clinical Research Limited; Dr. Atri is a consultant/advisor for and receives research support from AbbVie Inc., Avid Technology, Inc., Biogen, and Eli Lilly and Company, Lundbeck, Merck Sharp & Dohme Corp., a subsidiary of Merck & Co., Inc., Novartis AG, and VTV Therapeutics; Dr. Atri is a consultant/advisor for and earns royalties and/or holds patents with Oxford University Press.
Amaal J. Starling, MD, FAHS: serves as a consultant or on advisory boards for Alder Biopharmaceuticals, Inc, Amgen Inc, Eli Lilly and Company, and eNeura Inc.

UNAPPROVED/OFF-LABEL USE DISCLOSURE
The EOCME requires CME faculty to disclose to the participants;
1. When products or procedures being discussed are off-label, unlabelled, experimental, and/or investigational (not US Food and Drug Administration [FDA] approved); and
2. Any limitations on the information presented, such as data that are preliminary or that represent ongoing research, interim analyses, and/or unsupported opinions. Faculty may discuss information about pharmaceutical agents that is outside of FDA-approved labelling. This information is intended solely for CME and is not intended to promote off-label use of these medications. If you have any questions, contact the medical affairs department of the manufacturer for the most recent prescribing information.

TO ENROLL

To enroll in the *Medical Clinics of North America* Continuing Medical Education program, call customer service at 1-800-654-2452 or sign up online at http://www.theclinics.com/home/cme. The CME program is available to subscribers for an additional annual fee of USD $300.90.

METHOD OF PARTICIPATION

In order to claim credit, participants must complete the following;

1. Complete enrolment as indicated above.
2. Read the activity.
3. Complete the CME Test and Evaluation. Participants must achieve a score of 70% on the test. All CME Tests and Evaluations must be completed online.

CME INQUIRIES/SPECIAL NEEDS

For all CME inquiries or special needs, please contact elsevierCME@elsevier.com.

ISSUE OF RELATED INTEREST

Neurologic Clinics, February 2018 (Vol. 36, No. 1)
Multiple Sclerosis
Darin T. Okuda, *Editor*
Available at: http://www.neurologic.theclinics.com/

Contributors

CONSULTING EDITOR

BIMAL H. ASHAR, MD, MBA, FACP
Associate Professor of Medicine, Division of General Internal Medicine, The Johns Hopkins University School of Medicine, Baltimore, Maryland

EDITOR

TRACEY A. MILLIGAN, MD, MS, FAAN
Assistant Professor, Department of Neurology, Harvard Medical School, Vice Chair for Education, Department of Neurology, Distinguished Clinician, Brigham and Women's Hospital, Boston, Massachusetts

AUTHORS

ALIREZA ATRI, MD, PhD
Director, Banner Sun Health Research Institute, Banner Health, Sun City, Arizona; Lecturer, Department of Neurology, Center for Brain/Mind Medicine, Brigham and Women's Hospital, Harvard Medical School, Boston, Massachusetts

KELSEY BARRELL, MD
Assistant Professor of Neurology, University of Utah School of Medicine, Salt Lake City, Utah

SHAMIK BHATTACHARYYA, MD, MS
Assistant Professor, Department of Neurology, Brigham and Women's Hospital, Harvard Medical School, Boston, Massachusetts

MICHAEL P. BOWLEY, MD, PhD
Assistant in Neurology, Massachusetts General Hospital, Instructor, Harvard Medical School, Boston, Massachusetts

REBECCA BURCH, MD
Staff Physician, Assistant Professor, Department of Neurology, John R. Graham Headache Center, Brigham and Women's Hospital, Harvard Medical School, Jamaica Plain, Massachusetts

FAN Z. CAPRIO, MD
Assistant Professor of Neurology, Division of Stroke and Neurocritical Care, Northwestern University Feinberg School of Medicine, Chicago, Illinois

CHRISTOPHER T. DOUGHTY, MD
Department of Neurology, Associate Neurologist, Brigham and Women's Hospital, Instructor, Harvard Medical School, Boston, Massachusetts

KRISTIN M. GALETTA, MD
Resident, Department of Neurology, Brigham and Women's Hospital, Harvard Medical School, Department of Neurology, Massachusetts General Hospital, Boston, Massachusetts

WILLIAM T. JACKSON, MD
Resident, Department of Neurology, Mayo Clinic College of Medicine, Scottsdale, Arizona

EMILY L. JOHNSON, MD
Assistant Professor, Department of Neurology, The Johns Hopkins School of Medicine, Baltimore, Maryland

TRACEY A. MILLIGAN, MD, MS, FAAN
Assistant Professor, Department of Neurology, Harvard Medical School, Vice Chair for Education, Department of Neurology, Distinguished Clinician, Brigham and Women's Hospital, Boston, Massachusetts

STEPHEN G. REICH, MD
Professor, The Frederick Henry Prince Distinguished Professor, Department of Neurology, University of Maryland School of Medicine, Baltimore, Maryland

PAUL B. RIZZOLI, MD, FAAN, FAHS
Assistant Professor, Department of Neurology, Brigham and Women's Hospital, Clinical and Fellowship Director, John R. Graham Headache Center, Brigham and Women's Faulkner Hospital, Harvard Medical School, Boston, Massachusetts

MICHAEL RONTHAL, MBBCh, FRCP, FRCPE, FCP (SA)
Professor of Neurology, Harvard Medical School, Beth Israel Deaconess Medical Center, Boston, Massachusetts

JOSEPH M. SAVITT, MD, PhD
Associate Professor of Neurology, University of Maryland School of Medicine, Baltimore, Maryland

A. GORDON SMITH, MD
Professor and Chair of Neurology, Virginia Commonwealth University, Richmond, Virginia

FARZANEH A. SOROND, MD, PhD
Professor of Neurology, Chief, Division of Stroke and Neurocritical Care, Northwestern University Feinberg School of Medicine, Chicago, Illinois

AMAAL J. STARLING, MD, FAHS
Assistant Professor, Department of Neurology, Mayo Clinic College of Medicine, Scottsdale, Arizona

ANGELIKI VGONTZAS, MD
Department of Neurology, Brigham and Women's Hospital, Neurology Staff, John R. Graham Headache Center, Brigham and Women's Faulkner Hospital, Harvard Medical School, Boston, Massachusetts

GREGORY T. WHITMAN, MD
Instructor of Otolaryngology, Harvard Medical School, Massachusetts Eye and Ear Infirmary, Massachusetts Eye and Ear Balance and Vestibular Center, Braintree, Massachusetts

Contents

The diagnosis of neurologic disease is relevant to the non-neurologist because neurologic symptoms are a common reason patients present to their health care provider and most of these patients are never referred to a neurologist. The diagnosis of a neurologic disease is a rewarding endeavor because it requires intellectual rigor, skill, and is of paramount importance to patient care. A tailored history and examination lead to localization and differential diagnosis. Diagnostic testing often involves neuroimaging and serum testing and also may involve lumbar puncture, electroencephalogram, nerve conduction studies, and electromyography. In the modern era, all neurologic diagnoses lead to treatments.

Dizziness and imbalance are common and challenging chief complaints carrying high morbidity, due to their association with falls, injuries, and loss of quality of life. The physical examination represents an opportunity to collect objective clinical data that facilitate an understanding of symptoms that might otherwise be enigmatic and ineffable. This review focuses on the examination techniques used routinely by physicians who provide specialized care for patients with dizziness and imbalance.

Gait disorders in the elderly may be based on a neurologic deficit at multiples levels, or may be secondary to nonneurologic causes. The physiology and pathophysiology of gait problems are reviewed and bedside examination and investigative tools are discussed. The reader will have an excellent working knowledge of the subject and will know how to diagnose and treat gait disorders and falls.

Migraine and tension-type headache are highly prevalent. Migraine is associated with significant work- and family-related disability. Migraine is underdiagnosed; it reasonable to err on the side of migraine when choosing between primary headaches. Barriers to appropriate treatment of migraine include lack of access to providers, misdiagnosis, and acute and preventive therapies not being prescribed. Acute, rescue, and preventive treatment options are extensive, and new classes of treatments are either available or in development. This review addresses diagnostic challenges including recognizing migraine with aura. It also summarizes nonpharmacologic, acute, rescue, and preventive treatment options for migraine and treatment of tension-type headache.

The vast majority of headache patients encountered in the outpatient general medicine setting will be diagnosed with a primary headache disorder, mostly migraine or tension-type headache. Other less common primary headaches and secondary headaches, related to or caused by another condition, are the topic of this article. Nonmigraine primary headaches include trigeminal autonomic cephalalgias, primarily cluster headache; facial pain, primarily trigeminal neuralgia; and miscellaneous headache syndromes, such as hemicrania continua and new daily persistent headache. Selected secondary headaches related to vascular disease, cerebrospinal fluid dynamics, and inflammatory conditions are also reviewed.

Concussion is a public health crisis affecting vulnerable populations including youth athletes. As awareness increases, more patients with acute concussion are seeking medical evaluations. Internists are frontline medical providers and thus should be able to identify, diagnose, manage, and know when to refer patients with concussion. Management of concussion includes rapid removal from play, symptomatic treatment, and return to learn/play recommendations. Inappropriate management may lead to recurrent concussions, prolonged recovery, and potential long-term consequences. Understanding the key features of diagnosis, postinjury assessment tools, symptomatic treatment, and management of concussion, including return to learn/play recommendations, is essential for primary care providers.

Alzheimer's disease (AD) care requires timely diagnosis and multidisciplinary management. Evaluation involves structured patient and caregiver history and symptom-function reviews, examination, and testing (laboratory and neuroimaging) to delineate impairment level, determine the cognitive-behavioral syndrome, and diagnose cause. Clinical biomarkers are available to aid high confidence in etiologic diagnosis. Management uses psychoeducation, shared goal setting, and patient-caregiver dyad decision making. When combined, pharmacologic and nonpharmacologic therapies mitigate symptoms and reduce clinical progression and care burden. AD biopathologic processes develop over decades before symptoms manifest; this period is increasingly targeted in research as an opportunity to best delay or prevent AD dementia.

Despite advances in earlier diagnosis and available aggressive treatments for vascular risk factors, stroke remains a leading cause of death and long-term disability worldwide. Disparities exist in stroke risk, rates of stroke, and treatment. Stroke is a heterogeneous disease with multiple additive risk factors and causes. Primary prevention of stroke focusing on risk factor modification plays an important role in reducing the burden of stroke in an aging population. Secondary prevention of recurrent strokes relies on the workup and a tailored treatment targeted at the mechanisms responsible for the incident stroke or transient ischemic attack.

Epilepsy affects 65 million people worldwide, and is a leading neurologic cause of loss of quality-adjusted life years. The diagnosis of seizures and epilepsy often depends on a careful history, and is supported with electroencephalogram and imaging. First-line treatment of epilepsy includes medical management. Antiepileptic drugs must be chosen with the patient's particular comorbidities in mind. Drug-resistant epilepsy cases should be referred to an epilepsy specialist and may be evaluated for additional medications, epilepsy surgery, neurostimulation, or dietary therapy. When caring for women, providers must take into account needs for contraception or pregnancy safety where applicable.

Autoimmune disorders of the central nervous system are common and often affect people in the most productive years of their lives. Among primary autoimmune diseases of the central nervous system, multiple sclerosis is most prevalent in the United States. Many other autoantibody-mediated neurologic syndromes have been identified within the past 2 to 3 decades, including neuromyelitis optica and anti-N-methyl-D aspartate receptor encephalitis. Finally, the central nervous system can also be affected by systemic autoimmune diseases such as sarcoidosis. Many of these diseases are treatable when detected early.

The diagnosis of Parkinson's disease (PD) is based on the presence of bradykinesia and either resting tremor or rigidity and there should be no features from the history or examination to suggest an alternative cause of parkinsonism. In addition to the motor manifestations of PD, there is a long list of nonmotor symptoms, several of which occur before motor signs and are considered "prodromal" PD. These are classified as neuropsychiatric, autonomic, sleep, and sensory. There are many medical options for the treatment of PD but levodopa remains the mainstay. Deep brain stimulation and other advanced therapies are also available.

Foreword
Dads and Moms

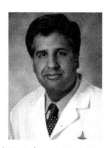

Bimal H. Ashar, MD, MBA, FACP
Consulting Editor

My father grew up in India. At the age of 22, he excitedly accepted an opportunity to continue his education at the University of Michigan. With $20 in his pocket, he traveled to the United States on a cargo ship, suffering from severe motion sickness throughout his journey. Through hard work, perseverance, and an adventurous spirit, he and my mother ultimately immigrated to America and were able to provide my brother and me with a middle class upbringing. At the time (1970s), I had little understanding of what it must have been like for them to raise two sons in a culture in which they had limited familiarity. I can remember my father driving an hour, struggling to find parking, and then sitting through a double-header baseball game between the Orioles and the Yankees, despite having little knowledge of the game. Over the subsequent years, my father endured the deaths of his son (at the age of 21) to a brain tumor, his older brother to Parkinson's disease, and a younger brother to an acute stroke.

My father is now 85 years old and is one of the more than 5.7 million Americans suffering from Alzheimer disease. He has trouble formulating and expressing his thoughts and is completely dependent on my mother to direct his daily activities. At times, he is completely cognizant of his limitations and expresses his frustration with his mental deterioration and his progressive loss of control over his life.

In this issue of the *Medical Clinics of North America*, Dr Milligan and her colleagues discuss the impact, diagnosis, and treatments of neurologic diseases such as Alzheimer. Many (but not all) of the conditions discussed affect older individuals: our patients, our mothers, and our fathers. I hope that readers will find this issue to be

Med Clin N Am 103 (2019) xiii–xiv
https://doi.org/10.1016/j.mcna.2018.11.002
0025-7125/19/© 2018 Published by Elsevier Inc.

an invaluable resource in dealing with these common and debilitating disorders. I know I have.

Bimal H. Ashar, MD, MBA, FACP
Division of General Internal Medicine
Johns Hopkins University School of Medicine
601 North Caroline Street
#7143
Baltimore, MD 21287, USA

E-mail address:
Bashar1@jhmi.edu

Preface

The Importance of Neurology for the Non-Neurologist

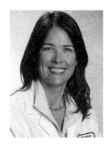

Tracey A. Milligan, MD, MS, FAAN
Editor

Neurology is fascinating for neurologists and non-neurologists alike. Not only does our nervous system control all bodily functions but also our brain is the essence of who we are and how we think, perceive, feel, behave, and remember. Diseases of the nervous system are common, and all diseases of the nervous system have available treatment. Treatment is occasionally curative, often disease modifying, and there are always symptomatic treatments available. There has been remarkable progress in understanding diseases of the nervous system. Every year there is a greater number of new therapeutics available in neurology than almost any other field of medicine.

Non-neurologists commonly diagnose and treat neurologic diseases. This issue of *Medical Clinics of North America* is directed to the non-neurologist, and its primary aim is to improve the care of the patient with a neurologic problem. This issue contains all the most important neurologic topics for non-neurologists. The information is presented in a way that reviews the neuroscience and neuropathology and provides high-yield, clinically relevant, and practical information for patient care. Neurologic disease is increasingly prevalent, and many physicians and other health care providers are on the frontlines of caring for patients with neurologic concerns. Familiarity with the epidemiology, pathophysiology, diagnosis, management, and prognosis associated with neurologic conditions is essential for all health care providers.

This issue begins with a thoughtful and comprehensive overview to the approach to diagnosis in neurologic conditions (Milligan) and continues with expert perspective on the approach to patients with one of the most common symptoms, dizziness (Whitman), and gait disorders (Ronthal). The issue continues with the most common neurologic disease and one that is associated with pain and lost income, headache, with articles on migraine (Burch), nonmigrainous headache (Vgontzas and Rizzoli), and concussion (Jackson and Starling).

Med Clin N Am 103 (2019) xv–xvi
https://doi.org/10.1016/j.mcna.2018.11.001
0025-7125/19/© 2018 Published by Elsevier Inc.

The number of Americans affected by Alzheimer disease (AD) has reached 5.7 million, making it the sixth leading cause of death in the country. By 2050, this number is likely to double or even triple. Atri provides an outstanding and comprehensive review of AD that is pertinent to the care of the patient with dementia. Stroke is the leading cause of disability and the fourth leading cause of death. One in six people worldwide will have a stroke in their lifetime. Caprio and Sorond have done an excellent job describing the primary and secondary prevention of stroke. Epilepsy is highly prevalent, affecting people of all ages. In the United States, there are 3.4 million people with epilepsy, and there are 65 million people worldwide with epilepsy. Johnson provides a compelling and modern overview of seizures and epilepsy. Multiple sclerosis and autoimmune neurology of the central nervous system are increasingly important topics due to the novel therapeutics and new diseases that are being recognized. Galetta and Bhattacharyya provide an extremely interesting contribution regarding these topics. Parkinson's disease is a feared diagnosis for many older people, and Reich and Savitt provide a highly informative and practical overview regarding the diagnosis and treatment of Parkinson's disease and essential tremor. Rounding out this issue's topics are informative and comprehensive articles on entrapment neuropathies of the upper extremity and lower extremity by Doughty and Bowley and peripheral neuropathy by Barrell and Smith.

This important issue of *Medical Clinics of North America*, Neurology for the Nonneurologist, comprises the most significant neurologic topics for the non-neurologist and contains incredibly well-written pieces that cover the full scope of neurology. The authors are all highly respected experts and provide a state-of-the-art update and perspective for each topic. Collectively, these contributions will provide health care providers with an invaluable resource as they treat patients facing neurologic conditions.

Tracey A. Milligan, MD, MS, FAAN
Harvard Medical School
Brigham and Women's Hospital
60 Fenwood Road
Boston, MA 02115, USA

E-mail address:
tmilligan@bwh.harvard.edu

Diagnosis in Neurologic Disease

Tracey A. Milligan, MD, MS

KEYWORDS

- Neurologic diagnosis • Neurologic history • Neurologic examination • Localization
- Neurologic testing

KEY POINTS

- Neurologic diagnosis is dependent on the history and physical examination, which are used to localize the lesion.
- The neurologic examination consists of a structured manner of examining the nervous system. It is divided into examination of the following areas: mental status, cranial nerves, motor, sensory, coordination, gait, and reflexes.
- Lesion localization, time course, and pattern of symptoms lead to a differential diagnosis.
- The topography of the neurologic axis from peripheral to central is a helpful structure to use in localizing a lesion.
- Diagnostic testing used in neurologic diseases includes neuroimaging, lumbar puncture, electroencephalogram, and nerve conduction studies and electromyography.

INTRODUCTION

The diagnosis of neurologic disorders is complex and is dependent on the history and physical examination. This review discusses key features relevant to the non-neurologist to allow for successful diagnosis and, when necessary, appropriate referral to the neurologist.

This topic is relevant to the non-neurologist because more than 40% of patients who present to their primary care provider have symptoms referable to the neurologic disease.[1] Up to 10% of patients seen by family practitioners present with neurologic symptoms and pose neurologic questions to their physicians. Only 16% of the 45 million Americans who visit a physician for a chief complaint referable to the nervous system are ever evaluated by neurologists.[2-5] Initiation of appropriate therapy is dependent on identifying the early signs and symptoms of neurologic disease, including subtle signs that may be overlooked. Many neurologic diseases are more

Disclosure Statement: The author has nothing to disclose.
Department of Neurology, Harvard Medical School, Brigham and Women's Hospital, 60 Fenwood Road, Boston, MA 02115, USA
E-mail address: tmilligan@bwh.harvard.edu

Med Clin N Am 103 (2019) 173–190
https://doi.org/10.1016/j.mcna.2018.10.011
0025-7125/19/© 2018 Elsevier Inc. All rights reserved.

easily treated when identified early. Patients with a disease in which there is no disease-modifying treatment benefit from early and accurate diagnosis, as the uncertainty can be more troubling than the disease.[6]

OVERALL PROCESS

The overall process to the diagnosis of a neurologic disease is primarily the clinical method used in all of medicine. The history is used to form a set of hypotheses that guide the physical examination. Signs may be found in the examination that lead to further probing of the history. The signs and symptoms elicited through the history and physical examination are interpreted in the context of anatomy and physiology and knowledge of pathophysiology and disease processes. A differential diagnosis is formulated, and tests are selected that are most likely to rule in or out various diseases in a way that is most accurate, bares the lowest risk to the patient, and is most economical. The diagnosis of the disease allows for initiation of treatment and counseling the patient as to the overall prognosis.

There are a few key differences and added steps when diagnosing a neurologic disease. This difference begins with the history, because neurology is the only discipline in which the physician is interviewing the diseased organ (except for psychiatry); in brain disorders, the physician is relying on the impaired organ to provide information about itself. This challenge requires more time and collateral information to obtain reliable and valid data.

A cornerstone of the neurologic diagnostic process is to use the patient's signs and symptoms to localize the lesion: the area(s) of the nervous system that is affected by the disease. Symptoms are integrated with the abnormal findings on examination to predict the anatomic area of pathology. The differential diagnosis incorporates localization with the speed of onset and time (time-intensity profile).

It can be challenging to determine the diagnosis in a patient with a neurologic disease; there can be uncertainty or disagreement about the diagnosis. Sometimes the patient does not respond to the treatment for a diagnosed disease. In these situations, it is paramount for the physician to return to the initial steps of the process and repeat the history and examination and reinterpret the facts obtained (**Fig. 1**).

HISTORY

Obtaining an accurate history is the most effective way of diagnosing disease.[7] As Osler[8] would remark, "Listen to your patient, he is telling you the diagnosis." However, in neurologic disease, particularly that affecting the brain, collateral history is needed to increase the accuracy of the history. When assessing a patient for dementia, time

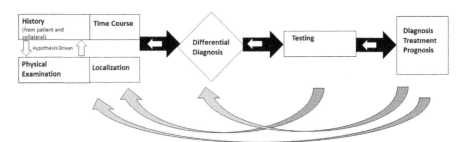

Fig. 1. The overall process to the diagnosis of a neurologic disease.

obtaining a history must be spent with a close family member or friend as well as with the patient. In assessing a patient with a possible seizure, it may be necessary to call someone who has witnessed the event and obtain a report of the event first-hand. It is important to use open-ended questions and avoid suggesting or labeling symptoms prematurely. Commonly used terms may also mean different things to different people. For example, learning what a patient means by "numb" (weakness or loss of sensation or paresthesia), "dizzy" (lightheadedness or imbalance or vertigo or anxiety), or difficulty speaking (slurred speech or word-finding problems) is necessary. The most common presenting problems in neurologic disease are found in **Box 1**.

An important part of the history is the mode of onset and the time course. The setting and situation of onset, symptom evolution, and time course can be typical of specific neurologic diseases. For example, a patient who gets dizzy when arising from bed, cannot walk due to imbalance, and feels nauseated could have a stroke or benign paroxysmal positional vertigo (BPPV). Other associated symptoms (eg, double vision for stroke) and time course (rapid resolution and recurrence with head turn for BPPV) are important historical factors for determining the diagnosis. The differential diagnosis of neurologic disease is based on the rate of symptom onset and the manner of progression. It is important to obtain the earliest symptoms, as they may have been ignored at the time and are only relevant in retrospect. The time-intensity profile of symptoms leads to the differential diagnosis. For example, symptoms that develop over seconds to hours are *acute-maximal at onset* and occur with ischemia, seizure, trauma, and hemorrhage. Symptoms developing over days to weeks to months are *subacute* and can be *smooth, stair-step,* or *crescendo.* This pattern suggests an expanding lesion or dysfunction, such as in tumors, infection, and demyelination. Symptoms developing and worsening over many months to years are *chronic-progressive;* this pattern is seen with neurodegenerative diseases such as dementia. *Recurring-episodic* attacks of sudden-onset symptoms with resolution to normal function are often referred to as "spells," such as spells of dizziness, spells of confusion, or other altered neurologic function. This pattern leads to a specific differential diagnosis that includes seizure, migraine, transient ischemic attacks, cerebral

---

Box 1
The most common symptoms of a neurologic disease

Headache

Memory loss

Loss of consciousness and seizures

Dizziness

Visual disturbances

Weakness

Partial or complete loss of sensation

Pain

Imbalance

Trouble walking

Tremor

Difficulty speaking or change in speech

Decreased alertness or attention

hypoperfusion such as in syncope, and amyloid angiopathy (only in the older adult). The timing and pattern of symptoms (diurnal, fluctuating, relapsing-remitting, progressive) can also lead to diagnosis of the disease (eg, ptosis and diplopia at the end of the day only: myasthenia gravis; vision loss with recovery and paresis with recovery: multiple sclerosis; cognitive change progressing to dementia in a month: prion disease).

One must be wary of the so-called pseudo-acute presentation. This occurs in neurodegenerative diseases when the progression has been slow and insidious, often misattributed to normal aging, and then there is sudden recognition of the patient's decline, either by another illness (acute on chronic) or a change in the patient's environment, for example, the death of a spouse or a move. The pseudo-acute presentation is analogous to a pen slowly and progressively rolling off a table, which can be ignored or is unapparent until it suddenly, "acutely," falls to the floor.[9]

PHYSICAL EXAMINATION

The diagnosis of a neurologic disease requires a general physical examination as well as a hypothesis-driven neurologic examination. The general physical examination may reveal signs that are relevant to the neurologic disease. Vital signs and examination of the neck, lymph nodes, skin, and cardiovascular system can be of particularly high yield.

The neurologic examination consists of a structured manner of examining the nervous system. It is divided into examination of the following areas: mental status, cranial nerves, motor, sensory, coordination, gait, and reflexes (**Table 1**). There are a variety of examination maneuvers to test these areas and entire textbooks devoted to the subject.[10–12]

The neurologic examination begins on meeting the patient and perhaps even earlier if the examiner is attuned to the sound of the patient's gait or the patient's manner of interacting with other staff members. During the history, the patient's mental status is examined. An examination of affect, attention, thought process, language, recall, and insight occur throughout the history. In patients with noncognitive complaints, the physician can often be relatively reassured of normal cognition by a clear, organized, and accurate history of the present illness, detailed past medical history, and the patient's knowledge of their medications and dosages. Vagueness, inconsistencies, disorganization, confusion, and aphasia can become apparent early in the history taking. In addition, the examiner can make note of eye and facial movement abnormalities, speech and voice dysfunction, hyperkinetic and hypokinetic movements, and ataxia even before the detailed examination has begun. For example, in a patient with more advanced Parkinson's disease, the diagnosis is apparent before beginning a formal physical examination. The observational skills of the physician are crucial part of performing a neurologic examination.

The neurologic examination in its entirety is detailed and lengthy. Therefore, before beginning the examination, the physician must have a specific hypothesis as to the etiology(ies) of the patient's presentation. The neurologic examination serves to test those hypotheses and is tailored to that purpose.[13] The neurologic examination also can serve as a screening examination to detect deficits that the patient may not be aware of or complain about. The screening examination varies depending on the specific patient demographic. In the patient with diabetes mellitus, it may focus on sensory function in the feet, whereas in a patient prescribed neuroleptics, it will focus on mental status, affect, tone, speed of movement, assessment of tremor, and gait. In the older adult, a wellness visit should include a screening test for cognitive function, such as the Mini-Cog test (3-word registration, clock drawing, and 3-word recall).[14]

Table 1
The neurologic examination

Mental Status	Cranial Nerves	Motor	Reflexes	Coordination and Gait	Sensory
• Observation • Orientation • Attention • Memory • Language • Visuospatial	• II • III, IV, VI • VII • Other cranial nerves	• Observation • Test for drift • Finger tapping • Bulk • Tone • Strength	• Deep tendon reflexes • Pathologic reflex (Babinski sign)	• Finger-nose-finger • Heel-knee-shin • Eye movements • Gait including tandem gait	• Tactile • Thermal • Pinprick • Vibration • Joint position (proprioception) • Romberg testing

Box 2 provides a general framework for a screening neurologic examination that can be performed in less than 5 minutes.

Of special note, it is important to document what was done in the neurologic examination, so it is clear whether any abnormalities noted in the future are new versus not previously tested.

Mental Status

Structured assessment of the mental status includes both psychiatric and neurologic components. The psychiatric components of mood, affect, thought process, and content are assessed and documented. The neurologic components that are foundational to the rest of the mental status examination are level of

---

Box 2
Neurologic screening examination checklist

5-Minute Neurologic Screening Examination Checklist
  With practice, this examination should take no more than 5 minutes. This is a screening examination only and is best suited to patients who DO NOT have a neurologic complaint and when a neurologic condition in NOT suspected.

Mental state
- Oriented to place and time
- Test of attention
- Test of memory
- Test of naming one high-frequency and low-frequency item
- Follow L/R multistep command across midline

Cranial nerves
- Pupils
- Eye movements
- Visual fields in all 4 quadrants 1 eye at a time
- Facial movement
- Elevation of palate
- Tongue protrusion

Motor functions
- General muscle bulk and tone
- Proximal and distal strength (deltoid, elbow extension, wrist extension, hip flexion, knee flexion, ankle dorsiflexion)
- Pronator drift
- Fast and fine finger movements

Sensory functions
- Touch
- Pin or temperature
- Vibration in toes

Reflexes
- Reflexes in arms and legs including ankle jerks
- Plantar response

Cerebellar function
- Finger-nose-finger testing

Station and gait
- Romberg
- Stance
- Gait (walking and turning)
- Tandem gait

consciousness, orientation, and attention. If there is impairment of those 3 elements, it will be difficult to interpret deficits in language, memory, and visuospatial testing. At the most extreme end of the spectrum, a comatose patient cannot be assessed for language function. Along the same lines, it is worth remembering that the delirious patient has impaired attention and therefore testing of memory will not be valid until the delirium has resolved. **Table 2** lists some of the common tests used to examine mental status.

Cranial Nerves

There are 12 cranial nerves (CNs), but they are all not equally relevant in diagnosing a neurologic disease.[15,16] Vision, extraocular eye movements, and facial movements have a higher sensitivity in detecting dysfunction of the neurologic system. In deference to the high sensitivity of these components of the CN examination, they are discussed first and therefore out of numerical order.

Optic nerve (cranial nerve II)

Pupillary size, shape, and reactivity are important to assess in neurologic diseases. For example, a large pupil may signify herniation of a mass in the temporal lobe or an intracerebral aneurysm. A small pupil with ipsilateral ptosis is seen with Horner syndrome, which has a long and specific localization pathway in the sympathetic nervous system. With the fundoscopic examination, the examiner can literally see the central nervous system, as the optic nerve (optic disc) is CN II and is part of the central nervous system. The fundus can provide information regarding intracranial pressure (ICP) (papilledema seen with elevated ICP) and demyelination (optic neuritis). Visual acuity provides information about the lens, retina, and the optic nerve. The visual pathway runs from front (the retina) to back (the occipital lobe) and can be tested and the lesion localized by visual field testing.

Table 2 Commonly used tests of mental status	
General behavior and appearance	Grooming, dress, posture, eye contact
Mood and affective responses	Emotional state and observable expression
Process and content of thought	Logical, organized, or racing; and poverty, delusions, obsessions, hallucinations
Speech characteristics	Fluent, pressured, halting
Consciousness	Awake, somnolence, obtundation, stupor, coma
Orientation	Person, place, and time
Attention span	Digit span forward and backward; Serial 7s; WORLD backward; months of the year or days of the week backward; register 3 words
Memory, recent and remote	Recall the 3 words; discuss current events and prior historical event (eg, death of JFK or 9/11)
Language	Follow commands, name objects, repeat sentence, read and follow command, write a sentence
Insight, judgment, and planning	Awareness of deficits and limitations; solve hypothetical problem
Visuospatial	Draw clock, copy cube or intersecting pentagons
Praxis	Pantomime brushing teeth, throwing a ball, hanging a picture

Extraocular movements (cranial nerves III, IV, VI)
Extraocular movements require the coordinated function of CNs III (oculomotor), IV (trochlear), and VI (abducens) with the frontal lobe, basal ganglia, cerebellum, brainstem, and the nerves themselves. There are characteristic abnormalities that can localize to a specific location in the nervous system. Examination of the extraocular movements is exquisitely sensitive to dysfunction of any of these pathways. With abnormalities in this system, the patient may describe diplopia or oscillopsia. The examiner can quickly become attuned to abnormal movements through observation; observing the eyes of another individual is a common behavior and requires only refining observations through careful examination maneuvers. Extraocular movements are one of the most sensitive tests in the physical examination.

Facial nerve (cranial nerve VII)
Examination of the facial nerve functions can be quite sensitive in detecting weakness involving the face. How peoples' faces move normally is highly learned by physicians and observed throughout the visit, therefore abnormalities are more easily detected. The patient often has access to an old photograph to demonstrate whether or not the finding is new or chronic. The pattern of facial weakness determines whether the weakness is peripheral or lower motor neuron or central and upper motor neuron/corticobulbar tract. The pattern of weakness distinguishes between Bell palsy and stroke. A Bell palsy will involve the forehead muscles and the patient will have difficulty closing the eye fully. A stroke involving the corticobulbar fibers will show relative preservation of the wrinkling of the forehead.

The other cranial nerves
Olfactory nerve (cranial nerve I) Olfaction is rarely tested, but can be one of the first impairments in Alzheimer and Parkinson's disease.

Trigeminal nerve (cranial nerve V) Sensation of the face and the movement of the muscles of mastication are supplied by the trigeminal nerve. As with the sensory examination elsewhere, it can only serve to complement other findings and is rarely of use in isolation.

Vestibulocochlear (cranial nerve VIII) The vestibulocochlear nerve is tested through hearing and reflexive eye movements that rely on intact vestibular input (eg, oculovestibular reflex and head thrust maneuver).

Glossopharyngeal (cranial nerve IX) and vagus (cranial nerve X) The nasal resonance of speech and the quality of the voice can provide information regarding CNs IX and X. A voice that is wet in quality (possibly signifying poor swallow), hoarse or breathy (impaired vocal fold function), or a weak cough should trigger a more detailed examination of the functions of these CNs, including observation of palatal movement and potentially direct visualization of the vocal folds.

Spinal accessory nerve (cranial nerve XI) The examination of this nerve is rarely helpful in the diagnosis of neurologic disease, but can be best accomplished by asking the patient to shrug the shoulders and observing the amount and symmetry of shoulder movement.

Hypoglossal nerve (cranial nerve XII) The most sensitive examination of the hypoglossal nerve is through listening to the patient's speech. Precise articulation of sounds requires normal movement of the tongue. If there is any slurring of sounds, a more focused examination of the appearance and function of the tongue is required.

Motor Examination

The motor examination begins with observing the patient for too much movement (hyperkinetic findings: tremor, tics, chorea) or too little movement (hypokinetic findings: masked facies, bradykinesia).[17] The motor system is examined differently depending on the purpose of the examination. Components of the motor examination include examination of muscle bulk, tone, and strength. The pattern of muscle weakness can narrow the differential diagnosis. For example, a patient with weakness at the shoulder and hip girdles may have a myopathy, such as polymyositis. Lesions of the corticospinal tract have a classic upper motor neuron pattern of weakness: in the upper extremities, elbow extension is weaker than flexion; wrist extension is weaker than flexion; and shoulder abduction is weaker than adduction. In the lower extremities, the hip abduction is weaker than adduction; knee flexion is weaker than extension; ankle dorsiflexion is weaker than plantar flexion; and ankle eversion is weaker than inversion. **Table 3** reviews the common signs of upper motor neuron versus lower motor neuron lesions.

In diagnosing weakness, checking for a pronator drift by asking the patient to hold both arms in front palms up ("like holding a pizza box") and then asking the patient to close his or her eyes, can reveal subtle weakness by one arm drifting down and pronating slightly. Testing fine and fast finger movements by tapping the index finger in the first crease of the ipsilateral thumb can assess for speed (corticospinal function), excursion (pyramidal function), and rhythm/accuracy (cerebellar function).

Reflexes

The most sensitive reflex to check is the ankle jerk (Achilles reflex). This is the most length-dependent of the reflexes and the one most likely to be abnormal in the general patient population. This reflex should be compared with other more easily elicitable reflexes, such as the patellar reflex and biceps reflex. **Table 4** lists the common reflexes and the nerve root that is being tested. Upper motor neuron lesions will result in hyperreflexia on the side contralateral to the lesion and are often accompanied by a positive Babinski sign ("upgoing toe").

Coordination

Testing of coordination involves finger-nose-finger and heel-knee-shin maneuvers.[18] These maneuvers test the cerebellar networks that include not only the cerebellum, but the fibers in the brainstem and the input from the dorsal root ganglia. The cerebellar networks are also examined by checking for nystagmus and assessing tandem gait.

Table 3
Common signs of upper motor neuron (UMN) versus lower motor neuron (LMN) lesions

UMN	LMN
Hyperreflexia	Hyporeflexia
Increased tone (spasticity)	Normal or flaccid tone
Positive Babinski sign (upgoing toe)	Negative Babinski sign

UMN pattern of weakness:
  UE- extensors weaker than flexors
  LE - flexors weaker than extensors
	Atrophy and fasciculations

Table 4 Reflex testing		
Reflex	**Nerve**	**Root Level**
Jaw	Trigeminal	Pons
Biceps	Musculocutaneous	C5-C6
Brachioradialis	Radial	C6-C7
Triceps	Radial	C6-C7
Patella	Femoral	L3-L4
Achilles	Tibial	S1-S2

Sensory Examination

The sensory examination is by its very nature subjective, as it is only attainable through the subjective response of the patient.[19] The sensory findings are very suggestible. If the sensory examination remains unreliable despite repeated efforts, it is better to move on to other parts of the examination. The sensory examination serves only to complement the other aspects of the history and physical examination. The key technique is to focus on differences between the 2 sides of the body, proximal versus distal, and to assess for a level below which there is sensory loss or a zone of sensory loss. Moving from a zone of abnormality to normality improves the patient's ability to perceive a difference. The Romberg test assesses proprioception by asking the patient who is stable with feet together to close his or her eyes. A step backward by the patient signifies loss of proprioceptive input because without visual input this patient loses balance.

Gait

Examination of gait is not only a sensitive way of detecting neurologic disease (eg, the parkinsonian tremor that is more apparent when walking), but can also be the only abnormality in a serious neurologic disease (eg, impaired tandem gait in a patient with a midline cerebellar hemorrhage on the verge of causing herniation or obstructive hydrocephalus).[18]

Specific Assessments

Coma examination

Many non-neurologists are intimidated by the coma examination, but it is actually the simplest version of the neurologic examination. The depth of coma is examined by attempting to awaken the patient through loud voice, then noxious stimulation (sternal rub or shoulder squeeze) and assessing the patient's ability to follow simple commands (look up, squeeze hand). CN examination focuses on pupil size and reactivity, corneal reflex, oculocephalic reflex, facial grimace, gag, cough. Motor examination consists of tone and presence and type of withdrawal to noxious stimulation. Reflex examination complements the findings of the motor examination looking for presence, quality, and symmetry of reflexes and for Babinski sign. An excellent resource for how to perform a coma examination is The Cleveland Clinic's Death by Neurologic Criteria (DNC) course, which is available online.[20] It explains how to properly assess cerebral function in patients in a coma and details the elements included in the clinical coma examination. In addition, it outlines the accepted medical standards for determining DNC.

Acute stroke

The National Institutes of Health Stroke Scale is the most widely used deficit assessment tool in neurology. It is required by the Joint Commission within 12 hours of admission for all patients with stroke admitted to a stroke center.[21] This scale is used for scoring severity of acute stroke assessment and is reliable when used by non-neurologists who undergo training. Training is easily available online.[22,23]

LOCALIZATION AND DIFFERENTIAL DIAGNOSIS

The process of localization involves using the information obtained during the history and during the tailored neurologic examination to determine to location of the lesion causing the patient's symptoms and signs.[24] Localization begins during the history and is refined through the examination. Correct localization requires a knowledge of neuroanatomy and physiology, vascular territories, and of the diseases that affect the nervous system. Localization leads to a differential diagnosis and selection of tests, but is also repeated following diagnostic tests to ensure the abnormalities found in testing are relevant to the patient's presentation. Localization involves an attempt to determine a single anatomic lesion or neuroanatomical pathway that is involved. Localization also involves determining whether the process must be multifocal or is part of a specific syndrome or disease. Topographic localization can be approached by starting from the periphery and moving centrally, considering each site as a possible source of the lesion. For example, when a patient presents with weakness, consider possible sources of muscle, neuromuscular junction, peripheral nerve, plexus, spinal nerve root, anterior horn of the spinal cord, corticospinal tract/pyramidal tract through the spinal cord, brain stem, internal capsule, corona radiata, and motor cortex (**Table 5**).

The localization and time course in combination with the specific patient characteristics obtained in the history lead to the differential diagnosis (**Fig. 2**). For example, in a patient who presents with right-sided weakness, a history of vascular risk factors, sudden onset, and weakness involving the right face, arm, and leg and aphasia, we can recognize a syndrome of left middle cerebral artery thromboembolic stroke. If the patient worsened after presentation with nausea and vomiting, we would include a differential of intracerebral hemorrhage. A more challenging localization would occur in a patient presenting with a foot drop (impaired dorsiflexion of the foot). The history of prolonged leg crossing (for peroneal), back pain (for L5 radiculopathy), or history of parasagittal meningioma (for central cause) would all lead to specific maneuvers on the examination to localize the lesion (impaired eversion and spared inversion for peroneal neuropathy; weak inversion and eversion and hip abduction and L5 sensory change for L5 radiculopathy; brisk ipsilateral reflexes and positive Babinski sign for a central cause). A precise localization leads to a differential diagnosis. Only the history, examination, and localization process are necessary to diagnose some diseases (eg, essential tremor, BPPV, Parkinson's disease), whereas other diseases require more testing based on the differential diagnosis. The process of differential diagnosis includes consideration of the major categories of neurologic disease, which can be recalled by using the acronym VINDICATE, with a slight modification for the purpose of neurologic differential diagnosis VIND Ψ CATE (**Box 3**). The localization is often repeated after diagnostic testing to ensure findings obtained on testing are relevant to the clinical presentation.

DIAGNOSTIC TESTS

There are standard and specialized tests that are used in ruling in and out various neurologic conditions. The advances in technology and genetic testing have

Table 5
Localization and typical signs and symptoms

Location (Disease)	Typical Signs and Symptoms
Muscle (myopathy)	Proximal weakness (motor only)
Neuromuscular junction (myasthenia)	Fatigable weakness (motor only)
Peripheral nerve (neuropathy)	Pain; motor, sensory, and reflex loss in specific nerve distribution, OR distal symmetric sensory loss (stocking/glove) and/or weakness
Plexus (brachial or lumbosacral) (plexopathy)	Mixed nerve and root distribution
Spinal nerve root (radiculopathy)	Radicular pain; motor, sensory and reflex loss in specific root distribution
Anterior horn cell (LMN disease)	LMN weakness and reflex loss
Dorsal root ganglion (sensory neuronopathy)	Sensory loss and reflex loss
Spinal cord (myelopathy)	Sensory level; UMN weakness below level of the lesion (LMN weakness at level of lesion); neurogenic bladder; dissociated sensory loss
Brainstem	Contralateral long tract signs (UMN weakness and/or sensory deficits); ipsilateral cranial nerve deficits; impaired level of consciousness
Cerebellum	Ataxia; tremor; nystagmus
Thalamus	LOC or memory disturbance; hemisensory loss and/or pain; hemiataxia; neglect or aphasia
Basal ganglia (hyperkinesia or hypokinesia)	Rigidity; tremor; chorea; athetosis; dystonia
Cerebral cortex (encephalopathy)	Hemiplegia (UMN) and/or hemisensory loss; aphasia (L); neglect (R); hemianopia; dementia; seizure

Abbreviations: L, left; LMN, lower motor neuron; R, right; UMN, upper motor neuron.

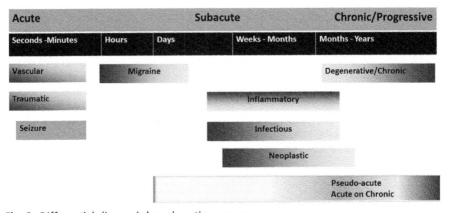

Fig. 2. Differential diagnosis based on time course.

| Box 3 |
Major categories of neurologic disease VIND Ψ CATE
Vascular
Infectious
Neoplastic
Degenerative
Ψ Psychogenic
Congenital/Genetic
Autoimmune
Trauma
Endocrine/Toxins/Metabolic/Drugs

expanded the types of tests available for use in diagnosis. The goal is to choose the test(s) that best confirms or refutes the diagnosis in the most economical, safest, and least invasive manner. Serum testing for metabolic, inflammatory, infectious, endocrine, and autoantibody measurement is tailored to the differential diagnosis. Some of the other commonly used tests are reviewed here. Increasingly, it is possible to use targeted genetic testing or whole exome sequencing to achieve a diagnosis.

Neuroimaging

The availability of increasingly sophisticated neuroimaging is transforming the field of neurologic diagnosis. Although the neurologic history and examination remain the best tools in the accurate diagnosis of neurologic illness, many diseases are diagnosed more easily and quickly with neuroimaging. Neuroimaging, however, has led to a new type of problem for the physician: the incidental finding. In many cases it cannot be clear whether or not a finding is truly incidental or is actually meaningful without the proper history and examination.

Computerized tomography

Computed tomography (CT) allows for imaging of the brain and spinal cord as well as the surrounding soft tissues and bone. It is best used in cases of trauma or suspected hemorrhage or when MRI is not possible due to unavailability or when the patient has metal in the body precluding MRI. CT is inexpensive and widely available. It is fast and does not require screening for metallic foreign bodies and can be more easily arranged for acutely ill patients. The principal disadvantages of CT are the use of ionizing radiation and difficulty imaging specific regions of the nervous system, such as the brainstem and cerebellum. It is not as sensitive or diagnostic as MRI for many neurologic diseases. But CT is best for seeing acute bleeding and is equivalent or superior in visualizing calcium, fat, and bone, particularly in skull base and vertebrae.

CT angiography (CTA) and venography can be used to visualize the arteries and veins in the head and neck, but require contrast to do so. CTA has a high sensitivity for detecting cerebral aneurysms and is also used to diagnose vascular stenoses in the neck and brain. Contrast studies also can be used to detect a breakdown of the blood-brain barrier.

MRI

For the visualization of most neurologic diseases, MRI is superior to CT. In nonacute situations, it is usually better to test with MRI rather than CT; MRI allows for much better resolution and detection of lesions. MRI involves placing the patient in a strong magnetic field that aligns hydrogen protons, and radiofrequency pulses are manipulated and stimulate the protons to emit a signal. This is visualized through various sequences. Gadolinium, a paramagnetic agent that enhances the process of proton relaxation during T1 sequences, highlights regions with blood-brain barrier disruption and is used as a contrast agent. Patients with renal disease are at risk for nephrogenic systemic sclerosis and gadolinium is avoided in this population, as well as in pregnant women.

Diffusion-weighted imaging (DWI) can be prioritized when acute stroke is suspected because it takes only a minute to accomplish and detects the earliest stages of ischemic stroke, generally within 2 hours or less of the onset. Restricted diffusion of water in cerebral infarction appears as a bright white signal on DWI and dark on apparent diffusion coefficient.

Magnetic resonance angiography (MRA) and venography are noninvasive techniques for visualizing the main intracranial and cervical arteries and veins. Like CTA, this technique can reliably detect intracranial vascular lesions and extracranial artery stenosis.

The advantages of MRI over CT include the use of nonionizing energy and ability to obtain better resolution of different structures within the brain and other organs (spinal cord, nerves, and muscles). The main drawback to MRI is the strong magnetic field it generates. It is also less widely available, takes longer, and is more expensive than CT. Patients can find it claustrophobic.

Ultrasonography

Ultrasonography is inexpensive, readily available, portable, and safe. It can be used to document and follow the severity of vascular stenoses of the head and neck. It is also used to detect vasospasm from subarachnoid hemorrhage and monitor for microemboli if it is not clear whether or not a more proximal lesion is symptomatic. Ultrasound is also used to guide temporal artery biopsy and visualize some peripheral nerves. It can also be used to guide lumbar puncture.

Catheter angiography

Catheter angiography is an invasive procedure with increased risks, but it provides high spatial resolution. It can be used when suspecting vascular lesions, such as vascular malformations in the brain and spinal cord and for assessing for a small vessel vasculitis. MRA and CTA are supplanting conventional angiography except when there is a need to image distal small vessels, document fine details of vascular lesions, and is part of a therapeutic intervention (eg, coiling of aneurysms).

Nuclear medicine imaging

PET measures regional cerebral concentration of systemically administered radioactive tracers. Concentration in various parts of the brain is determined. This technique was originally and is still used for research purposes, but is also approved by the Food and Drug Administration for use in clinical practice. PET with fludeoxyglucose F 18 is approved for clinical use for determining epileptic foci, assessing glucose metabolism of potential tumors, and for distinguishing Alzheimer disease from frontotemporal dementia. Radiotracers for tau and amyloid are being used for research purposes in the quest to detect those at higher risk for Alzheimer disease.

Single-photon emission computerized tomography (SPECT) is used for diagnosis in neurologic disease as well. SPECT perfusion is used to detect epileptic foci and can be used as an aid to diagnose brain death. DaTscan (ioflupane I 123) uses SPECT imaging to assess if there is an abnormality in the dopamine transporter and can distinguish between Parkinson's disease, other causes of parkinsonism, and essential tremor.

Lumbar Puncture

Lumbar puncture (LP) is one of the oldest diagnostic tests. It is used to detect ICP as well as to diagnose brain inflammation and infection. It can be an important part of the assessment of thunderclap headache when CT fails to show subarachnoid hemorrhage. The analyses of the fluid can lead to diagnosis of a specific infection. The greatest risk is a post-LP headache. In rare cases, typically those with a mass lesion already causing hydrocephalus or herniation, LP can lead to transtentorial or cerebellar herniation. Therefore before an LP, fundoscopic and neurologic examination and/or head CT should be performed. A summary of possible LP findings is found in **Table 6**.

Electroencephalogram

Electroencephalogram (EEG) is a measurement of brain electrical activity. It is easily performed, inexpensive, and has no intrinsic risks associated with it. Electrodes are placed in a standardized way on the scalp of a patient and brain activity is recorded. For routine EEGs, the ideal recording consists of 20 or more minutes in relaxed awake, drowsy, and asleep states with hyperventilation and photic stimulation. Sleep, hyperventilation, and photic stimulation are considered activating procedures meaning they can bring out or accentuate abnormalities. EEG is without risk and is inexpensive. It is indicated when there is a suspected or confirmed diagnosis of seizure or epilepsy. It can demonstrate abnormalities even when neuroimaging is normal. It also can classify the type of epilepsy and lead to information that guides best treatment and prognosis. It is important to note that a normal EEG does not rule out epilepsy because the sensitivity is only approximately 30%. Some abnormalities are fairly nonspecific, such as generalized theta or delta slowing. EEG sensitivity can be increased by repeating the study, performing a sleep-deprived EEG, performing the study within 24 hours of the event, using ambulatory EEG monitoring, and using video-EEG monitoring.

Nerve Conduction Studies and Electromyogram

Nerve conduction studies (NCSs) and needle electromyography (EMG) provide physiologic assessment of peripheral nerves and muscles. NCSs are performed on both motor and sensory nerves. In motor NCSs, an electrical stimulus is delivered to a skin location overlying a motor peripheral nerve and the response is recorded from muscles supplied by that nerve (compound motor action potential [CMAP]). The motor conduction velocity can be calculated by measuring the distance between 2 different stimulated sites and the difference between the latency of onset of the CMAPs. In sensory NCSs, a sensory nerve action potential is measured by stimulating sensory axons and recording proximal or distal to the site of stimulation. Sensory NCSs examine only the larger and faster axons and therefore do not reliably detect a small fiber neuropathy. NCSs can be used to identify focal lesions and distinguish axonal and demyelinating neuropathies as well as distinguish neuropathy from myopathy and motor neuron disease. Needle EMG includes assessment of muscle electrical activity by insertion activity, spontaneous activity, and the recruitment pattern of the muscle. It can diagnose acute axonal loss, demyelinating neuropathy, acute myopathy, and chronic myopathy.

Table 6
Characteristic CSF findings

Etiology	Appearance	Pressure cm H$_2$O	WBC/μL	Protein mg/dL	Glucose mg/dL (CSF:Serum Ratio)
Normal CSF	Clear	5–20 mm	0–4 (lymphocytes)	23–38	50–80 (0.6)
Acute bacterial	Turbid	Increased	1000–10,000 (PMN)	100–500	<40
Viral	Clear (RBCs in HSV encephalitis)	Normal to mildly increased	5–300 (rarely >1000) (lymphocytes)	Normal to mildly increased	Normal
Tuberculosis	Slightly opaque	Increased	100–600 (mixed or lymphocytes)	Increased	Decreased
Fungal	Cloudy	Increased	40–400 (mixed)	Increased	Decreased
Subarachnoid hemorrhage	Xanthochromia	Often increased	Slightly increased	Increased	Normal
Idiopathic intracranial hypertension	Clear	Increased	Normal	Normal	Normal

Abbreviations: CSF, cerebrospinal fluid; HSV, herpes simplex virus; PMN, polymorphonuclear neutrophil; RBC, red blood cell; WBC, white blood cell.

SUMMARY

The diagnosis of neurologic disease is a rewarding endeavor because it requires intellectual rigor, skill, and is of paramount importance to patient care. A tailored history and examination lead to localization and differential diagnosis. Diagnostic testing often involves neuroimaging. Many neurologic diseases lead to disability or death and early identification and treatment can be life changing. In the modern era, all neurologic diagnoses lead to treatments. All neurologic diseases have either targeted treatment toward the disease or to the symptoms. Some diseases can be cured. Neurotherapeutics is a rapidly expanding field and there are many new and exciting therapeutics that include not only pharmacologic and biologic agents, but also genetic treatment, brain-computer interfaces, and neurostimulators.

REFERENCES

1. Neurology AAo. Neurology clerkship core curriculum. Available at: https://www.aan. com/siteassets/home-page/tools-and-resources/academic-neurologist–researchers/ clerkship-and-course-director-resources/neurology-clerkship-core-curriculum-guide lines.new.pdf. Accessed October 1, 2018.
2. Ashman JJ, Rui P, Okeyode T. Characteristics of office-based physician visits, 2015. NCHS Data Brief 2018;(310):1–8.
3. Hirtz D, Thurman DJ, Gwinn-Hardy K, et al. How common are the "common" neurologic disorders? Neurology 2007;68(5):326–37.
4. Miller JQ. The neurologic content of family practice. Implications for neurologists. Arch Neurol 1986;43(3):286–8.
5. Stone J, Carson A, Duncan R, et al. Who is referred to neurology clinics? The diagnoses made in 3781 new patients. Clin Neurol Neurosurg 2010;112(9):747–51.
6. Johnson Wright L, Afari N, Zautra A. The illness uncertainty concept: a review. Curr Pain Headache Rep 2009;13(2):133–8.
7. Thrush D. How to do it: take good history. Pract Neurol 2002;2:113–6.
8. Gandhi JS. William Osler: A life in medicine. BMJ 2000;321(7268):1087.
9. TA M. Pseudoacute presentation of neurologic disease. 2018. Available at: https://www.youtube.com/watch?v=cZTCN9cf788&feature=youtu.be. Accessed October 1, 2018.
10. Blumenfeld H. Neuroanatomy through clinical cases. 2nd edition. Sunderland (MA): Sinauer Associates; 2010.
11. Boes CJ. History of neurologic examination books. Proc (Bayl Univ Med Cent) 2015;28(2):172–9.
12. Campbell WW, DeJong RN. DeJong's the neurologic examination/William W. Campbell. 7th edition. Philadelphia: Lippincott Williams & Wilkins; 2013.
13. Hillis JM, Milligan TA. Teaching the neurological examination in a rapidly evolving clinical climate. Semin Neurol 2018;38(4):428–40.
14. Kuslansky G. The Mini-Cog compares well with longer screening tests for detecting dementia in older people. Evid Based Ment Health 2004;7(2):38.
15. Milligan TA, Kaplan TB. Cranial Nerve Examination I. Journal of Visualized Experiments Science Education 2016. Available at: https://www.jove.com/science-education/10091/cranial-nerves-exam-i-i-vi. Accessed November 9, 2018.
16. Milligan TA, Kaplan TB. Cranial Nerve Examination II. Journal of Visualized Experiments Science Education 2016. Available at: https://www.jove.com/science-education/10005/cranial-nerves-exam-ii-vii-xii.

17. Milligan TA, Kaplan TB. Motor Examination I. Journal of Visualized Experiments Science Education 2016. Available at: https://www.jove.com/science-education/10052/motor-exam-i. Accessed November 9, 2018.
18. Milligan TA, Kaplan TB. Motor Examination II. Journal of Visualized Experiments Science Education 2016. Available at: https://www.jove.com/science-education/10095/motor-exam-ii. Accessed November 9, 2018.
19. Milligan TA, Kaplan TB. Sensory examination. Journal of Visualized Experiments Science Education 2016. Available at: https://www.jove.com/science-education/10113/sensory-exam. Accessed November 9, 2018.
20. Clinic C. Death by neurologic criteria DNC. 2011. Available at: https://www.cchs.net/onlinelearning/cometvs10/dncPortal/default.htm. Accessed October 1, 2018.
21. Leifer D, Bravata DM, Connors JJ 3rd, et al. Metrics for measuring quality of care in comprehensive stroke centers: detailed follow-up to Brain Attack Coalition comprehensive stroke center recommendations: a statement for healthcare professionals from the American Heart Association/American Stroke Association. Stroke 2011;42(3):849–77.
22. American Heart Association. NIH Stroke scale. 2014. Available at: https://learn.heart.org/nihss.aspx. Accessed October 1, 2018.
23. The International Electronic Education Network. NIH Stroke scale. 1999. Available at: http://www.nihstrokescale.org/. Accessed October 1, 2018.
24. Goldberg S. Principles of neurologic localization. Am Fam Physician 1981;23(4):131–41.

Examination of the Patient with Dizziness or Imbalance

Gregory T. Whitman, MD

KEYWORDS

- Examination • Dizziness • Vertigo • Balance • Vestibular • Nystagmus • Gait

KEY POINTS

- Because of the multisensory nature of balance and vestibular function, the clinician seeing a dizzy patient, must perform a comprehensive neurological assessment.
- Altered mental status and abnormalities of vision may disturb balance and gait.
- The direction and duration of any nystagmus should be recorded, and one should note whether nystagmus is spontaneous, gaze evoked, or positional.
- Past pointing tests, Romberg tests, and the Fukuda stepping test may disclose imbalance.

INTRODUCTION

"Dizziness" may signify vertigo (an illusory sense of movement of the environment or self), lightheadedness (eg, a floating sensation), or other sensations that defy description. Many people with dizziness have an abnormality of gait or postural stability, necessitating inclusion of gait and balance in the clinical approach to dizziness.

Assessment of dizziness in US emergency rooms reportedly costs $4 billion per year.[1] Annual medical expenses due to falls in the United States were reported to be $50.0 billion.[2] Despite these high costs, many patients with dizziness or imbalance are discharged from the hospital without a clear diagnosis, suggesting the need for improved physical examination approaches.

One might reasonably ask: What is the rationale for combining dizziness and imbalance into one category? Some patients with dizziness report their symptoms are localized within or around the head and that their gait is normal. For others, the main problem is abnormality of gait, the head feels normal. In practice, though,

Disclosure Statement: Dr G.T. Whitman has nothing to disclose with respect to relationships with any commercial company that has a direct financial interest in subject matter or materials discussed in article or with a company making a competing product.
Department of Otolaryngology, Harvard Medical School, Massachusetts Eye and Ear Infirmary, Massachusetts Eye and Ear Balance and Vestibular Center, 250 Pond Street, Braintree, MA 02184, USA
E-mail address: gtw3@cornell.edu

Med Clin N Am 103 (2019) 191–201
https://doi.org/10.1016/j.mcna.2018.10.008
0025-7125/19/© 2018 The Author. Published by Elsevier Inc. This is an open access article under the CC BY-NC-ND license (http://creativecommons.org/licenses/by-nc-nd/4.0/).
medical.theclinics.com

most patients with dizziness or imbalance fall on a spectrum between the patient with head-related symptoms alone, and the patient with balance and gait symptoms alone.

The reader is assumed to be familiar with the basic neurologic examination. This topic will not be reviewed in detail. The routine neurologic examination, though, is critical, because of the extensive differential diagnosis. The differential diagnosis of dizziness is reviewed elsewhere.[3] The primary goals of this review are as follows:

1. To outline a systematic approach to physical examination of the patient with dizziness or imbalance,
2. To discuss useful and frequently overlooked neurologic signs that are useful in clinical practice for making a diagnosis.

First and foremost, one has to acknowledge the multisensory nature of balance and vestibular function. Balance function may remain surprisingly normal (compensated), until a large number of neurons and systems have been lost. One is surprised to encounter patients with substantially absent peripheral vestibular reflexes but near normal gait. Although the latter situation may be surprising, it is also common in otherwise young, healthy patients who have lost vestibular function.

At the same time, a diverse array of neurologic disturbances may contribute to imbalance. That is, gait disorders are commonly "multifactorial." Consider a set of 3 disorders, as follows:

1. Unilateral benign paroxysmal positional vertigo (BPPV),
2. Mild diabetic peripheral neuropathy,
3. Bilateral impairment of visual acuity, due to cataracts.

It is by no means clear that any of the formerly mentioned 3 problems in isolation would greatly disturb balance. Combined, however, the set of all 3 diagnoses would almost assuredly cause imbalance. A critical principle, then, is that one must maintain a high index of suspicion that imbalance is multifactorial.

As elsewhere in Neurology, the assessment of multiple coincident lesions is challenging and benefits from the experience of the examiner. For the nonspecialist, the best approach to the possibility of multiple lesions may be to carefully catalog as many abnormal neurological findings as possible, in as much detail as possible, acknowledging that in the end, the combination of objective abnormalities may add up to an explanation.

ORTHOSTATIC VITAL SIGNS

Orthostatic vital signs are most useful when viewed as a stress test. The basic routine of checking vitals lying down and then sitting up is insufficient. Prolonged action of gravity may be necessary to cause enough pooling of blood below the heart to elicit orthostatic intolerance, except in cases where orthostatic vital sign measurements are hardly necessary. The patient who says, "When I stand up, I get lightheaded," should be encouraged to stand, for a few minutes, for example, while history taking is continued. The examiner should ask about symptoms (including blurred vision and dizziness) while the patient stands. Note should be made of any deterioration in cognitive function while upright, and serial sets of standing vital signs may be informative. It is common knowledge that a sustained fall in systolic blood pressure of at least 20 mm Hg, after moving from the sitting (or lying down) position to the standing position, is evidence for orthostatic hypotension; however, one must not overlook the patient with possible orthostatic cerebral hypoperfusion, and marked clinical symptoms in the standing position, but who may not manifest overt hypotension. Although many approaches to orthostatic vital signs would be acceptable, it is wise to routinely observe dizzy patients, in the standing position, for at least 3 minutes, while monitoring for symptoms and/or changes of vital signs. If overwhelming dizziness develops during such a test, the patient should, for safety, be placed back into a sitting or lying down position and allowed to recover.

CERVICAL SPINE

The neck provides proprioceptive information to the brain and is thus a potential substrate for dizziness. Pain specialists are familiar with the dizziness occasionally elicited with performance of bilateral cervical spine injection procedures.[4] It is likely that application of a combination of tests involving error in position sense of the neck and nystagmus upon turning of the neck would improve diagnosis of patients with cervical spine disorders plus dizziness.[5,6] The best approach to the use of such methods, in practice, remains to be clarified. At present, the best the busy clinician can hope for with respect to diagnosing cervicogenic dizziness may be to perform range-of-motion testing in the yaw (horizontal), pitch (sagittal), and roll tilt (coronal) planes and ask the patient whether any of the "dizziness" symptoms are reproduced with certain neck positions or motions. If so, the clinician can then look for treatable cervical spine disorders. One should remember to consider the differential diagnosis of cervical artery dissection, of which neck pain is a common early feature. For that reason, along with the possibility of cervical myelopathy, the clinician considering a diagnosis of cervicogenic dizziness must be sure to look for abnormal findings on the basic neurologic examination that might lead one in a different direction.

MENTAL STATUS

Although the central vestibular system is often conceptualized in terms of posterior fossa structures, widespread brain areas are needed to integrate multisensory information in such a way as to create cues and impressions pertaining to space and motion. Such integrative function inevitably involves the cerebral cortex.

One should at least consider in passing the possibility that a chief complaint of "dizziness" may be localized to the cerebral cortex. Indeed, it is not unusual for a patient with Alzheimer disease to report "dizziness" that defies explication, even in the best of hands. This being the case, one should identify and record abnormal cognitive behaviors such as repetitive questioning. If present, these suggest short-term memory impairment. Cognitive function can be screened for by asking the patient to spell the word "world" backward. If there is any doubt about the patient's cognition, the clinician can assess further with a brief cognitive test battery such as the Montreal Cognitive Assessment.[7]

As part of the mental status examination, one should assess for anxiety. A common clinical conundrum is anxiety, or more properly an anxiety disorder, may be formulated as a cause of dizziness, a consequence of an inner ear disorder that causes dizziness, or a product of aggravation of an underlying anxiety disorder by an inner ear disorder.[8] In some cases, the anxiety is an important therapeutic target. A qualitative notation on the chart about the examiner's impressions of the patient's mood and affect contributes to tracking of this component.

VISION

Isolated loss of vision seldom causes a marked disturbance of balance. Like other sensory channels, however, vision does contribute to balance, and visual impairment contributes to imbalance. In particular, visual field cuts may be unobvious to the patient and may aggravate imbalance and increase fall risk.[9] The standard confrontation tests of visual fields are familiar to most physicians. In addition, visual fields can be assessed in detail at the bedside, using a laser pointer and a wall.[10] For patients who are users of bifocal, trifocal, or progressive lenses, walking should be assessed with and without the use of glasses. Declines in performance with the use of certain lenses should be noted.

FACIAL NERVE FUNCTION

The Ramsay Hunt syndrome consists of facial nerve palsy, combined with a painful rash involving the pinna or external auditory canal, plus vestibular and hearing deficits in varying proportions. This syndrome is presumed to often be due to latent virus reactivation. Treatment, which is beyond the scope of this review, is modeled after that used in the setting of Bell palsy. It is important to recognize the facial palsy, which may be relatively subtle in the context of severe dizziness. On examination, eye closure is less vigorous on the involved side, and the ipsilesional nasolabial fold is relatively flat. After some recovery, synkinesis may be noted, such that closure of the eye on the affected side is associated with aberrant twitching of facial muscles.

OTOSCOPY AND HEARING

Although a detailed ear examination is beyond the scope of this review, a few points warrant brief discussion. Applying positive and negative pneumatic pressure during otoscopy may elicit dizziness in pressure-sensitive disorders. These pressure-sensitive disorders, including the superior semicircular canal dehiscence syndrome[11] and occasionally Meniere syndrome.[12] In the instance of Ramsay Hunt syndrome (see earlier), otoscopy may disclose vesicles in the external auditory canal.

Hearing loss is a key feature of some disorders that cause dizziness. One must not, however, immediately assume that hearing loss is sensorineural. For example, cerumen blocking the external auditory canal may cause hearing impairment. At the same time, one should try to make a diagnosis of sensorineural hearing loss as early as possible, because of the potential need to treat sudden sensorineural hearing loss with corticosteroid medication. Sensorineural hearing loss that involves loss of acuity for low-frequency sound is a component of the diagnostic criteria for Meniere disease. Interestingly, there are also emerging data suggesting that hearing loss of any form may contribute to imbalance due to loss of sound cues about the spatial environment.[13,14]

The well-known Rinne test is typically performed with a 512-Hz tuning fork. If the patient reports that sound is heard louder through bone than air, the result suggests either a component of conductive hearing loss or a pseudoconductive hearing loss, due to a third mobile window, such as superior semicircular canal dehiscence.[15] It is helpful to have a low-frequency (128 or 64 Hz) tuning fork, because hearing asymmetries tend to be marked for this frequency when testing patients with Meniere. If whispered speech is poorly understood in either ear, a retrocochlear lesion, for example, vestibular schwannoma, should be considered.

NYSTAGMUS

The most common type of nystagmus, called jerk nystagmus, is a rhythmic eye movement having well-defined slow and fast phases. One should observe for the presence of spontaneous nystagmus, while the patient is sitting, looking straight ahead. In the case of acute unilateral peripheral vestibulopathy, and/or vestibular neuritis, and/or labyrinthitis, spontaneous nystagmus is predominantly horizontal and unidirectional with fast phases away from the lesion (a smaller torsional component may be evident). The amplitude of spontaneous, unidirectional nystagmus typically increases with gaze in the direction of fast phases.

The nystagmus of acute peripheral vestibulopathy becomes coarser when one eliminates fixation, using Frenzel video goggles. Alternatively, to eliminate fixation, one of the patient's eyes can be covered while the other eye is viewed with an ophthalmoscope and observed for nystagmus.

Smooth pursuit should be tested by asking the patient to slowly follow a finger to the right and left, and up and down, noting smoothness of eye movements. Saccadic smooth pursuit localizes to the brain. The specificity of the latter sign, however, is greater in younger patients.[16] Despite the high prevalence of saccadic smooth pursuit with increasing age, excessive degeneration of smooth pursuit function is reported to be associated with neurodegenerative brain diseases.[17]

Gaze-evoked and/or gaze-holding nystagmus may be defined as nystagmus that is absent when looking straight but is present when looking (maintaining gaze) in some directions. Gaze-evoked nystagmus may be seen in normal people with extreme eye deviation, for example, all the way to the right, but there is no widely accepted consensus on a definition of "extreme." Suffice it to say that the specificity of gaze-evoked nystagmus is highest when small deviations of eye position away from straight ahead elicit nystagmus.

Direction switching nystagmus (eg, right beating with right gaze, and left beating with left gaze) is a red flag for a possible brain lesion, as is pure vertical nystagmus, or vertical nystagmus with only a subtle torsional component. If direction switching nystagmus is asymmetric, that is, coarser with gaze in one particular direction, this suggests a focal, structural brain lesion.

Persistent downbeat nystagmus may be spontaneous, but it tends to be coarser on gaze to the right or left. It can be due to lesions of the cerebellum or at the craniocervical junction, as in the case of Arnold Chiari malformations. Rebound nystagmus localizes to the cerebellum. It is recognized as follows: the patient first is asked to follow a target such as the examiner's finger to an eccentric position, for example, all the way to the right, and then to make a saccade back to the midline, at which point a burst of nystagmus is seen, in the direction of the saccade back toward the midline.

An important type of nystagmus is that observed in patients with BPPV. As implied by the name of this condition, the nystagmus that is the hallmark of BPPV is paroxysmal and occurs in certain positions. The nystagmus occurs within seconds after moving into a provocative position. The latency between adopting a provocative position and the onset of nystagmus is typically less than 15 seconds, but it can be longer.

If all evidence points to BPPV, but nystagmus cannot be easily elicited, it may be worth a try to maintain the patient in each provocative position for a longer period, for example, 30 seconds, and observe for nystagmus. The latency between movement of the head and onset of nystagmus is presumably due to a combination of the time needed for freely floating particles to move around a semicircular canal and then subsequently into and through the ampulla.

The best single test for BPPV is the Dix-Hallpike test,[18] which was originally described by Dix and Hallpike.[19] In brief, while the patient is seated, the head is turned 30° to 45° in the horizontal plane toward the ear to be tested. The patient next lies down with the neck extended about 30° below the level of the examining surface. The examiner observes for a paroxysmal burst of nystagmus. With the onset of nystagmus, most patients feel anxious, some more than others. If the clinician anticipates such reactions, anticipation of such reactions may facilitate counseling of the patient and talking the patient through particle repositioning maneuvers, in a calm and reassuring manner.

In the most common form of BPPV, where debris is trapped in a posterior semicircular canal, the nystagmus is a combination of upbeat and torsional with the upper poles of the eyes beating toward the ground. The technical method of performance of the Dix-Hallpike test has been described elsewhere in great detail.[20,21]

It is important to note that the Dix-Hallpike test will only be positive if there is debris in one or more of the semicircular canals. If debris is instead primarily within the utricle, the Dix-Hallpike test may be negative. The patient may, however, experience vertigo again within a short timeframe, if the debris is transported from the utricle into a semicircular canal. The moral is that if BPPV is strongly suspected, but the Dix-Hallpike test is negative, it may be advisable to repeat the test on a different day. Selected nystgamus types and associated abnormalities may be found in (**Table 1**).

VERTICAL OCULAR MISALIGNMENT

The search for skew deviation is becoming a routine part of the neurologic examination in some emergency departments.[22] The key point for the nonspecialist is that any new vertical misalignment of the eyes should be considered a potential central sign, for example, due to involvement of the brainstem. To probe for ocular misalignment, one can simply ask the patient whether there is a history of double vision. Ocular misalignment can be revealed on examination through use of the alternate cover test, in which a patient fixates on a target, such as the examiner's nose, while each of the patient's eyes is alternately covered. This procedure is repeated several times, alternating between the right and left eye. The examiner should observe for readjustment of eye position when either eye is uncovered.

ABNORMAL SACCADIC EYE MOVEMENTS

Fixation may be derailed by inappropriate saccades referred to as saccadic intrusions. One common saccadic intrusion is the square wave jerk. The square wave jerk is an

Table 1	
Selected abnormal examination findings and the differential diagnosis	
Examination Finding	**Differential Diagnosis**
Dix-Hallpike test shows paroxysmal upbeat torsional (or horizontal or downbeat) nystagmus	BPPV involving the posterior (or horizontal or anterior) semicircular canal, respectively
Spontaneous, unidirectional, predominantly horizontal nystagmus	Acute peripheral vestibulopathy and/or vestibular neuritis and/or labyrinthitis
Gaze evoked, direction switching nystagmus	Posterior fossa lesion
Skew deviation	Posterior fossa lesion
Facial palsy and vesicles in the external auditory canal	Ramsay Hunt syndrome
Asymmetric loss of hearing acuity	Meniere syndrome, vestibular schwannoma

eye movement in which a small, single saccade, in random direction, is followed by a saccade back to the direction of fixation. Square wave jerks are nonspecific. Their presence may signify basal ganglia or cerebellar disease, but they are also seen in older people without evident neurologic disease. Unlike jerk nystagmus, saccades may be distinguished by the absence of well defined, rhythmic fast and slow phases.

VESTIBULO-OCULAR REFLEX TESTS

A focused assessment of the semicircular canal function, at least for the horizontal canal, can be performed at the bedside. The head impulse test was developed to assess the horizontal angular vestibulo-ocular reflex. The technical method of the head impulse test has been described in detail elsewhere.[23] In brief, the patient fixates on the examiner's nose, typically starting with the patient's head turned about 10° to the right or left of midline. The head is then abruptly, passively, and unpredictably turned by the examiner, toward one side or the other, through about 20°, using caution to avoid injury. The examiner watches for catch up saccades back toward the midline. In the case of peripheral vestibulopathy, the eyes move passively with the head during head impulses, resulting in the need for a catch up saccade, away from the weak ear, toward the examiner's nose. An assumption of this test, and a fairly good one, is that in some disorders, such as acute vestibular neuritis, peripheral vestibular involvement is substantially diffuse and would thus be expected to involve the horizontal semicircular canals.

Like the head impulse test, dynamic visual acuity tests assess the vestibulo-ocular reflex. First, the patient's best near vision is determined. Then, the examiner passively oscillates the patient's head to the right and left in the yaw (horizontal) plane at about 2 Hz. If the patient loses more than 2 lines of vision, vestibular weakness should be suspected. It is best to use a near card, because the demands on the vestibulo-ocular reflex are greater with near viewing.[24]

LIMB MOTOR TESTS

The title of this section is deliberately noncommittal and meant to encompass what physicians typically call motor and cerebellar tests. Labeling tests as "motor" (by which many neurologists would mean muscle bulk, tone, and strength) or "cerebellar," as is often done in practice, belies the inherent multisystem and poorly localized nature of the functions being tested.

Moreover, many techniques involving limbs depend on substantial sensory inputs for which any test interpretation must (but usually does not) account. Thus, it is wise to choose tests that are as simple as possible, on both the afferent and efferent sides, in order to limit the amount of information given to the patient and increase the sensitivity of the test.

The finger-to-nose tests familiar to every medical student are flawed. They give the patient abundant sensory information, potentially disguising deficits. More sensitive for detection of peripheral vestibulopathy are past pointing tests. These past pointing tests that require a patient (with eyes closed) to extend both arms and repeatedly touch the examiner's fingers approaching the examiner's fingers either from above or below. Past pointing tests were studied by Róbert Bárány,[25] who described his method as follows[26]:

> The patient is asked to close his eyes and touch the doctor's finger with…index finger, then…keeping the arm outstretched…lower it to knee-level, then raise it again and touch the doctor's finger once more…The direction of…deviation will

differ according to the direction of the nystagmus...always in an opposite direction to the nystagmus...

The muscle power examination has obvious relationships to balance and gait. Particularly important is to test both foot dorsiflexor[27] and plantarflexor[28] power. Deficits of either may cause critical gait and balance impairment. Strength can be assessed either with manual muscle power examination, or at times more revealingly, by asking the patient to perform tasks using the patient's own body weight, such as standing on the toes, while the examiner observes the vigor with which this maneuver is completed.

BALANCE AND GAIT TESTS

The Romberg sign is a well-known indicator of visual dependence that implies loss of normal proprioception or loss of peripheral vestibular function.[29] Originally developed for diagnosis of myelopathy, namely tabes dorsalis, the Romberg sign is also encountered in clinical practice when testing patients with bilateral peripheral vestibular hypofunction,[30] and those with vitamin B12 deficiency, copper deficiency, or hyperzincemia.[31]

The Romberg test can be made more difficult and thus more sensitive to balance-related issues by asking the patient to stand in tandem with eyes closed. The examiner should note whether the patient can confidently maintain this posture for several seconds. There are many variations of the Romberg test. In general, these tests have been somewhat unduly criticized, as a result of their less than excellent sensitivity (due in part to vestibular compensation) and specificity (many different types of disorders and aging affect balance).

As is the case with respect to other clinical neurologic tests, any one isolated abnormality must be interpreted with caution. Combined with other tests, though, the Romberg test contributes sensitivity to the neurologic examination. For example, a patient who presents after an acute vertiginous illness, and who falls strongly to the left, has mild left-sided hearing loss and has right beating nystagmus on extreme rightward gaze, might be suspected to have had left-sided labyrinthitis. Any one of these findings alone, in isolation, might be discounted, but together, they form an important pattern.

Similar comments might be made about the Fukuda stepping test. In this test, a patient is asked to march in place with arms outstretched and eyes closed for about 1 minute, and the examiner observes for abnormal turning toward the right or left greater than 20°.[32] If used as a stand-alone test, it is not likely to have high sensitivity or specificity for any particular disorder. However, when combined with other tests described in this review, the Fukuda test increases the likelihood of recognition of a diagnostically useful pattern.

In the examination of gait, one should ask the patient to walk outside the examination room and look for potential signs of central nervous system dysfunction, for example, small step length, irregular step length, and asymmetric arm swing. The "walking Romberg" test gauges postural stability during a 5-m walk with the patient's eyes closed. Most patients with clinically significant cervical myelopathy were reported to manifest either a Romberg sign or a walking Romberg sign.[33]

Recently, there has been increasing interest in dual-task paradigms that simultaneously assess cognition and gait.[34] Balance places phenomenal demands on attention. If a patient has an underlying cognitive disorder, an abnormality of gait, or both, the gait and balance dysfunction can in some cases be unmasked by placing cognitive demands on the patient while simultaneously also asking the patient to perform a balance or gait task. The breakdown of gait function during a cognitively challenging task may be expressed in terms of the dual task cost (DTC) of walking while performing a cognitively demanding task, for example:

DTC = ([single-task gait velocity – dual-task gait velocity]/single-task gait velocity) $\times$ 100.[35]

One of the first reported clinical tests in this category was the "Stops walking when talking" test that was reported to predict fall risk.[36] The clinician can glean helpful information through careful observation of the patient's gait in the hallway during conversation, in comparison to that when the patient is concentrating on walking. One definition of high DTC that might reasonably be used in practice would be a decrease in gait velocity of greater than 20% when performing a cognitive task, such as counting backward from 100 while walking.[37] If a patient's performance declines markedly during conversation or performance of a cognitive task such as counting backward (reflecting a high DTC), then cognitive impairment and a risk for falls[38] should both be suspected.

SUMMARY

Through performance of a neurologic and ear examination, objective data can be gleaned that narrow the differential diagnosis of "dizziness." The multisensory and integrative nature of balance places distinct demands on the diagnostic process. Accordingly, the combination of multiple types of physical examination methods may be expected to increase the sensitivity of one's approach to detection of disorders.

REFERENCES

1. Saber Tehrani AS, Coughlan D, Hsieh YH, et al. Rising annual costs of dizziness presentations to U.S. emergency departments. Acad Emerg Med 2013;20: 689–96.
2. Florence CS, Bergen G, Atherly A, et al. Medical costs of fatal and nonfatal falls in older adults. J Am Geriatr Soc 2018;66(4):693–8.
3. Whitman GT. Dizziness [review]. Am J Med 2018. https://doi.org/10.1016/j. amjmed.2018.05.014.
4. Zhu X, Grover MJ. Cervicogenic dizziness successfully treated with upper cervical medial branch nerve radiofrequency ablation: a case report. A A Pract 2018; 10(6):150–3.
5. L'Heureux-Lebeau B, Godbout A, Berbiche D, et al. Evaluation of paraclinical tests in the diagnosis of cervicogenic dizziness. Otol Neurotol 2014;35(10): 1858–65.
6. Reiley AS, Vickory FM, Funderburg SE, et al. How to diagnose cervicogenic dizziness. Arch Physiother 2017;7:12.
7. Hobson J. The montreal cognitive assessment (MoCA). Occup Med (Lond) 2015; 65(9):764–5.
8. Staab JP, Ruckenstein MJ. Which comes first? Psychogenic dizziness versus otogenic anxiety. Laryngoscope 2003;113(10):1714–8.
9. Mihailovic A, Swenor BK, Friedman DS, et al. Gait implications of visual field damage from glaucoma. Transl Vis Sci Technol 2017;6(3):23.
10. Stark R. Clinical testing of visual fields using a laser pointer and a wall. Pract Neurol 2013;13(4):258–9.

11. Shuman AG, Rizvi SS, Pirouet CW, et al. Hennebert's sign in superior semicircular canal dehiscence syndrome: a video case report. Laryngoscope 2012;122(2): 412–4.
12. Nadol JB Jr. Positive Hennebert's sign in Meniere's disease. Arch Otolaryngol 1977;103(9):524–30.
13. Zhong X, Yost WA. Relationship between postural stability and spatial hearing. J Am Acad Audiol 2013;24(9):782–8.
14. Vitkovic J, Le C, Lee SL, et al. The contribution of hearing and hearing loss to balance control. Audiol Neurootol 2016;21(4):195–202.
15. Bance M. When is a conductive hearing loss not a conductive hearing loss? Causes of a mismatch in air-bone threshold measurements or a "pseudoconductive" hearing loss. J Otolaryngol 2004;33(2):135–8.
16. Maruta J, Spielman LA, Rajashekar U, et al. Visual tracking in development and aging. Front Neurol 2017;8:640.
17. Shakespeare TJ, Kaski D, Yong KXX, et al. Abnormalities of fixation, saccade and pursuit in posterior cortical atrophy. Brain 2015;138(Pt 7):1976–91.
18. Bhattacharyya N, Gubbels SP, Schwartz SR, et al. Clinical practice guideline: benign paroxysmal positional vertigo (update). Otolaryngol Head Neck Surg 2017;156(3_suppl):S1–47.
19. Dix MR, Hallpike CS. The pathology, symptomatology and diagnosis of certain common disorders of the vestibular system. Proc R Soc Med 1952;45(6):341–54.
20. Muncie HL, Sirmans SM, James E. Dizziness: approach to evaluation and management. Am Fam Physician 2017;95(3):154–62.
21. Kim JS, Zee DS. Clinical practice. Benign paroxysmal positional vertigo. N Engl J Med 2014;370(12):1138–47.
22. Newman-Toker DE, Kerber KA, Hsieh YH, et al. HINTS outperforms ABCD2 to screen for stroke in acute continuous vertigo and dizziness. Acad Emerg Med 2013;20(10):986–96.
23. Spiegel R, Kirsch M, Rosin C, et al. Dizziness in the emergency department: an update on diagnosis. Swiss Med Wkly 2017;147:w14565.
24. Viirre E, Tweed D, Milner K, et al. A reexamination of the gain of the vestibuloocular reflex. J Neurophysiol 1986;56(2):439–50.
25. Behrman W. The pointing test of barany. Br Med J 1938;1(4033):898.
26. Robert Bárány - Nobel Lecture. Available at: https://www.nobelprize.org/nobel_prizes/medicine/laureates/1914/barany-lecture.html. Accessed June 6, 2018.
27. Poppler LH, Groves AP, Sacks G, et al. Subclinical peroneal neuropathy: a common, unrecognized, and preventable finding associated with a recent history of falling in hospitalized patients. Ann Fam Med 2016;4(6):526–33.
28. Macgilchrist C, Paul L, Ellis BM, et al. Lower-limb risk factors for falls in people with diabetes mellitus. Diabet Med 2010;27(2):162–8.
29. Cheng HM, Park JH, Hernstadt D. Subacute combined degeneration of the spinal cord following recreational nitrous oxide use. BMJ Case Rep 2013. https://doi.org/10.1136/bcr-2012-008509.
30. Strupp M, Kim JS, Murofushi T, et al. Bilateral vestibulopathy: diagnostic criteria consensus document of the classification Committee of the Bárány Society. J Vestib Res 2017;27(4):177–89.
31. Verma R, Praharaj HN, Khanna VK, et al. Study of micronutrients (copper, zinc and vitamin B12) in posterolateral myelopathies. J Neurol Sci 2013;329(1–2): 11–6.
32. Dai M, Cohen B, Smouha E, et al. Readaptation of the vestibulo-ocular reflex relieves the mal de debarquement syndrome. Front Neurol 2014;5:124.

33. Findlay GF, Balain B, Trivedi JM, et al. Does walking change the Romberg sign? Eur Spine J 2009;18(10):1528–31.
34. Fritz NE, Cheek FM, Nichols-Larsen DS. Motor-cognitive dual-task training in persons with neurologic disorders: a systematic review. J Neurol Phys Ther 2015; 39(3):142–53.
35. Montero-Odasso MM, Sarquis-Adamson Y, Speechley M, et al. Association of dual-task gait with incident dementia in mild cognitive impairment: results from the gait and brain study. JAMA Neurol 2017;74(7):857–65.
36. Hyndman D, Ashburn A. Stops walking when talking as a predictor of falls in people with stroke living in the community. J Neurol Neurosurg Psychiatry 2004;75(7): 994–7.
37. Sakurai R, Bartha R, Montero-Odasso M. Entorhinal cortex volume is associated with dual-task gait cost among older adults with MCI: results from the gait and brain study. J Gerontol A Biol Sci Med Sci 2018. https://doi.org/10.1093/gerona/gly084.
38. Yamada M, Aoyama T, Arai H, et al. Dual-task walk is a reliable predictor of falls in robust elderly adults. J Am Geriatr Soc 2011;59(1):163–4.

Gait Disorders and Falls in the Elderly

Michael Ronthal, MBBCh, FRCP, FRCPE, FCP (SA)

KEYWORDS

- Elderly gait disorders • Falls • Gait physiology • Bedside diagnosis

KEY POINTS

- Gait is a complex function, and dysfunction at multiple levels can affect normal walking and predispose to falls.
- Diagnosis of the basic pathophysiology comes from a hands-on bedside examination.
- Once the abnormal signs are defined further study is rationally indicated.
- Not infrequently the cause of a gait disorder is multifactorial.

INTRODUCTION

Walking is part of daily living and in normal subjects it is easy. The physiology of walking is complex and diagnosis of a gait disorder requires a working knowledge of normal physiology. When this complex control system fails, the risk of falls increases.

The prevalence of gait and balance disorders increases with age and is 10% between 60 and 69 years and is more than 60% in those older than 80 years. The prevalence increases to 82% in those older than 85 years.[1]

In the United States, 30% of people older than 65 years fall each year and in people older than 80 years, falls occur in as often as 50% of people.[2] Seventy-five percent of deaths due to falls occur in 13% of the population older than 65 years.[3]

Gait and complex cognitive functioning are closely related, and walking should no longer be considered a simple motor activity independent of cognition. Walking involves the integration of attention, planning, and memory and other motor and perceptual and cognitive processes.[4] Worse executive function has been correlated with decrease in gait velocity, slower pace, reduced cadence, and gait variability.[5-7]

PHYSIOLOGY OF GAIT

The control of walking is a complicated affair, but a basic understanding of the normal control system guides diagnosis when walking is disordered.

Disclosure Statement: No Disclosures.
Department of Neurology, Harvard Medical School, Beth Israel Deaconess Medical Center, 330 Brookline Avenue, Boston, MA 02215, USA
E-mail address: mronthal@bidmc.harvard.edu

Med Clin N Am 103 (2019) 203–213
https://doi.org/10.1016/j.mcna.2018.10.010
0025-7125/19/© 2018 Elsevier Inc. All rights reserved.

Sherrington remarked: all parts of the nervous system are connected together and no part of it is probably ever capable of reaction without affecting and being affected by various other parts.[8] Normal gait requires a delicate balance between various interacting neuronal systems and consists of 3 primary components: locomotion including initiation and maintenance of rhythmic stepping; balance; and ability to adapt to the environment. All levels of the nervous system are needed for normal gait.[9]

Spinal Cord Level

Repetitive, alternating, and coordinated movements of the arms and legs are triggered by central pattern generators (CPGs) segmentally organized in the spinal cord. Newborn infants exhibit automatic stepping and placing movements. Experimentally decerebrate and spinal cat preparations provide support for the notion of CPGs in the cord, when the spinal animal can be induced to walk on a treadmill.[10,11] This basic motor pattern is modified by sensory feedback and supraspinal control, which overwhelms the CPG with maturation.

Supraspinal Locomotor Centers

Spinal CPGs are controlled by descending input from specific locomotor command regions in the brain stem and cerebellum.[12] If a brain stem region contains neurons that, when activated chemically or electrically, leads to the production of locomotion, that area is called a "locomotor region" (LMR). Stimulation of the brain stem at various levels in the decerebrate cat produces different movement patterns depending on the level of stimulation.[13] Locomotor regions include the subthalamic LMR, the mesencephalic LMR including the pedunculopontine nucleus in the dorsal midbrain, the cerebellar LMR in the cerebellar midline, and the pontine LMR. The cerebellar vermis integrates proprioceptive, vestibular, and visual afferent information into the locomotor program.[14]

The basal ganglia output nuclei have connections to the mesencephalic LMR.[15]

The frontal cortices have connections with the cerebellum via the thalamus and pontine nuclei and with the basal ganglia via the basal ganglia thalamocortical circuit.[16] Cortical executive function plays a role in willed walking,[17] strategic planning of the best route, and continuous interaction with the environment.[18,19]

Classification

One classification of gait disorders relates to the level of the sensorimotor deficit, that is, low, middle, and high. Low deficits are defects in peripheral sensory and peripheral motor systems. On the sensory side consider vestibulopathy, neuropathy, and visual deficits. On the motor side include nonneurologic deficits such as arthritis, as well as motor neuropathy and myopathy. Patients adapt well and compensate by limping or using assistive devices.

Middle deficits result in spasticity, parkinsonism, and cerebellar ataxia, each of which produces a classic gait disorder.

High deficits, often with cognitive impairment, result in frontal gait patterns and behavioral aspects such as fear of falling and cautious gait.

There may be deficits at more than one level.[20]

Many gait disorders are of multifactorial origin, but a simple etiologic classification is clinically most useful. One should start by deciding if the problem is primarily neurologic or the cause is outside the nervous system. Based on gait observation and a detailed physical examination the site of the malfunction is diagnosed. Further study such as MRI helps to define the pathology.

In a survey of patients referred because of abnormal gait, by Sudarsky and Ronthal, and follow-up by Sudarsky,[21,22] the classification according to cause is detailed in **Table 1**. Deficit, in about 14% of elderly patients presenting with a gait disorder, despite an excellent examination and sophisticated investigations, the cause remains unknown.

Much as in a detective story, one should have a theoretic list of possible suspects and based on the physical examination narrow down the list as to the site of physiologic dysfunction, which will dictate the further work up. Although most texts emphasize the value of a detailed history, in the gait disorder patient, the history is usually of little help.

The suspects include weakness, deafferentation, vestibular dysfunction, cerebellar ataxia, extrapyramidal disease, and higher-level dysfunction, psychogenic and non-neurologic. Each suspect will now be described in detail.

Weakness

The pattern of weakness can be diagnostic of the cause. Weakness may reflect dysfunction of central descending motor pathways—upper motor neuron (UMN)—or be the result of dysfunction of peripheral nerve from anterior horn cell to myoneural junction or of muscle itself.

Muscles vary in strength from site to site, and it may be difficult to differentiate mild weakness from normal. If the examiner can overcome muscle power exerting resistance close to the joint that the muscle moves, using an equivalent examiner muscle (eg, fingers test toe strength), that muscle is by definition weak. One should record the degree of weakness.

In UMN weakness there is usually added spasticity. The pattern of weakness in the lower limb or limbs makes the diagnosis: muscles particularly affected are hip flexors, foot dorsiflexors, and knee flexors.

In lower motor neuron weakness, the pattern of weakness is different, depending on the site of pathology. Additional clues may be a sensory segmental level or a dropped reflex.

In proximal weakness that affects the limb girdles only, suspect a myopathy. An important clue is weakness of neck flexors and extensors. The gait is waddling.

Isolated quadriceps weakness supports the diagnosis of a femoral nerve lesion and the leg may give way at the knee on standing.

Table 1
Gait disorders in 120 patients

Cause	Total	Percentage
Sensory deficits	22	18.3
Myelopathy	20	16.7
Multiple infarcts	18	15
Unknown cause	17	14.2
Parkinsonism	14	11.7
Cerebellar degeneration	8	6.7
Hydrocephalus	8	6.7
Other	6	5
Psychogenic	4	3.3
Toxic/metabolic	3	2.5

In foot drop due to a lesion of the common peroneal nerve, the gait is high stepping to clear the toes; the hip flexors are normal.

If weakness is triggered by repetitive exercise, myasthenia is likely. Diffuse weakness with muscle fasciculations and hyperreflexia points to motor neuron disease.

Deafferentation

Sensory input allows for monitoring of motor output. The critical feedback modality is position sense or proprioception.[23] Spinocerebellar feedback is of theoretic importance, but, with the exception of the spinocerebellar ataxias, it is hard to demonstrate that this is a frequent or potent cause of elderly gait dysfunction.

Vision and vestibular feedback are other sensory input systems.

Loss of position sense can, rarely, be seen in patients with very severe peripheral neuropathy as in diabetic pseudotabes but usually reflects dysfunction of the posterior columns of the spinal cord. Dorsal root ganglionopathy can cause loss of position sense and should be considered if the spinal cord workup is negative.

Lesions above the foramen magnum rarely cause proprioceptive loss, but sensory cortical pathology should also be considered if the spinal cord is normal.

The gait is usually described as "stamping." After heel strike, the foot slaps down on the ground forcefully in order to increase sensory stimulation. Position sense is defective in the toes and in severe cases even at the ankle. The Romberg sign is positive — the patient is steady standing with the feet together and eyes open, but on closing the eyes there is sway. Vision is compensatory, and the patient should be advised to keep the lights on at night in an attempt to prevent falling.

Loss of position sense in the upper limbs is usually due to a very high myelopathy. In hand postural testing, if the eyes are closed, aimless spontaneous movement of the fingers is labeled pseudoathetosis.

Vestibular dysfunction

Dizziness as such is a nonspecific complaint of multiple causes but could imply imbalance or dysequilibrium.[24] Consider cardiovascular pathology, neck spasm, a focal seizure if intermittent, ocular pathology, and psychogenic causes. Motion sickness can be regarded as physiologic dizziness.

An abnormal sensation of rotation or spinning implies dysfunction in the vestibular system, either peripheral or central. It is almost always episodic, and compensation occurs in weeks.

Vestibular reflexes allow for normal gait and posture. Feedback from the peripheral vestibular system, semicircular canals, and utricle induces reflex body muscle contraction to compensate for head movement and to maintain equilibrium with movement under the influence of steady changes in the force of gravity. The vestibular ocular reflex maintains eye movement stability in the face of any kind of head movement.

The most important sign of vestibular dysfunction is nystagmus, and its subjective symptom, oscillopsia. Unilateral nystagmus usually implies unilateral peripheral pathology. Bilateral horizontal, vertical, or rotary nystagmus implies central pathology.[25]

The gait disturbance varies from an occasional stumble through veering to one side or another to frank ataxia and staggering. The patient veers to the pathologic side. Stride length is shortened.

A short-lived spinning sensation with positional change can be tested for by provoking the symptoms. With the patient supine, the head is tilted 30° below the horizontal and twisted to one or other side. In paroxysmal positional vertigo, after a short latent period the patient complains of spinning and the eyes show rotary nystagmus, which spontaneously fatigues. The Epley positional physiotherapy exercises are usually curative.

The differential diagnosis of peripheral vestibular dysfunction includes acute vestibular neuronitis, Meniere disease, positional vertigo, postconcussional syndrome, and perilymph fistula.

Central causes are usually brain stem located, and an occasional patient with focal seizures arising in the temporal lobe will complain of episodic spinning sensation as part of a focal seizure.

If the history and examination are not contributory, consider hyperventilation syndrome.[26] Forced hyperventilation may reproduce the dizziness.

Cerebellar ataxia

Gait ataxia or lack of coordination in the legs implies dysfunction in the cerebellum, usually vermis, and cerebellar connections in the brain stem. Occasionally bifrontal dysfunction causes an ataxic gait. Cerebellar ataxia is restricted to active complex movements and is not improved by vision.

The cerebellum projects back to the spinal cord via the lateral vestibular nucleus and reticular formation, which allows for control of alpha and gamma motor neurons.

The gait is wide based, staggering, reeling, drunken. The patient cannot walk a straight line. Stride length is slightly shortened. The patient may miss a step and stagger, particularly on turning. There may be truncal ataxia—the trunk muscles cannot be coordinated in the interest of immobilization. A light tap on the chest or back causes a stagger or fall. The "finger-nose" and "heel-shin" tests are clumsy and dysmetric. There is generalized hypotonia. Speech may be slurred and scanning.

The cause is varied. Consider metabolic dysfunction, for example, hypothyroidism, vitamin E deficiency, alcoholism, paraneoplastic syndrome, repeated head injuries, repeated strokes, demyelination, encephalitis from chicken pox, autoimmune pathogenesis, and neoplasm.

Cerebellar degeneration on a genetic basis is now classified by genotype rather than the phenotype.[27]

Consequent to the abovementioned, a fairly extensive workup is required.

Extrapyramidal disorders

Hypokinetic disorders are characterized by slowness, akinesia, and disequilibrium. Hyperkinetic disorders such as chorea seldom interfere with gait.

The caudate and putamen make up the striatum and the other components of the basal ganglia include the globus pallidus, the substantia nigra, the subthalamic nucleus, and the thalamus.[28] The cortex activates or inhibits the basal ganglia by various pathways, dubbed direct and indirect. In Parkinson's disease, dopamine-producing neurons degenerate, particularly in the substantia nigra compacta. The normal inhibitory dopaminergic input to D2 striatal neurons, which project to the globus pallidus externa decreases. The inhibitory output from the globus pallidus to the subthalamic nucleus is therefore reduced and the subthalamic nucleus becomes hyperactive, which increases activation of the globus pallidus interna, which together with decreased input from the direct pathway results in overall decreased activation of the thalamic nuclei and their cortical projection areas.[29]

Gait abnormalities are the presenting complaint of 12% to 18% of parkinsonian patients.

In Parkinson's disease, the gait is narrow based and stride length is markedly reduced. The feet barely clear the floor (marche a petit pas). Posture is stooped. The arms do not swing. With the fixed posture the center of gravity is thrown forwards and the trunk precedes the lower limbs. The patient takes increasingly faster short steps to give the appearance of running or hurrying—festination. There is a tendency to fall backwards—retropulsion. When asked to turn about on a dime or about-face, multiple small steps are taken—"en bloc" turning. Start hesitation is present and the patient cannot initiate gait with large strides. The same phenomenon may occur when walking through a doorway—freezing of gait.[30,31]

Lower-half parkinsonism is a syndrome sparing the arms but with severe parkinsonian gait and freezing. The pathology is white matter degeneration on the basis of small vessel disease, so called "vascular parkinsonism."[32]

Some degenerative pathologies have mild or more prominent parkinsonian signs as part of the clinical presentation. In Lewy body dementia, there is progressive and fluctuating cognitive impairment, early visual hallucinations, and motor parkinsonism. Falls are more common in Lewy body dementia than Alzheimer dementia, and these falls are not related to the parkinsonian features. If dementia occurs within 12 months of the onset of parkinsonian motor signs the diagnosis should be dementia with Lewy bodies.

Frontotemporal dementia[33] with frontal lobe signs, sometimes with aphasia, may have parkinsonian signs or involuntary trunk movements that may influence gait stability.[34]

Multiple system atrophy[35] is characterized as a combination of parkinsonism, autonomic failure, ataxia, and pyramidal signs. Progressive akinesia and rigidity predominate in 80% of cases. Sometimes freezing of gait is seen.

Progressive supranuclear palsy is characterized by early postural instability, supranuclear vertical gaze palsy, L-DOPA–resistant parkinsonism, pseudobulbar palsy, and mild dementia. Falls occur early.[36]

Corticobasal degeneration is a clinically heterogenous disorder with some overlap to other neurodegenerative disorders.[37] Unilateral limb rigidity or bradykinesia, postural imbalance, unilateral limb dystonia, and dementia occur, but unilateral levodopa-resistant parkinsonism and alien limb are the hallmarks.

Higher-level gait disorders
Support for neural integration of the temporal lobes, the hippocampus that has a functional relationship with the prefrontal cortex, and the nigrostriatal system comes by way of modern imaging techniques, and the periventricular white matter plays a crucial role in connectivity of gait centers.[6,38,39]

Gait dysfunction can independently predict cognitive decline and adverse outcomes such as disability, cardiovascular disease, and survival.[5] In older people without dementia a gait disorder predicts institutionalization and death.[40]

Frontal gait disorders are seen in the context of frontal cognitive deficits. Frontal lobe dysfunction can result in 2 broad syndromes: one characterized by slowness of thought, loss of initiative, apathy, and emotional blunting and the other with disinhibition, impulsivity, and loss of judgment and insight. Orbito frontal and medial frontal lesions are likely to cause disinhibition, and dorsolateral lesions are likely to cause abulia.

The gait disorder may take the form of ignition failure: at gait initiation the patient takes 3 or 4 steps on the spot, the feet barely clearing the floor, and then he steps forward on a narrow base, with shortened stride length. Freezing sometimes occurs, but when well started the gait normalizes.

Frontal ataxia looks somewhat like a cerebellar syndrome. The feet may cross or move in a direction inappropriate to the center of gravity. The gait looks bizarre.

In "apraxia" of gait there may be some difficulty with initiation, there may be freezing, and the gait is narrow based with shortened stride length and shuffling. There is hesitation on turns, disequilibrium, loss of righting reflexes with falls, and frontal cognitive loss.

Although the only sign on imaging may be brain atrophy, on occasion a mass lesion or hydrocephalus is found.

Psychogenic gait disorders

An exaggeration of the normal gait of elderly people has been called a cautious gait.[41,42] There is normally an increase in foot-floor clearance during the early swing phase, reduction in stride length, increased stance time, stooped posture, reduced stride, and loss of the normal heel-to-toe sequence of foot-floor contact. No akinesia is present.[43]

Exaggeration of the abovementioned, often with conscious awareness of the need for caution, to adjust for balance and avoid falls is regarded as a compensatory adaptation with an appropriate response to real or perceived disequilibrium.[38]

Fear of falling is strongly associated with a history of recent falls and is present in about 50% of patients who have recently fallen.[44] The anxiety can be so severe to qualify as a phobia, and the patient may resort to crawling on hands and knees.

The characteristics of a psychogenic gait disorder include astasia-abasia, which is a fairly gross presentation of hysteria, defined as the inability to stand or walk in the absence of other neurologic abnormalities. There is maintenance of postural control on a narrow base with flailing arms and excessive trunk sway without falling (tightrope walking).

One study demonstrated 6 characteristic features of psychogenic gait disorder alone or in combination in 97% of patients with psychogenic gait disorder.[45] These include the following:

1. Momentary fluctuations of stance and gait, often in response to suggestion;
2. Excessive slowness or hesitation of locomotion incompatible with neurologic disease;
3. A "psychogenic" response to the Romberg test with a buildup of swaying amplitudes after a silent latency or with improvement with distraction;
4. Uneconomic postures with wastage of muscular energy;
5. "Walking on ice" characterized by small cautious steps with fixed ankle joints;
6. Sudden buckling of the knees, usually without falls.

In depression, psychomotor retardation results in lack of propulsive thrust at the moment the stance leg pushes off from the floor. Rather the foot seems to lift from the floor. Velocity is decreased with a shorter stride length. Cadence is slowed.[46]

Nonneurologic gait disorders

Gait disorders are frequently of multifactorial origin and a neurologic deficit may or may not be accompanied by nonneurologic factors or nonneurologic pathology may be the prime cause. The evaluation of a gait disorder therefore requires a finely tuned general medical examination as well as a neurologic evaluation.

Nonneurological factors are best classified in terms of orthopedic pathology, including arthritis, bursitis, and tendinitis, all of which cause pain, cardiovascular pathology, such as cardiac failure, lumbar vascular claudication, exposure to drugs, and visual failure.[47–49]

Falls

In the United States, falls are directly or indirectly related to 1,800,00 admissions to emergency departments and 16,000 deaths annually.[50] In a year 30% of those older than 65 years and 50% of those older than 80 years will experience at least one fall. Of those living at home about 1 in 40 will be hospitalized and of those admitted to hospital after a fall only about half will be alive 1 year later.[3]

Accordingly, efforts to prevent falls are topical and an American Academy of Neurology practice parameter[51] can be summarized as follows: "There is an increased risk of falls among persons with diagnoses of stroke, dementia and disorders of gait and balance. There is a probable increased risk among patients with Parkinson's disease, peripheral neuropathy, lower extremity weakness or sensory loss and substantial vision loss. A history of falling in the past year strongly predicts the likelihood of future falls."

All of the gait disorders discussed previously, both neurologic and nonneurologic, could play a role in a fall in an elderly person, which implies a thorough and exhaustive physical examination in the hope of finding something treatable. Among them, the definition of "idiopathic faller" (ie, no overt cause for falling in a given subject) represents a new milestone in building the "science of falling."[52]

It is useful to classify falls into those with or without loss of consciousness. If there is loss of consciousness a syncope workup is in order; syncope is a symptom and not a diagnosis.[53] Syncope is common with a 10-year cumulative incidence of 11.1% for both genders, and 16.9% female and 19.5% male incidence for those aged 80 years or older.[54]

Seizure in those with loss of consciousness is the next consideration. Older patients usually do not present with the well-known classic features of complex partial seizures and tend not to generalize. A short stare or long-lasting confusional state may be the sole manifestation in this age group.[55] An normal electroencephalogram does not deny the diagnosis.[56]

On occasion the fall itself results in a head strike with concussion, which lends complexity to the workup.

The differential diagnosis of falls without loss of consciousness includes cataplexy, drop attacks, and psychogenic pseudosyncope. Consider also metabolic disorders such as intoxication and hypoglycemia.

SUMMARY

The diagnosis of gait disorders can be a complicated business compounded by the fact that multiple causes in the same patient are common, giving rise to the label "multifactorial gait disorder." Only a meticulous examination and further workup where indicated will lead to an accurate diagnosis and, if possible, appropriate treatment.

REFERENCES

1. Bloem BR, Haan J, Lagaay AM, et al. Investigation of gait in elderly subjects over 88 years of age. J Geriatr Psychiatry Neurol 1992;5:78–84.
2. Tinetti ME, Williams CS. Falls, injuries due to falls and the risk of admission to a nursing home. N Eng J Med 1997;337:1279–84.
3. Rubensatein LZ. Falls in older people: epidemiology, risk factors and strategies for prevention. Age Ageing 2006;35-S2:ii37–41.
4. Mulder T, Hochstenbach J, Barnes MP, et al. Motor control and learning: implications for neurological rehabilitation. In: Greenwood RJ, et al, editors. Handbook of neurological rehabilitation. New York: Psychology Press; 2003. p. 143–57.
5. Valknova V, Ebmeier KP. What can gait tell us about dementia? Review of epidemiological and neuropsychological evidence. Gait Posture 2017;53:215–23.
6. Scherder E, Eggermont L, Swaab D, et al. Gait in ageing and associated dementias; its relationship with cognition. Neurosci Biobehav Rev 2007;31:485–97.

7. Kearney FC, Harwood RH, Gladman JRF, et al. The relationship between executive function and falls and gait abnormalities in older adults: a systematic review. Dement Geriatr Cogn Disord 2013;36:20–35.

8. Sherrington CS. The integrative action of the nervous system. New Haven (CT): Yale University Press; 1906.

9. Nielsen JB. How we walk: central control of muscle activity during human walking. Neuroscientist 2003;9:195–204.

10. Dietz V. Spinal cord pattern generators for locomotion. Clin Neurophysiol 2003; 114:1379–89.

11. Grillner S. Control of locomotion in bipeds, tetrapods and fish. In: Brooks VB, editor. Handbook of physiology, the nervous system, vol. 11. Bethesda (MD): American Physiological Society; 1981. p. 1179–236. Motor control, part 2.

12. Armstrong DM. The supraspinal control of mammalian locomotion. J Physiol 1988;405:1–37.

13. Whelan PJ. Control of locomotion in the decerebrate cat. Prog Neurobiol 1996;49: 481.

14. Mori S, Matsuyama K, Mori F, et al. Supraspinal sites that induce locomotion in the vertebrate central nervous system. Adv Neurol 2001;87:25–40.

15. Inglis WL, Winn P. The peduncularpontine tegmental nucleus: where the striatum meets the reticular formation. Prog Neurobiol 1995;47:1–29.

16. Hashimoto T. Speculation on the responsible sites and pathophysiology of freezing of gait. Parkinsonism Rel Dis 2006;12:S55–62.

17. Jahanshahi M, Frith CD. Willed action and its impairments. Cogn Neuropsychol 1998;15:483–533.

18. Woollacott M, Shumway-Cook A. Attention and control of posture and gait: a review of an emerging area of research. Gait Posture 2002;16:1–14.

19. Snijders AH, Van de Warrenburg BP, Giladi N, et al. Neurological gait disorders in elderly people: clinical approach and classification. Lancet Neurol 2007;6:63–74.

20. Alexander NB, Goldberg A. Gait disorders: search for multiple causes. Cleve Clinic J Med 2005;72(7):586–600.

21. Sudarsky L, Ronthal M. Gait disorders among elderly patients: a survey study of 50 patients. Arch Neurol 1983;40:740–3.

22. Sudarsky L. Clinical approach to gait disorders of aging: an overview. In: Masdeu J, Sudarsky L, Wolfson L, editors. Gait disorders of aging: falls and therapeutic strategies. Philadelphia: Lippincott-Raven; 1997.

23. Cook AW, Browder EJ. Function of posterior columns in man. Arch Neurol 1965; 12:72.

24. Dix M, Hallpike C. The pathology, symptomatology, and diagnosis of certain common disorders of the vestibular systems. Ann Otol Rhinol Laryngol 1952;61:987.

25. Drachman DA, Hart CW. An approach to the dizzy patient. Neurology 1972;22: 323.

26. Magerian GJ. Hyperventilation syndromes: infrequently recognized common expressions of anxiety and stress. Medicine 1982;61:219.

27. Klockgether T, Ludtke R, Kramer B, et al. The natural history of degenerative ataxia: a retrospective study in 466 patients. Brain 1998;121:589.

28. Levy R, Hazrati LN, Herrero MT, et al. Revaluation of the functional anatomy of the basal ganglia in normal and parkinsonian states. Neuroscience 1997;76:335.

29. Obeso LA, Rodriguez MC, DeLong MR. Basal ganglia pathophysiology: a critical revue. Adv Neurol 1997;74:3.

30. Giladi N, Nieuwboer A. Understanding and treating freezing of gait in Parkinsonism, proposed working definition and setting the stage. Mov Disord 2008; 23(suppl):S423-5.
31. Snijders AH, Takakusaki K, Debu B, et al. Physiology of freezing of gait. Ann Neurol 2016;80:644-59.
32. Demirkiran M, Bozdemir H, Sarica Y. Vascular parkinsonism: a distinct heterogenous clinical entity. Acta Neurol Scand 2001;104:63-7.
33. Sjogren M, Andersen C. Frontotemporal dementia – a brief review. Mech Ageing Dev 2006;127:180-7.
34. Pijnenburg YA, Gillissen F, Jonker C, et al. Initial complaints in fronto temporal lobar degeneration. Dement Geriatr Cogn Disord 2004;17:302-6.
35. Wenning GK, Colosimo F, Geser F, et al. Multiple system atrophy. Lancet 2004;3: 93-103.
36. Litvan I, Campbell G, Mangone CA, et al. Which clinical features differentiate progressive supranuclear palsy (Steele-Richardson-Olszewski syndrome) from related disorders. A clinicopathological study. Brain 1997;120:65-74.
37. Schneider JA, Watts RL, Gearing M, et al. Corticobasal degeneration: neuropathologic and clinical heterogeneity. Neurology 1997;48:959-69.
38. Nutt J, Marsden C, Thompson P. Human walking and higher-level gait disorders, particularly in the elderly. Neurology 1993;43:268-79.
39. Bhadelia RA, Price LL, Tedesco KL, et al. Diffusion tensor imaging, white matter lesions, the corpus callosum and gait in the elderly. Stroke 2009;40:3816-20.
40. Verghese J, LeValley A, Hall CB, et al. Epidemiology of gait disorders in community-residing older adults. J Am Geriatr Soc 2006;54:255-61.
41. Sudarsky L. Psychogenic gait disorders. Semin Neurol 2006;26:351-6.
42. Keane JR. Hysterical gait disorders. Neurology 1989;39:586-9.
43. Elble RJ, Hughes L, Higgens C. The syndrome of senile gait. J Neurol 1992;239: 71-5.
44. Jette A, Assman S, Peterson EW. Fear of falling and activity restriction: the survey of activities and fear of falling in the elderly (SAFE). J Gerontol B Psychol Sci Soc Sci 1998;53:43-50.
45. Lempert T, Brandt T, Dietrich M, et al. How to identify psychogenic disorders of stance and gait. A video study in 37 patients. J Neurol 1991;238:140-6.
46. Sloman L, Berridge M, Homatidis S, et al. Gait patterns of depressed patients and normal subjects. Am J Psychiatry 1982;139:94-7.
47. Gerster JC. Plantar fasciitis and Achilles tendinitis among150 cases of seronegative spondylarthris. Rheumatol Rehabil 1980;19:218.
48. Cumming RG, Miller JP, Kelsey JL, et al. Medications and multiple falls in elderly people. The St Louis OASIS study. Age Ageing 1991;20:455.
49. Rosaasignol S. Visuomotor regulation of locomotion. Can J Physiol Pharmacol 1996;74:418.
50. Alexander BH, Rivara FP, Wolf ME. The cost and frequency of hospitalization for fall related injuries in older adults. Am J Public Health 1992;82(7):1020-3.
51. Thurman DJ, Stevens JA, Rao JK. Practice parameter: assessing patients in a neurology practice for risk of falls (an evidence-based review). Report of the Quality Standards Subcommittee of the American Academy of Neurology. Neurology 2008;70(6):1-27.
52. Fasano A, Plotnik M, Bove F. The neurobiology of falls. Neurol Sci 2012;33: 1215-23.
53. Brignole M. Distinguishing syncopal from non-syncopal causes of falls in older people. Age Ageing 2006;35(Suppl.2):ii46-50.

54. Soteriades ES, Evans JC, Larson MG, et al. Incidence and prognosis of syncope. N Eng J Med 2002;347:878–85.
55. Hauser CJ, Towne A, Ramsay R, et al. Medical aspects of epilepsy in the elderly. Epilepsy Res 2006;68(Suppl 1):39–48.
56. Ramsay RE, Rowan AJ, Pryor FM. Special considerations in treating the elderly patient with epilepsy. Neurology 2004;62:S24–9.

Migraine and Tension-Type Headache

Diagnosis and Treatment

Rebecca Burch, MD

KEYWORDS

- Headache • Migraine • Migraine with aura • Tension-type headache • Treatment
- Prevention • Nonpharmacologic treatment • Rescue treatment

KEY POINTS

- The prevalence of migraine or severe headache in the last 3 months is 15.3% in the United States; this includes 20.7% of women and 9.7% of men.
- Migraine may be misdiagnosed as tension-type headache, sinus headache, or other headache types. A diagnosis of migraine should be strongly considered for recurrent, disabling headaches without red flags for secondary headache.
- Tension-type headache typically responds to nonsteroidal antiinflammatory drugs or simple analgesics for acute treatment and tricyclic antidepressants for prevention.
- Triptans are the mainstay of acute treatment for migraine and may be used in combination with nonsteroidal antiinflammatory drugs, simple analgesics, or antiemetics.
- Prevention should be offered when headaches are frequent or disabling, or when acute treatments are overused or contraindicated. Topiramate, valproate, propranolol, metoprolol, and amitriptyline have the best evidence for efficacy. A new class of preventive treatments, the calcitonin gene related peptide monoclonal antibodies, is now available.

INTRODUCTION

Migraine is a recurrent, often disabling headache with neurovascular pathophysiology. It is highly prevalent in the United States and around the world, affecting an estimated 37 million people in the United States and 1 billion people worldwide.[1] Migraine or severe headache in the last 3 months is reported by 15.3% of people in the United States.[2] Migraine is more common in women compared with men, with a prevalence of 20.7% in women and 9.7% in men.[2] Migraine is most common during the ages of 18 to 50, a time of high potential work productivity and family caregiving responsibilities.[3] Migraine-related disability

Conflicts of Interest Statement: The author has no relevant conflicts of interest to disclose.
Department of Neurology, John R. Graham Headache Center, Brigham and Women's Hospital, Harvard Medical School, 1153 Centre Street, Suite 4H, Jamaica Plain, MA 02130, USA
E-mail address: rburch@partners.org

Med Clin N Am 103 (2019) 215–233
https://doi.org/10.1016/j.mcna.2018.10.003
0025-7125/19/© 2018 Elsevier Inc. All rights reserved.

can therefore be significant. Economic losses owing to migraine-related disability are attributable to both absenteeism and presenteeism, or decreased productivity even during work days.[4] US population-based studies suggest that lack of access to care, incorrect diagnosis, and failure to prescribe acute and preventive treatments are all barriers to optimal management of migraine.[5]

Tension-type headache is more prevalent than migraine. The epidemiology of tension-type headache is less well-studied than that of migraine. The best available estimates suggest that about 40% of people in the United States have experienced tension-type headache in the last year.[6] Because it is less severe, however, it is less likely to be seen in health care settings and is associated with less disability.[7]

DIAGNOSIS OF MIGRAINE AND TENSION-TYPE HEADACHE

The diagnostic criteria for migraine and tension-type headache are found in **Table 1**.[8] Migraine is frequently mistaken for tension-type headache, and the Spectrum study found that this was a common headache-related diagnostic error in primary care settings.[9] There are several sources of diagnostic confusion. The International Classification of Headache Disorders criteria for migraine require only 2 of the 4 commonly seen pain characteristics, which means that a bilateral and nonthrobbing headache can meet the criteria for migraine if it is moderate to severe, worsens with physical activity, and has the appropriate migraine accompanying features. Neck pain and provocation by stress, which are sometimes thought to be associated with tension-type headache, are common features of migraine as well. Neck pain is present in about two-thirds of people with migraine and stress is one of the most commonly reported migraine triggers.[10,11]

Migraine should also be considered when patients report a history of sinus headache, "sick headaches" or headaches that have a strong menstrual relationship. The Sinus, Allergy, and Migraine study found that 86% of patients who self-reported a history of sinus headache met the criteria for migraine or probable migraine.[12] The authors noted that reported triggers were a common reason for misdiagnosis, with common triggers of migraine in this population including weather changes, seasonal variation, and exposure to allergens.

Because migraine is common and frequently misdiagnosed, it is reasonable to err on the side of diagnosing migraine if a headache is recurrent, disabling, and does not have any red flags for secondary headache.[9] Making an accurate diagnosis of migraine leads to appropriate disease-specific treatment, which is more likely to be effective.

Tension-type and migraine are both divided into subtypes according to headache frequency.[8] The headache is classified as episodic if present on fewer than 15 days per month, or chronic if present 15 or more days per month. Episodic migraine may increase in frequency and become chronic over time, a process called migraine chronification or transformation. Chronic migraine has been associated with a higher burden of comorbidity and disability.[4]

MIGRAINE WITH AURA

About one-third of people with migraines have at least some attacks associated with migraine aura.[3] The diagnostic criteria for migraine aura are found in **Box 1**. Aura is a focal neurologic event with a discrete time course, typically preceding the development of migraine headache.[13] Migraine aura can also occur in the absence of headache.[8] Visual aura is the most common aura subtype and is

Table 1
Diagnostic criteria for migraine and tension-type headache

Headache Type	Migraine	Tension-Type Headache
Number of attacks	At least 5	At least 10
Duration	4–72 h (untreated or unsuccessfully treated)	30 min to 7 d
Pain characteristics	At least 2 of the 4: Unilateral location Pulsating quality Moderate or severe pain intensity Aggravation by or causing avoidance of routine physical activity (eg, walking or climbing stairs)	At least 2 of the 4: Bilateral location Pressing or tightening (nonpulsating) quality Mild or moderate intensity Not aggravated by routine physical activity such as walking or climbing stairs
Accompanying features	During headache at least 1 of the following: Nausea and/or vomiting Photophobia and phonophobia	Both of the following: No nausea or vomiting No more than one of photophobia or phonophobia

Adapted from International Headache Society (IHS). The International Classification of Headache Disorders, 3rd edition (ICHD-3). Available at: https://www.ichd-3.org/. Accessed June 24, 2018; with permission.

present in about 95% of people who get aura of any type.[14] In addition to visual aura, typical aura also includes sensory changes or dysphasic speech. Hemiplegic migraine presents with an aura including motor weakness, and should be differentiated from numbness by neurologic examination during the event. Aura should be distinguished from migraine prodromal symptoms, such as mood changes, increase or decrease in appetite, fatigue, or systemic autonomic symptoms.[15] Blurry vision is frequently reported by patients as a migraine accompanying symptom, but can be differentiated from visual aura in that it typically lasts throughout the headache or develops in association with worsened pain, and in that it typically involves the whole visual field.[16]

Patients should not be given a diagnosis of migraine with aura if there is uncertainty about symptoms, owing to treatment and cardiovascular risk implications. Women with migraine with aura have a 2-fold increase in the risk of ischemic stroke compared with women without aura.[17] Because exogenous estrogen also increases the risk of stroke, use of estrogen containing contraceptives (also called combined hormonal contraceptives [CHCs]) is contraindicated in women with migraine with aura.[18,19] It is not clear whether modern, lower estrogen dose CHCs are associated with the same level of risk.[20] In the absence of data supporting safety, it is reasonable to follow current guidelines. It is worth noting that the absolute risk of stroke in this population remains low even with use of CHCs, and an individualized assessment of risks and benefits is appropriate. Situations in which it may be reasonable to use CHCs include a lack of reliable or effective contraceptive alternatives, medical conditions that benefit from hormonal regulation, or limiting side effects from progesterone-only formulations.[18]

Box 1
Diagnostic criteria for migraine aura

1. Aura symptoms may be visual, sensory, speech and/or language, motor, brainstem, retinal
2. Symptoms should have at least 3 of the following characteristics
   - At least 1 aura symptom spreads gradually over 5 minutes or longer
   - Two or more aura symptoms occur in succession
   - Each individual aura symptom lasts 5 to 60 minutes
   - At least 1 aura symptom is unilateral
   - At least 1 aura symptom is positive
   - The aura is accompanied, or followed within 60 minutes, by headache

Adapted from International Headache Society (IHS). The International Classification of Headache Disorders, 3rd edition (ICHD-3). Available at: https://www.ichd-3.org/. Accessed June 24, 2018; with permission.

WORKUP

Migraine and tension-type headache are primary headache disorders, or those that are not caused by or attributed to another disorder. These are primarily clinical diagnoses and there is currently no available serum, cerebrospinal fluid, or imaging test to confirm a diagnosis of migraine or tension-type headache. Testing is instead used to rule out potential underlying causes of secondary headache.[21] A list of red flags that should raise concerns for secondary headache is given in **Box 2**.[22] There is no expert consensus on a panel of serum tests for headache, but some considerations might include an erythrocyte sedimentation rate and C-reactive protein in patients over 50 years of age, thyroid-stimulating hormone, vitamin B_{12} levels, testing for Lyme disease or other regional tick-borne illnesses, or iron studies where appropriate.[21] The yield of these tests is generally low and the possibility of false-positive results should be considered. The most appropriate diagnostic test is typically neuroimaging.[23] MRI is preferred to computed tomography scanning owing to better assessment of

---

Box 2
Red flags that suggest secondary headache

History
  "First or worst" headache
  Risk factors for prothrombotic or immunocompromised state (eg malignancy, human immunodeficiency virus infection, pregnancy)
  Age less than 5 or greater than 50 years
  Abrupt onset (thunderclap headache)
  Change in headache character
  Progressive worsening with lack of response to treatment
  Positional worsening or improvement
  Worsening with Valsalva or straining

Examination
  Papilledema
  Cognitive impairment
  Fever, stiff neck
  Focal neurologic deficits

Modified from Cady RK. Red flags and comfort signs for ominous secondary headaches. Otolaryngol Clin North Am 2014;47(2):294; with permission.

conditions that may mimic migraine such as intracranial neoplasm.[23] The accumulated radiation risk associated with multiple head computed tomography scans may also not be negligible.[24]

TREATMENT OF TENSION-TYPE HEADACHE

Tension-type headache is by definition a mild to moderate headache and as such often responds to over-the-counter analgesics.[25] Guidelines from the European Federation of Neurologic Societies found that the over-the-counter treatments acetaminophen, aspirin, ibuprofen, and naproxen had level A evidence (effective) for acute treatment of tension-type headache, as did the prescription nonsteroidal antiinflammatory drugs (NSAIDs) ketoprofen and diclofenac.[26] Caffeine, typically used in combination preparations with NSAIDs, was rated level B (probably effective). Butalbital combination analgesics and the acetaminophen, dichloralphenazone, and isomethemptene combination are also used for refractory tension-type headaches.[27] Butalbital-containing medications may contribute to increasing headache frequency when used more than 2 days a week.[28] Triptans are not effective for pure tension-type headache. Some patients have headaches that meet criteria for migraine as well as headaches that are phenotypically consistent with tension-type headaches. In these patients, the tension-type headaches are most likely a forme fruste of migraine and often do respond to triptans.[29]

There are no guidelines to suggest when prevention should be started for tension-type headache. It seems reasonable to consider starting prevention when headache frequency reaches 2 days a week or more, but this largely depends on the level of disability associated with the headaches and patient preference. Tricyclic antidepressants including amitriptyline have the best evidence for prevention of tension-type headaches.[26] Selective serotonin reuptake inhibitors have been studied but have not been shown to have benefit over placebo or tricyclic antidepressants.[30] The muscle relaxant tizanidine has also been shown to have some benefit.[31] When these treatments fail, preventives with evidence for efficacy in migraine are sometimes tried.

NONPHARMACOLOGIC TREATMENT AND LIFESTYLE MANAGEMENT FOR MIGRAINE

Nonpharmacologic treatments with evidence for efficacy for prevention of migraine include thermal or electromyography biofeedback, relaxation training, and cognitive–behavioral therapy.[32] Some patients find that relaxation and biofeedback practices may also help abort an early attack. The use of mindfulness-based stress reduction, meditation, and acceptance and commitment therapy for the prevention of migraine are also active areas of research.[33]

Positive lifestyle habits including regular exercise, maintaining adequate hydration, eating regular meals, and avoiding known triggers may reduce headache frequency.[34,35] Of these, sleep often has the greatest impact, and sleep duration and quality should be assessed in any patient with bothersome headaches.[36] Dietary interventions for the prevention of migraine are widely reported in the lay literature. Despite this, there are very few scientific studies supporting dietary restriction or modification as a preventative strategy.[37,38] If patients have noticed particular food triggers, or are interested in trying a broader dietary intervention, dietary modifications can be made while keeping a headache diary to provide objective evidence.[39]

Over-the-counter vitamin supplements and herbal preparations are often considered nonpharmacologic treatments. American Academy of Neurology guidelines found that magnesium, feverfew, and vitamin B_2 (riboflavin) had level B evidence for efficacy and coenzyme Q10 was a level C for prevention of migraine.[40] Petasites, an extract from the butterbur plant, had level A evidence, but use of butterbur is currently not recommend owing to reports of liver toxicity.[41] Nonpharmacologic treatments for migraine are summarized in **Table 2**.

There is increasing interest, particularly among patients, in medical cannabis and cannabinoid treatments for migraine and other headache types. There is a paucity of good quality evidence in this area, although some positive case reports have been published.[42] Anecdotally, many patients report an analgesic benefit from marijuana use or the widely available cannabidiol oil. Marijuana use has been reported as a risk factor for reversible cerebral vasoconstriction syndrome, which causes cerebral vasospasm and can lead to ischemic or hemorrhagic stroke.[43,44] There is also a lack of good information about safety in psychiatrically vulnerable populations. Given this, it seems premature to recommend marijuana as a treatment for migraine. At this time, the author does not recommend against use for patients who find benefit from it, but does not recommend it as a treatment either.

ACUTE TREATMENT OF MIGRAINE

Acute treatment, also called abortive or symptomatic treatment, is taken to relieve the pain of a migraine attack. Classes of medications used for acute treatment of migraine include simple analgesics such as acetaminophen, NSAIDs (both over the counter and prescription), combination analgesics including the over-the-counter aspirin/acetaminophen/caffeine combination and the prescription analgesics containing butalbital, serotonin receptor agonists (triptans), ergot derivatives (particularly dihydroergomatine), and antiemetics.[45] Several antiemetics have intrinsic antimigraine properties, including metoclopramide, prochlorperazine, and promethazine.[46] Butalbital and/or caffeine-containing combination analgesics are not recommended as first-line agents owing to the risk of medication overuse headache.[47,48] Opioids are

Table 2 Nonpharmacologic and behavioral treatments for migraine		
Treatment	Dose and Frequency	AHS or US Headache Consortium Level of Evidence[a]
CoQ10	75 mg TID or 100 mg BID	C
Feverfew	6.25 mg TID	B
Magnesium	500–600 mg/day	B
Riboflavin	400 mg/day	B
Thermal biofeedback combined with relaxation training		B
Relaxation training		B
Electromyographic biofeedback		B
Cognitive–behavioral therapy		B

Abbreviations: AHS, American Headache Society; BID, 2 times per day; TID, 3 times per day.
[a] B = probably effective; C = possibly effective.

not recommended as a treatment for migraine except in very limited circumstances, discussed elsewhere in this article.[49] A summary of acute medication options for treatment of migraine is listed in **Table 3**.

Many patients with migraine have milder subforms of the disease that respond well to over-the-counter or nonspecific treatments.[50] Most patients with more frequent and severe migraine also have some less severe headaches that also respond to these treatments.[29] Patients with more severe migraines, which includes most patients who present to clinical settings, will require a prescription for a migraine-specific therapy such as a triptan, or a prescription NSAID.[50] Triptans are the first-line treatments for migraine in most cases.[51] Triptans should not be prescribed to patients with a history of coronary artery disease or multiple risk factors for coronary artery disease, patients who have coronary vasospasm, or who have poorly controlled hypertension.[52] selective serotonin reuptake inhibitor/serotonin and norepinephrine reuptake inhibitor use is not necessarily a contraindication to starting a triptan. Although concerns for serotonin syndrome led to a black box warning on coprescription of these medication classes, the evidence for the existence of this as a practical concern is very sparse.[53] A recent large database study failed to show a meaningful risk of serotonin syndrome in patients coprescribed a selective serotonin reuptake inhibitor/serotonin and norepinephrine reuptake inhibitor and a triptan.[54]

There have been few head-to-head studies among triptans. Studies have found that patients who do not respond to 1 triptan may have a better response to another.[55] It is not possible to predict which triptan will be most effective for a given patient and some trial and error may be necessary. It is reasonable to try 3 or 4 different triptans before switching to a different type of abortive therapy.

Triptans are generally well-tolerated. They may produce "triptan sensations," feelings of pressure, tightness, or flushing in the head, neck, or chest.[56] Patients should be counseled about the potential for triptan sensations when a triptan is initially prescribed.

The goal of acute treatment, regardless of agent, is pain freedom.[57,58] Many patients will report that their acute treatment "takes the edge off" or provides only partial relief. This incomplete response to acute treatment is a risk factor for migraine chronification and also increases the disability associated with a migraine attack.[59] If a patient reports an incomplete response, treatment should be optimized by increasing the dose of the acute treatment, recommending earlier use of treatment, switching agents within or between classes, or combining different classes of treatments (such as combining a triptan with an NSAID, antiemetic, or both). In patients with nausea, migraine disability may also be reduced by use of an antiemetic.[60] Although many patients report improvement of nausea with relief from the headache, this is not always the case and treatment of migraine pain and nausea should be considered separately.

Many patients with migraine have both more and less severe headaches, particularly as headache frequency increases. Two treatment approaches have been proposed in this scenario. Stepped care is the practice of starting with a nonspecific treatment such as acetaminophen or an over-the-counter NSAID, followed by a migraine-specific therapy such as a triptan if the headache continues or escalates. In stratified care, the patient is asked to predict whether the headache is likely to be mild versus moderate or severe, and choose either a nonspecific treatment or a migraine-specific treatment based on this prediction.[61] Treatment outcomes are consistently better when stratified care is used.[62] Many patients still use stepped care despite this, often out of concern for running out of their limited number of

Table 3
Acute treatments for migraine headache

Medication	Dose and Frequency	AHS Level of Evidence for Migraine[a]	Notes
Simple analgesics and combination analgesics			
Acetaminophen	1000 mg	A	For nonincapacitating attacks
Aspirin/acetaminophen/ caffeine	500/500/ 130 mg	A	Risk of medication overuse, particularly with OTC availability
Isometheptene/ dichloralphenazone/ acetaminophen	65/100/ 325 mg	B (for isometheptine alone)	Intermittently available
Butalbital/acetaminophen/ caffeine	50/325/ 40 mg	C	High risk of medication overuse headache; risk of withdrawal seizure with daily use of high doses
Butalbital/caffeine/aspirin	50/325/ 40 mg	C	High risk of medication overuse headache; risk of withdrawal seizure with daily use of high doses
NSAIDs			
Aspirin	500 mg	A	
Diclofenac	50, 100 mg	A	Dissolving powder may be more effective than tablet form
Ibuprofen	200, 400, 800 mg	A	
Indomethacin	25–50 mg	N/A	High incidence of gastric discomfort
Ketoprofen	100 mg	B	
Naproxen	500, 550 mg	A	Naproxen sodium may be more effective than naproxen base
Triptans and ergot derivatives			
Almotriptan	12.5 mg	A	May have a more benign side effect profile
Eletriptan	20, 40 mg	A	
Frovatriptan	2.5 mg	A	Long acting; also used BID for menstrual migraine prophylaxis
Naratriptan	1.0, 2.5 mg	A	Long acting; also used BID for menstrual migraine prophylaxis
Rizatriptan	5, 10 mg	A	Also available in an orally dissolving tablet
Sumatriptan	PO 25, 50, 100 mg SQ 4, 6 mg NS 5, 10, 20 mg	A	Most broadly covered by insurance; also available as a rectal suppository

(continued on next page)

Table 3
(continued)

Medication	Dose and Frequency	AHS Level of Evidence for Migraine[a]	Notes
Zolmitriptan	PO 2.5, 5.0 mg NS 2.5, 5.0 mg	A	Also available as an orally dissolving tablet
Dihydroergotamine	NS 0.5– 2.0 mg	A	Pretreat with an antiemetic owing to a high incidence of nausea
Opioids			
Codeine/acetaminophen	25/400 mg	B	High risk of medication overuse headache
Other opioids		Other oral opioids not studied for acute treatment of migraine	High risk of medication overuse headache; avoid routine or first line use
Antiemetics			
Metoclopramide	5, 10 mg	N/A	Less sedating than phenothiazine antiemetics; risk of akathisia reaction; may reduce migraine pain
Ondansetron	4, 8 mg	N/A	Not sedating; no benefit for migraine pain
Prochlorperazine	PO 5, 10 mg PR 25 mg	N/A	Risk of sedation, akathisia reaction; may reduce migraine pain
Promethazine	12.5, 25.0 mg PR 25 mg	N/A	Risk of sedation, akathisia reaction; may reduce migraine pain

Abbreviations: AHS, American Headache Society; BID, 2 times per day; N/A, not applicable; NS, nasal spray; NSAIDs, nonsteroidal antiinflammatory drugs; OTC, over the counter; PO, orally; PR, rectal suppository; SQ, subcutaneously.

[a] A = established as effective; B = probably effective; C = possibly effective.

triptans each month. When possible, patients should be educated to treat with their triptan first line if there is a reasonable possibility that the headache will be moderate to severe.

Acute treatment is more effective when taken early in the attack.[63] Animal and human studies have found that triptans are less effective once central sensitization, or the progression of neuronal activation from the periphery to the brainstem pain nuclei as a migraine evolves, sets in. The clinical marker for central sensitization is cutaneous allodynia, the feeling of burning pain to light touch of the scalp.[64]

MEDICATION OVERUSE HEADACHE

The frequency of acute medication use should be limited to prevent the development of medication overuse headache.[65] Medication overuse is diagnosed when a patient has headache more than 15 days per month and is taking a medication that can cause medication overuse headache more than 10 days per month (ergot, triptans, opioids, combination analgesics including butalbital containing analgesics, or any combination of different types of acute medications) or 15 days per month (acetaminophen, NSAIDs).[8] Opioids and butalbital-containing medications are the medication classes most likely to contribute to medication overuse headache.[48] Many patients who have migraine or tension-type headache use acute treatment very frequently. It is worth noting that withdrawal of the overused medication will result in improvement of the headache, indicating that the overused medication is actually contributing to the headache, in only about 50% of cases.[66] Despite this finding, migraine or tension-type headache and medication overuse headache can be diagnosed in combination if the headache meets criteria for both conditions.

RESCUE THERAPY AND TREATMENT OF STATUS MIGRAINOSUS

Rescue therapy is an important component of the migraine treatment plan for many patients, particularly if accompanying nausea or vomiting are severe, symptoms escalate rapidly, the migraine is present upon awakening, or if first-line acute treatments are often unreliable.[45] Routine planning for rescue treatment may prevent unexpected days of migraine disability, emergency room visits, and the need for urgent management of migraines outside of office visits. **Box 3** lists rescue treatments for migraine.

Nonoral routes of administration are favored for rescue therapy.[67] The onset of action is typically faster and treatment effects are more robust for parenteral and rectally administered treatments than for oral treatments, and patients with severe vomiting are typically unable to absorb oral treatments.[68] Nasal sprays and orally dissolving tablets are largely absorbed through the gastrointestinal tract and some patients do not respond to them fully. Sumatriptan is available as a subcutaneous injection and rectal suppository. Promethazine and prochlorperazine suppositories are helpful for patients with vomiting or who find benefit from sleep, as sedation is a common side effect. Indomethacin is also available as a suppository and may be helpful for patients who respond well to NSAIDs. Dihydroergotamine nasal spray may be useful for patients who are not vomiting. Very rarely, it may be appropriate to use an opioid in a responsive patient for whom use is infrequent and in whom use prevents the need for urgent or emergency room care. There is no evidence to support use of any particular opiate for migraine. Butalbital combination medications may be used in the same way.

The American Headache Society Guidelines for the acute treatment of migraine in the emergency room found the best evidence for the use of subcutaneous sumatriptan as well as intravenous metoclopramide and prochlorperazine.[69] Steroids, including dexamethasone, do not seem to be effective for the acute treatment of migraine, but do decrease the risk of headache recurrence after discharge.[70] A patient who has not used a triptan for their migraine attack should be offered subcutaneous sumatriptan first line. If the patient has already taken a triptan, a combination of nonopioid treatments (migraine cocktail) such as metoclopramide or prochlorperazine with diphenhydramine and ketorolac may be used as the first-line treatment for migraine in the emergency room.[71] Diphenhydramine is not effective as monotherapy, but may prevent akathisia from other treatments.[69] Intravenous dihydroergotamine is an effective migraine-specific treatment that is underused in the emergency room setting. Intravenous magnesium also has level B

Box 3
Rescue and emergency room treatments for migraine

Sumatriptan SQ 4, 6 mg

DHE NS 1 to 2 mg or IV 1 mg ×1 or q8 hours, pretreated with an antiemetic, for several days

Promethazine or prochlorperazine PR 25 mg; prochlorperazine IV/IM 10 mg

Metoclopramide IV 10 mg

Indomethacin PR 50 mg

Sedating medications (diphenhydramine PO 25 mg, hydroxyzine PO 25–50 mg, benzodiazepines)

Ketorolac IV/IM 30 to 60 mg

Valproate IV 400 to 1000 mg

Magnesium sulfate IV 1000 to 2000 mg, for migraine with aura

Steroids, either as an oral taper or an IV dose ×1

Abbreviations: DHE, dihydroergotamine; IM, intramuscularly; IV, intravenously; NS, nasal spray; PO, orally; PR, rectal suppository; SQ, subcutaneously.

---

evidence for efficacy as an acute treatment specifically for migraine with aura.[69] Opioids, and particularly parenteral opioids, should be avoided as a first-line therapy.[49]

Unremitting migraine for at least 72 hours is termed status migrainosus. The treatment of refractory status migrainosus is not well-studied, but treatments sometimes used include steroids, intravenous dihydroergotamine repeated every 8 hours for several days (the Raskin protocol), or infusions of antiemetics such as valproate or levetiracetam.[72]

PREVENTIVE TREATMENT OF MIGRAINE

Preventive therapy should be considered when acute treatment is insufficient. The criteria for consideration of preventive therapy include moderate to severe headache more than 4 times a month, overuse of acute medications, poor response to acute treatment, situations where typical acute treatments are contraindicated, or if rarer headaches are unusually debilitating or alarming (such as headaches with prolonged severe aura).[73] Preventive therapies are typically chosen based on evidence for efficacy, side effect profile, and comorbidities. The goals of preventive treatment are to reduce headache frequency, duration, and severity; improve response to acute treatment; decrease the need for acute treatment; and reduce overall headache disability.[74]

Some patients may be hesitant to take a daily medication for treatment of an episodic condition. A shared decision-making model, where the clinician acts as an educator and patients are active partners in treatment decisions, is ideal when considering prevention.[75] Where appropriate, patients can be provided with several options, educated about evidence for efficacy and possible side effects, and given the opportunity to choose their treatment path. Obtaining patient buy in to treatment may improve adherence, which is typically quite poor for migraine preventives.[76] Patients should be educated that complete headache freedom is rarely an obtainable goal and that a decrease in headache-related disability is the target of treatment.

Table 4
Preventive treatments for migraine

Medication	Target Dose and Frequency	AAN/AHS Level of Evidence[a]	Notes
Antidepressants			
Amitriptyline	25–100 mg nightly	A	First line if comorbid insomnia; side effects include sedation and weight gain
Venlafaxine	75–150 mg/day	B	Consider if comorbid depression; withdrawal syndrome can be unpleasant and is probably underappreciated
Antihypertensives			
Atenolol	50–100 mg/day	B	Well-tolerated; may cause orthostasis and exercise intolerance; unlike other beta-blockers, contraindicated in pregnancy
Metoprolol	25–100 mg BID	A	Well-tolerated; may cause orthostasis and exercise intolerance
Propranolol[b]	40–120 mg BID (nightly dosing often used)	A	Well-tolerated; considered safest preventive in pregnancy; may cause orthostasis and exercise intolerance
Candesartan	16 mg/day	C	Generally well-tolerated; contraindicated during pregnancy (category D)
Lisinopril	20 mg/day	C	Generally well-tolerated; contraindicated during pregnancy (category D)
Verapamil	120–360 mg/day	U	Strong impression of clinical benefit despite level U rating; generally well-tolerated; may be particularly useful in migraine with aura
Antiepileptic drugs			
Topiramate[b]	50–200 mg/day (side effects higher above 100 mg/day)	A	First line if weight gain is a concern; contraindicated during pregnancy (category D)
Gabapentin	900–2400 mg total daily dose, divided BID-TID; higher doses more effective	U	Strong impression of clinical benefit despite level U rating; some patients also report benefit as an acute treatment
Sodium valproate[b]	500–1000 mg total daily dose	A	High side effect burden including weight gain, hair loss, hepatotoxicity, and bone marrow suppression; rarely used as a first-line treatment for this reason; contraindicated during pregnancy (category X)

(continued on next page)

Table 4
(continued)

Medication	Target Dose and Frequency	AAN/AHS Level of Evidence[a]	Notes
Other			
Onabotulinum toxin A[b]	155 units SQ, divided between 31 injection sites, every 12 wk	A (American Academy of Neurology Guideline)	FDA approved for chronic migraine only; trials for episodic migraine were conclusively negative
Memantine	10–20 mg/day or divided BID	N/A	Generally well-tolerated
Erenumab	70–140 mg SQ monthly	N/A	Approved in May 2018; data regarding long term safety in clinical practice not available yet; benign side effect profile in clinical trials
Fremanezumab	225 mg SQ monthly or 675 mg SQ quarterly	N/A	Approved in September 2018; data regarding long term safety in clinical practice not available yet; benign side effect profile in clinical trials
Galcanezumab	240 mg SQ first month, then 120 mg SQ monthly	N/A	Approved in September 2018; data regarding long term safety in clinical practice not available yet; benign side effect profile in clinical trials

Abbreviations: AAN, American Academy of Neurology; AHS, American Headache Society; BID, 2 times per day; FDA, US Food and Drug Administration; TID, 3 times per day.

[a] A = established as effective; B = probably effective; C = possibly effective; level U: evidence is conflicting or inadequate.

[b] FDA approved for prevention of migraine.

Adherence may also be improved by starting preventive medications at a low dose and increasing gradually to the target dose.[77] There is evidence to suggest that people with migraine may be particularly sensitive to medication side effects.[78] An adequate trial of prevention requires at least 2 months once the target dose is reached. Treatment response should be monitored using a headache and medication use diary, a disability scale, or other objective measure.

Most preventive treatments for migraine were originally developed as antidepressants, antihypertensives, or antiepileptic drugs. Other classes of treatments, such as neurotoxins and monoclonal antibodies to calcitonin gene related peptide (CGRP) or its receptor, are also used.[79] The CGRP monoclonal antibodies (mAbs) are the only class of currently used preventives developed specifically for treatment of migraine (methysergide was the first such treatment but is no longer in use).[80] CGRP is a widely distributed vasodilator that is intrinsically involved in the pathophysiology of migraine. The CGRP mAbs target either the CGRP molecule itself or the CGRP receptor. In a network metaanalysis, the CGRP mABs seemed to be about as effective as other available preventive treatments, but have fewer side effects and are more convenient to use.[81] There are some remaining uncertainties about the long-term safety of these treatments, because the role of CGRP in other organ systems is not fully known.[82] Owing to these concerns and the high cost of these treatments, the CGRP mAbs are currently typically used for refractory migraine patients rather than as first-line treatments.[83]

Evidence for the efficacy of preventive treatments for episodic migraine was assessed in a 2012 guideline from the American Academy of Neurology and American Headache Society.[84] Levels of evidence range from A (best) to U (unknown) based on the number of good quality studies supporting use.[84] Commonly used preventive therapies, doses, and notes about clinical use are given in **Table 4**. Canadian and European Neurologic societies have also produced guidelines on this topic.[85] There was agreement between the guidelines that valproate, topiramate, propranolol, and metoprolol had the best ratings, with amitriptyline close to the top of the list as well. These medications can therefore be considered good first-line treatments, although valproate has a high side effect burden and cannot be used in women of childbearing potential. In addition to the treatments described in the table, muscle relaxants such as cyclobenzaprine and tizanidine, agents commonly used for other pain disorders such as duloxetine and pregabalin, other tricyclic antidepressants, and the antihistamine cyproheptadine (particularly for children) are sometimes used as well.[79] Timolol, although approved by the US Food and Drug Administration for migraine prevention, is used very rarely in clinical practice.

CHRONIC OR REFRACTORY MIGRAINE

Patients with chronic migraine often have multiple comorbidities that contribute to migraine chronification or disability, and suboptimal lifestyle habits may contribute as well.[86] Factors that may contribute to migraine chronification or persistence are presented in **Box 4**. It is often necessary to address these comorbidities as a part of the migraine treatment plan, in addition to targeting migraine pain and accompanying symptoms.[87] Multimodality care, possibly including psychiatry, sleep medicine, physical therapy, and nutrition support, may be helpful. Treatment gains may initially be modest, but over time incremental gains can add up to significant improvements in quality of life.

Combinations of preventive measures may be considered in patients with refractory migraine.[88] This is particularly the case if a treatment is effective but has bothersome side effects. For example, adding topiramate may mitigate the weight gain caused by other preventives. In patients with chronic migraine, onabotulinum toxin A may also be

---

Box 4
Potentially modifiable factors that contribute to migraine chronification or persistence

High frequency of headache attacks

Poor response to acute treatment

Medication overuse

Excessive caffeine intake

Obesity

Obstructive sleep apnea

Stressful life events

Mood disorders

added.[89] Withdrawing other preventives with partial benefit is not necessary when starting onabotulinum toxin treatment.

SUMMARY

Migraine and tension-type headache are highly prevalent and migraine is associated with significant work and family related disability. Migraine is underdiagnosed and it reasonable to err on the side of migraine when there are diagnostic uncertainties. Barriers to appropriate treatment of migraine include lack of access to providers, misdiagnosis, and disease-specific therapies not being prescribed. Acute, rescue, and preventive treatment options are extensive, and new classes of treatments are either available or in development.

REFERENCES

1. GBD 2016 Disease and Injury Incidence and Prevalence Collaborators. Global, regional, and national incidence, prevalence, and years lived with disability for 328 diseases and injuries for 195 countries, 1990-2016: a systematic analysis for the Global Burden of Disease Study 2016. Lancet 2017;390(10100):1211–59.
2. Burch R, Rizzoli P, Loder E. The prevalence and impact of migraine and severe headache in the United States: figures and trends from government health studies. Headache 2018;58(4):496–505.
3. Lipton RB, Stewart WF, Diamond S, et al. Prevalence and burden of migraine in the United States: data from the American Migraine Study II. Headache 2001; 41(7):646–57.
4. Stewart WF, Wood GC, Manack A, et al. Employment and work impact of chronic migraine and episodic migraine. J Occup Environ Med 2010;52(1):8–14.
5. Dodick DW, Loder EW, Manack Adams A, et al. Assessing barriers to chronic migraine consultation, diagnosis, and treatment: results from the chronic migraine epidemiology and outcomes (CaMEO) study. Headache 2016. https://doi.org/10.1111/head.12774.
6. Schwartz BS, Stewart WF, Simon D, et al. Epidemiology of tension-type headache. JAMA 1998;279(5):381–3.
7. Saylor D, Steiner TJ. The global burden of headache. Semin Neurol 2018;38(2): 182–90.
8. International Classification of Headache Disorders (ICHD). ICHD-3 The International Classification of Headache Disorders 3rd edition. ICHD-3 The International Classification of Headache Disorders 3rd edition. Available at: https://www.ichd-3.org/. Accessed June 24, 2018.
9. Lipton RB, Cady RK, Stewart WF, et al. Diagnostic lessons from the spectrum study. Neurology 2002;58(9 Suppl 6):S27–31.
10. Andress-Rothrock D, King W, Rothrock J. An analysis of migraine triggers in a clinic-based population. Headache 2010;50(8):1366–70.
11. Ashina S, Bendtsen L, Lyngberg AC, et al. Prevalence of neck pain in migraine and tension-type headache: a population study. Cephalalgia 2015;35(3):211–9.
12. Eross E, Dodick D, Eross M. The sinus, allergy and migraine study (SAMS). Headache 2007;47(2):213–24.
13. DeLange JM, Cutrer FM. Our evolving understanding of migraine with aura. Curr Pain Headache Rep 2014;18(10):453.
14. Russell MB, Rasmussen BK, Fenger K, et al. Migraine without aura and migraine with aura are distinct clinical entities: a study of four hundred and eighty-four

male and female migraineurs from the general population. Cephalalgia 1996; 16(4):239–45.

15. Blau JN. Migraine prodromes separated from the aura: complete migraine. Br Med J 1980;281(6241):658–60.

16. Silberstein SD. Migraine symptoms: results of a survey of self-reported migraineurs. Headache 1995;35(7):387–96.

17. Mahmoud AN, Mentias A, Elgendy AY, et al. Migraine and the risk of cardiovascular and cerebrovascular events: a meta-analysis of 16 cohort studies including 1 152 407 subjects. BMJ Open 2018;8(3):e020498.

18. World Health Organization (WHO). Medical eligibility criteria for contraceptive use. 2016. Available at: http://www.who.int/reproductivehealth/publications/family_planning/Ex-Summ-MEC-5/en/. Accessed June 24, 2018.

19. ACOG Committee on Practice Bulletins-Gynecology. ACOG practice bulletin. No. 73: use of hormonal contraception in women with coexisting medical conditions. Obstet Gynecol 2006;107(6):1453–72.

20. Sheikh HU, Pavlovic J, Loder E, et al. Risk of stroke associated with use of estrogen containing contraceptives in women with migraine: a systematic review. Headache 2018;58(1):5–21.

21. Evans RW. Diagnostic testing for migraine and other primary headaches. Neurol Clin 2009;27(2):393–415.

22. Cady RK. Red flags and comfort signs for ominous secondary headaches. Otolaryngol Clin North Am 2014;47(2):289–99.

23. Holle D, Obermann M. The role of neuroimaging in the diagnosis of headache disorders. Ther Adv Neurol Disord 2013;6(6):369–74.

24. Radiation emissions from computed tomography: a review of the risk of cancer and guidelines. Ottawa (Canada): Canadian Agency for Drugs and Technologies in Health; 2014.

25. Kaniecki RG. Tension-type headache. Continuum 2012;18(4):823–34.

26. Bendtsen L, Evers S, Linde M, et al. EFNS guideline on the treatment of tension-type headache - report of an EFNS task force. Eur J Neurol 2010;17(11):1318–25.

27. Barbanti P, Egeo G, Aurilia C, et al. Treatment of tension-type headache: from old myths to modern concepts. Neurol Sci 2014;35(Suppl 1):17–21.

28. Monteith TS, Oshinsky ML. Tension-type headache with medication overuse: pathophysiology and clinical implications. Curr Pain Headache Rep 2009;13(6): 463–9.

29. Lipton RB, Stewart WF, Cady R, et al. 2000 Wolfe Award. Sumatriptan for the range of headaches in migraine sufferers: results of the Spectrum Study. Headache 2000;40(10):783–91.

30. Banzi R, Cusi C, Randazzo C, et al. Selective serotonin reuptake inhibitors (SSRIs) and serotonin-norepinephrine reuptake inhibitors (SNRIs) for the prevention of tension-type headache in adults. Cochrane Database Syst Rev 2015;(5):CD011681.

31. Fogelholm R, Murros K. Tizanidine in chronic tension-type headache: a placebo controlled double-blind cross-over study. Headache 1992;32(10):509–13.

32. Silberstein SD. Practice parameter: evidence-based guidelines for migraine headache (an evidence-based review): report of the quality standards subcommittee of the American Academy of Neurology. Neurology 2000;55(6):754–62.

33. Wells RE, Smitherman TA, Seng EK, et al. Behavioral and mind/body interventions in headache: unanswered questions and future research directions. Headache 2014;54(6):1107–13.

34. Woldeamanuel YW, Cowan RP. The impact of regular lifestyle behavior in migraine: a prevalence case-referent study. J Neurol 2016;263(4):669–76.
35. Hagen K, Åsberg AN, Stovner L, et al. Lifestyle factors and risk of migraine and tension-type headache. Follow-up data from the Nord-Trøndelag Health Surveys 1995-1997 and 2006-2008. Cephalalgia 2018. https://doi.org/10.1177/0333102418764888. 333102418764888.
36. Smitherman TA, Kuka AJ, Calhoun AH, et al. Cognitive-behavioral therapy for insomnia to reduce chronic migraine: a sequential Bayesian analysis. Headache 2018. https://doi.org/10.1111/head.13313.
37. Martin VT, Vij B. Diet and headache: part 1. Headache 2016;56(9):1543–52.
38. Martin VT, Vij B. Diet and headache: part 2. Headache 2016;56(9):1553–62.
39. Slavin M, Ailani J. A clinical approach to addressing diet with migraine patients. Curr Neurol Neurosci Rep 2017;17(2):17.
40. Holland S, Silberstein SD, Freitag F, et al. Evidence-based guideline update: NSAIDs and other complementary treatments for episodic migraine prevention in adults: report of the Quality Standards Subcommittee of the American Academy of Neurology and the American Headache Society. Neurology 2012; 78(17):1346–53.
41. Migraine preventative butterbur has safety concerns | Neurology Times. Available at: http://www.neurologytimes.com/headache-and-migraine/migraine-preventative-butterbur-has-safety-concerns. Accessed June 24, 2018.
42. Baron EP. Comprehensive review of medicinal marijuana, cannabinoids, and therapeutic implications in medicine and headache: what a long strange trip it's been .... Headache 2015;55(6):885–916.
43. Uhegwu N, Bashir A, Hussain M, et al. Marijuana induced reversible cerebral vasoconstriction syndrome. J Vasc Interv Neurol 2015;8(1):36–8.
44. Wolff V, Ducros A. Reversible cerebral vasoconstriction syndrome without typical thunderclap headache. Headache 2016;56(4):674–87.
45. Becker WJ. Acute migraine treatment. Continuum 2015;21(4 Headache):953–72.
46. Kelly A-M, Walcynski T, Gunn B. The relative efficacy of phenothiazines for the treatment of acute migraine: a meta-analysis. Headache 2009;49(9):1324–32.
47. Thorlund K, Sun-Edelstein C, Druyts E, et al. Risk of medication overuse headache across classes of treatments for acute migraine. J Headache Pain 2016; 17(1):107.
48. Bigal ME, Serrano D, Buse D, et al. Acute migraine medications and evolution from episodic to chronic migraine: a longitudinal population-based study. Headache 2008;48(8):1157–68.
49. Tepper SJ. Opioids should not be used in migraine. Headache 2012;52(Suppl 1): 30–4.
50. Diamond S, Bigal ME, Silberstein S, et al. Patterns of diagnosis and acute and preventive treatment for migraine in the United States: results from the American Migraine Prevalence and Prevention study. Headache 2007;47(3):355–63.
51. Pringsheim T, Becker WJ. Triptans for symptomatic treatment of migraine headache. BMJ 2014;348:g2285.
52. Loder E. Triptan therapy in migraine. N Engl J Med 2010;363(1):63–70.
53. Evans RW, Tepper SJ, Shapiro RE, et al. The FDA alert on serotonin syndrome with use of triptans combined with selective serotonin reuptake inhibitors or selective serotonin-norepinephrine reuptake inhibitors: American Headache Society position paper. Headache 2010;50(6):1089–99.
54. Orlova Y, Rizzoli P, Loder E. Association of coprescription of triptan antimigraine drugs and selective serotonin reuptake inhibitor or selective norepinephrine

reuptake inhibitor antidepressants with serotonin syndrome. JAMA Neurol 2018; 75(5):566–72.

55. Dodick DW. Triptan nonresponder studies: implications for clinical practice. Headache 2005;45(2):156–62.
56. Nappi G, Sandrini G, Sances G. Tolerability of the triptans: clinical implications. Drug Saf 2003;26(2):93–107.
57. Silberstein SD, Newman LC, Marmura MJ, et al. Efficacy endpoints in migraine clinical trials: the importance of assessing freedom from pain. Curr Med Res Opin 2013;29(7):861–7.
58. Lipton RB, Hamelsky SW, Dayno JM. What do patients with migraine want from acute migraine treatment? Headache 2002;42(Suppl 1):3–9.
59. Lipton RB, Fanning KM, Serrano D, et al. Ineffective acute treatment of episodic migraine is associated with new-onset chronic migraine. Neurology 2015;84(7): 688–95.
60. Lipton RB, Buse DC, Saiers J, et al. Frequency and burden of headache-related nausea: results from the American Migraine Prevalence and Prevention (AMPP) study. Headache 2013;53(1):93–103.
61. Lipton RB. Disability assessment as a basis for stratified care. Cephalalgia 1998; 18(Suppl 22):40–3 [discussion: 43–6].
62. Seng EK, Robbins MS, Nicholson RA. Acute migraine medication adherence, migraine disability and patient satisfaction: a naturalistic daily diary study. Cephalalgia 2017;37(10):955–64.
63. Goadsby PJ, Zanchin G, Geraud G, et al. Early vs. non-early intervention in acute migraine-'Act when Mild (AwM)'. A double-blind, placebo-controlled trial of almotriptan. Cephalalgia 2008;28(4):383–91.
64. Díaz-Insa S, Goadsby PJ, Zanchin G, et al. The impact of allodynia on the efficacy of almotriptan when given early in migraine: data from the "Act when mild" study. Int J Neurosci 2011;121(12):655–61.
65. Cheung V, Amoozegar F, Dilli E. Medication overuse headache. Curr Neurol Neurosci Rep 2015;15(1):509.
66. Scher AI, Rizzoli PB, Loder EW. Medication overuse headache: an entrenched idea in need of scrutiny. Neurology 2017;89(12):1296–304.
67. Matchar DB, Young WB, Rosenberg JH, et al. Evidence-based guidelines for migraine headache in the primary care setting: pharmacological management of acute attacks. Neurology 2000;54. Available at: http://tools.aan.com/professionals/practice/pdfs/gl0087.pdf.
68. Newman LC. Why triptan treatment can fail: focus on gastrointestinal manifestations of migraine. Headache 2013;53(Suppl 1):11–6.
69. Orr SL, Friedman BW, Christie S, et al. Management of adults with acute migraine in the emergency department: the American Headache Society evidence assessment of parenteral pharmacotherapies. Headache 2016;56(6):911–40.
70. Woldeamanuel YW, Rapoport AM, Cowan RP. The place of corticosteroids in migraine attack management: a 65-year systematic review with pooled analysis and critical appraisal. Cephalalgia 2015;35(11):996–1024.
71. Kelley NE, Tepper DE. Rescue therapy for acute migraine, part 3: opioids, NSAIDs, steroids, and post-discharge medications. Headache 2012;52(3): 467–82.
72. Rozen TD. Emergency department and inpatient management of status migrainosus and intractable headache. Continuum 2015;21(4 Headache):1004–17.
73. Silberstein SD, Goadsby PJ. Migraine: preventive treatment. Cephalalgia 2002; 22(7):491–512.

74. Dodick DW, Silberstein SD. Migraine prevention. Pract Neurol 2007;7(6):383–93.
75. Peters M, Abu-Saad HH, Vydelingum V, et al. Patients' decision-making for migraine and chronic daily headache management. A qualitative study. Cephalalgia 2003;23(8):833–41.
76. Hepp Z, Bloudek LM, Varon SF. Systematic review of migraine prophylaxis adherence and persistence. J Manag Care Pharm 2014;20(1):22–33.
77. Silberstein SD. Headache in clinical practice. 2nd edition. Abingdon (UK): Routledge; 2018.
78. Luykx J, Mason M, Ferrari MD, et al. Are migraineurs at increased risk of adverse drug responses? A meta-analytic comparison of topiramate-related adverse drug reactions in epilepsy and migraine. Clin Pharmacol Ther 2009;85(3):283–8.
79. Silberstein SD. Preventive migraine treatment. Continuum 2015;21(4 Headache): 973–89.
80. Edvinsson L, Haanes KA, Warfvinge K, et al. CGRP as the target of new migraine therapies - successful translation from bench to clinic. Nat Rev Neurol 2018; 14(6):338–50.
81. Migraine: Final Report - ICER. ICER. Available at: https://icer-review.org/material/cgrp-final-report/. Accessed September 22, 2018.
82. Deen M, Correnti E, Kamm K, et al. Blocking CGRP in migraine patients – a review of pros and cons. J Headache Pain 2017;18(1):96.
83. Loder EW, Burch RC. Who should try new antibody treatments for migraine? JAMA Neurol 2018;75(9):1039.
84. Silberstein SD, Holland S, Freitag F, et al. Evidence-based guideline update: pharmacologic treatment for episodic migraine prevention in adults: report of the Quality Standards Subcommittee of the American Academy of Neurology and the American Headache Society. Neurology 2012;78(17):1337–45.
85. Loder E, Burch R, Rizzoli P. The 2012 AHS/AAN guidelines for prevention of episodic migraine: a summary and comparison with other recent clinical practice guidelines. Headache 2012;52(6):930–45.
86. May A, Schulte LH. Chronic migraine: risk factors, mechanisms and treatment. Nat Rev Neurol 2016;12(8):455–64.
87. Diener H-C, Solbach K, Holle D, et al. Integrated care for chronic migraine patients: epidemiology, burden, diagnosis and treatment options. Clin Med 2015; 15(4):344–50.
88. Schwedt TJ. Chronic migraine. BMJ 2014;348:g1416.
89. Simpson DM, Hallett M, Ashman EJ, et al. Practice guideline update summary: botulinum neurotoxin for the treatment of blepharospasm, cervical dystonia, adult spasticity, and headache: report of the guideline development subcommittee of the American Academy of Neurology. Neurology 2016;86(19):1818–26.

Nonmigraine Headache and Facial Pain

Angeliki Vgontzas, MD, Paul B. Rizzoli, MD*

KEYWORDS

- Headache - Facial pain - Nonmigraine - Neuralgia - Trigeminal - Cluster - CSF
- Thrombosis

KEY POINTS

- The multiple nonmigraine primary headaches together constitute a fascinating group of conditions with important clinical and management implications for the patient.
- Secondary headache must be considered in every patient presenting with a new-onset or change in headache; selected more important or more common secondary headaches are reviewed here.
- Facial pain and neuralgias constitute a large and distinct group of head pains with separate evaluation and treatment approaches.

INTRODUCTION

Most headache patients encountered in the outpatient general medicine setting will be diagnosed with a primary headache disorder, mostly migraine or tension-type headache. Other less common primary headaches and secondary headaches, that is, those related to or caused by another condition (**Box 1**), are the topic of this article. Nonmigraine primary headaches include the trigeminal autonomic cephalalgias, primarily cluster headache; facial pain, primarily trigeminal neuralgia (TGN); and miscellaneous headache syndromes, such as hemicrania continua and new daily persistent headache (NDPH). Selected secondary headaches related to vascular disease, cerebrospinal fluid (CSF) dynamics, and inflammatory conditions are also reviewed.

OTHER PRIMARY HEADACHES
Trigeminal Autonomic Cephalalgias

Cluster headache
Cluster headache, although rare, is an important topic for the general medical reader due to the severe nature of the pain combined with the documented tendency for the

Disclosure Statement: No relevant disclosures.
Department of Neurology, Brigham and Women's Hospital, John R. Graham Headache Center, Brigham and Women's Faulkner Hospital, Harvard Medical School, 1153 Centre Street, Suite 4H, Boston, MA 02130, USA
* Corresponding author.
E-mail address: prizzoli@bwh.harvard.edu

Med Clin N Am 103 (2019) 235–250
https://doi.org/10.1016/j.mcna.2018.10.007
0025-7125/19/© 2018 Elsevier Inc. All rights reserved.

medical.theclinics.com

Box 1
Nonmigraine headache

1. Other primary headache
   Trigeminal autonomic cephalalgias
     Cluster
     Hemicrania continua
     SUNCT/SUNA
   Facial pain and neuralgias
     Trigeminal neuralgia
     Occipital neuralgia
     Atypical facial pain
     Other selected neuralgias
   New daily persistent headache
   Other miscellaneous primary headaches (**Table 1**)
     Primary stabbing headache
     Primary cough headache
     Exertional/exercise headache
     Headache associated with sexual activity
     Hypnic headache

2. Selected secondary headaches
   Vascular-related
     Cervical carotid/vertebral dissection
     Cerebral venous thrombosis
     Reversible cerebrovasoconstriction syndrome
     Posterior reversible encephalopathy syndrome
     Thunderclap headache
   CSF flow-related
     Idiopathic intracranial hypertension
     Low-pressure headache
     Chiari malformation
   Inflammatory-related
     Giant cell arteritis

---

condition to be misdiagnosed by the general practitioner.[1] Misdiagnosis may lead to years of unnecessary patient suffering, and increased familiarity with the condition may help prevent this.

Cluster is classified among the trigeminal autonomic cephalalgias, a group of headaches with unilateral pain symptoms closely tied to the sensory distribution of the trigeminal nerve and, in addition, associated with signs and symptoms of autonomic dysfunction. The prevalence of cluster in the population appears to be less than 0.4% with a male-to-female predilection of about 4 to 5:1.[2] There is usually no family history of similar headache, and risk factors for development of the headache may include smoking and excessive alcohol intake. The onset is usually between the ages of 20 and 40, and the pattern may display a cyclical appearance, for example, yearly at the same time of year. Chronic forms are described. Once a cluster episode is triggered, headaches often appear daily, one to 3 times daily for weeks to months followed by a period of many months without headache. Typically, an individual event is a unilateral, periorbital (trigeminal nerve, division V1) very severe pain with associated ipsilateral autonomic dysfunction manifesting as tearing, conjunctival injection, facial sweating, ptosis, or rhinorrhea. The pain peaks within 5 to 10 minutes and can last up to 3 hours (**Box 2**). Attacks may begin and end abruptly and can wake patients from sleep. Often reported with the attack is a sense of restlessness or agitation, manifesting as a pacing or rocking during the attack, in contrast to the behavior of the typical migraine patient who seeks a quiet, dark environment.

Table 1
Other miscellaneous primary headaches

Headache	Diagnosis Features	Age of Onset	Evaluation/Differential diagnosis	Treatments	Comments
Primary cough headache	Occurs moments after cough, straining, or other Valsalva maneuvers. Reaches its peak almost immediately, subsides over seconds to minutes (up to 2 h)	Patients >40	Associated with Arnold-Chiari malformation type 1; may also be associated spontaneous intracranial hypotension, carotid or vertebrobasilar diseases, middle cranial fossa or posterior fossa tumors, midbrain cyst, subdural hematoma, aneurysms and RCVS	Indomethacin (50–200 mg/d)	Cause possible perivascular inflammation
Primary exercise headache	Pulsating headache triggered by physical activity			Indomethacin 25 mg or other nonsteroidal anti-inflammatory drug (NSAID) in advance of activity. Propranolol may also be helpful. Reports of prevention by ergotamine tartrate	
Headache with sexual activity	Dull aching sensation in head and neck increased with sexual excitement and worse with orgasm	Any sexually active age	Subarachnoid hemorrhage, arterial dissection, RCVS	Indomethacin 25 mg or other NSAID in advance of activity. Propranolol may also be helpful	When seen after first event, evaluation is usually warranted (CT angiography/MR angiography, may consider lumbar puncture)

(continued on next page)

Table 1
(continued)

Headache	Diagnosis Features	Age of Onset	Evaluation/Differential diagnosis	Treatments	Comments
Nummular headache	Continuous or intermittent head pain in a fixed location on scalp, round or elliptical, 1–6 cm in diameter				
Hypnic headache	Mild-moderate bilateral or generalized headache waking the patient from sleep; most cases are daily or near daily headaches >3 mo	>50 years old	Could consider a primary sleep disorder, cluster headache, nocturnal hypertension, hypoglycemia; intracranial disorders must be excluded	Lithium 300–600 mg at nightly (hour of sleep), caffeine, melatonin, indomethacin	Consider sleep study
Primary stabbing headache	Short duration unilateral or bilateral stabs of pain in V1-2 distribution	Adults	No other evaluation needed	May not need specific treatment, otherwise treat as migraine	Also called sharp jabs and jolts; often seen in migraine patients

Data from Olesen J. International classification of headache disorders. Lancet Neurol 2018;17(5):396–7.

Box 2
International Classification of Headache Disorders cluster headache criteria

Severe or very severe unilateral orbital, supraorbital, and/or temporal pain lasting 15 to 180 minutes (when untreated)

Either or both of the following:
1. At least one of the following symptoms or signs, ipsilateral to the headache:
   a. Conjunctival injection and/or lacrimation
   b. Nasal congestion and/or rhinorrhea
   c. Eyelid edema
   d. Forehead and facial sweating
   e. Forehead and facial flushing
   f. Sensation of fullness in the ear
   g. Miosis and/or ptosis
2. A sense of restlessness or agitation
   Attacks have a frequency between one every other day and 8 per day for more than half of the time when the disorder is active

Data from Olesen J. International classification of headache disorders. Lancet Neurol 2018;17(5):396–7.

Diagnosis is clinical and based on the elicited history. Cluster is usually easily differentiated from other trigeminal autonomic cephalalgias, from sinus disease, and from migraine, although diagnostic dilemmas do occur. Secondary or symptomatic causes are reported; thus, imaging is recommended for new-onset or atypical symptoms. Functional imaging has shown changes in the ipsilateral posterior hypothalamus.

Cluster headaches may be aborted by breathing 100% oxygen for 15 minutes.[3] Supplemental, low-flow oxygen by nasal cannula is ineffective; high-flow oxygen through a tightly fitting, non-rebreather mask is required. Triptan medications, for example, sumatriptan injection, are also commonly beneficial. The total daily parenteral triptan dose commonly exceeds recommended dosing for migraine; however, medication overuse headache related to triptans appears to be less common in this population. Vasoconstrictive medications or ergotamine preparations may also be helpful. A short steroid taper early in the course of a bout of cluster may help shorten the cluster episode. Choices for preventive medication include calcium channel blockers and lithium. Verapamil may be required in quite high doses, such as 480 mg daily and higher to obtain benefit. Electrocardiographic monitoring of cardiac arrhythmias (such as prolonged PR intervals) may be required with these doses. Successful dosing for lithium is based on blood levels in the therapeutic range for the treatment of bipolar disorder. Occipital nerve blocks with short-acting anesthetics and steroid can be considered as initial treatment helping to provide relief until preventive medications can take effect. Topiramate, sodium valproate, and gabapentin have also shown some efficacy.[4,5] More recently, noninvasive neuromodulatory techniques, for example, gammaCore vagal nerve stimulator, have shown some benefit in treatment of individual attacks with only minor adverse effects.[6]

Hemicrania continua

Hemicrania continua is a unilateral, side-locked, continuous pain of moderate intensity with periods of severe exacerbation. Ipsilateral autonomic features, including conjunctival injection, tearing, nasal congestion, and even ptosis, are reported. A complete and striking response to indomethacin, and only indomethacin, is common. The importance of making the diagnosis is to avoid multiple evaluations and trials of ineffective therapies that can stretch over years if the correct diagnosis is not suspected.

***Short-lasting unilateral headaches: short-lasting unilateral neuralgiform headache
attacks with conjunctival injection and tearing /short-lasting unilateral neuralgiform
headache attacks with cranial autonomic symptoms***

Short-lasting unilateral headaches are very rare and are probably related headache
conditions (**Table 2**). They are characterized by ultra-short-lasting, side-locked, severe, and often periorbital pains (5- to 240-seconds duration). They occur very
frequently throughout the day and are associated with autonomic features. Short-
lasting unilateral neuralgiform headache attacks with conjunctival injection and tearing
(SUNCT) features ipsilateral lacrimation and conjunctival irritation. Short-lasting unilateral neuralgiform headache attacks with cranial autonomic symptoms (SUNA) have
one but not the other of these autonomic features and may, in addition, feature rhinorrhea or nasal congestion. Pain may be triggered by various forms of cutaneous stimulation. Generally, these are considered primary headaches, but secondary causes
have been documented, and imaging is warranted at onset. Both topiramate and
lamotrigine have shown benefit.[7]

Facial Pain and Neuralgias

Facial pain denotes a complex constellation of pain syndromes comprising multiple
neuralgias and neuropathies; ocular, aural, sinus, and dental causes of pain; central
causes of pain; and other more nonspecific forms of chronic pain termed atypical
facial pain.

Neuralgiform or neuropathic pain is distinguished from nociceptive pain in that it
represents the result of direct central or peripheral afferent nerve injury as opposed
to pain arising from a more "physiologic" stimulation of peripheral nociceptive receptors. The resulting symptoms are distinctive and include brief and paroxysmal or
steady burning or shooting pain, stimulation by normally nonpainful sensations (allodynia), and, in some instances, trigger points, and the presence of a refractory period
after stimulation, during which time the pain cannot be retriggered.

Table 2
Selected trigeminal autonomic cephalalgias

Name	Location	Duration	Attack Frequency/d	Associated Features	Treatment
Cluster	Unilateral orbital	15–180 min	1–8	Lacrimation, conjunctival injection, rhinorrhea	Verapamil, inhaled oxygen 15 L/min
Paroxysmal hemicrania	V1, ophthalmic division	2–30 min	2–40	Lacrimation, conjunctival injection, rhinorrhea	Indomethacin, with complete control
SUNCT	Unilateral orbital to temporal region	15 s to 4 min	3–200	Conjunctival injection AND lacrimation	Lamotrigine, intravenous (IV) lidocaine
SUNA	Unilateral orbital to temporal region	15 s to 4 min	3–200	Conjunctival injection OR lacrimation + rhinorrhea/nasal congestion	Lamotrigine, IV lidocaine

From Rizzoli P. Trigeminal autonomic cephalagias (TACs): cluster headache, paroxysmal hemicra-
nias, SUNCT, SUNA. In: Yong R, Nguyen M, Nelson E, et al, editors. Pain medicine. Cham
(Switzerland): Springer International Publishing; 2017. p. 537–8; with permission.

Multiple mechanisms of entrapment, trauma, disease invasion, or destruction of nerves may be envisioned as initiating neuropathic pain. From initiation, the subsequent changes related to inflammation may amplify the initial insult and help lead to secondary features, such as ectopic transmission and central sensitization. The combination of pathologic features in any given instance may give rise to different sets of symptoms, different sensory profiles,[8] for example, whether the pain is more burning or more episodic, more associated with numbness, or more tenderness to pressure. These profiles may account for variations in presentation of neuralgias and, furthermore, it has been suggested that appropriate management may be selected based on the symptom profile.[8]

Specific neuralgias are further characterized by pain in the distribution of the damaged cranial or cervical nerve. Two major cranial neuralgias, trigeminal and occipital, are discussed later. Selected, less commonly encountered neuralgias are presented in **Table 3**.

Trigeminal neuralgia
TGN is defined by brief recurrent paroxysms of severe neuropathic unilateral facial pain in the distribution of one or more divisions of the trigeminal nerve.[9] The prevalence of TGN is 15.5/100,000, being more common in women than men (3:1).[10,11] Pain attacks may be precipitated by innocuous stimuli (eg, chewing, talking). TGN may be distinguished from cluster headache by a lack of profound autonomic symptoms, no radiation beyond divisions of the trigeminal nerve, and short attack duration (<2 minutes). Classical TGN is secondary to neurovascular compression of the trigeminal nerve, with dislocation or atrophy in the trigeminal nerve root showing high specificity for the disease.[12] Secondary TGN may be caused by tumors in the

Table 3
Less common neuralgias

Neuralgia	Features	Nerve	Distribution	Comments
Glossopharyngeal[36]	Sharp, stabbing, severe	CN IX and X	Side of the throat, tonsillar area, base of tongue	First described in 1920; mostly idiopathic, rarely symptomatic
Supraorbital	Long-lasting attacks of moderate to severe frontal pain	SON (see **Fig. 1**)	Frontal and SO region	Tenderness over the SO notch
Supratrochlear[37]	Long-lasting or episodic pain and sensory disturbance	STN	Medial forehead	Tenderness in the SO rim medially over the nerve; distinguish from SON
Nervus intermedius	Paroxysmal brief shocklike	Sensory branch of VII	Deep auditory canal	
Auriculotemporal neuralgia	Paroxysmal, brief shocklike	ATN (see **Fig. 1**)	Anterior to the tragus	

Abbreviations: ATN, auriculotemporal nerve; CN, cranial nerve; SO, supraorbital; SON, supraorbital nerve; STN, supratrochlear nerve.

cerebellopontine angle, arteriovenous malformations, and multiple sclerosis plaques (which may result in the rare presentation of bilateral symptoms).[13] Idiopathic TGN is less common, occurring in 11% of patients. Treatment of TGN is typically initiated with either carbamazepine (200–1200 mg/d) or oxcarbazepine (600–1800 mg/d), which may reduce pain in up to 90% of patients.[14,15] Second-line medications include lamotrigine, baclofen, pregabalin or gabapentin, topiramate, and valproate.[16] It is not unusual to use several medications concurrently. Patients with classical TGN who are refractory to medical treatment should be referred for surgical treatments, including percutaneous procedures on the ganglion, gamma knife, and microvascular decompression.

Occipital neuralgia

Occipital neuralgia is an important cause of head and neck pain first described in the early 1800s. It can be debilitating but generally responds well to treatment. The prevalence is unknown; however, depending on the referral pattern, it may appear to be common in some practices. It is characterized by a rather distinctive pattern of symptoms, with associated physical findings, that, when present, can provide a fairly high index of clinical diagnostic confidence (**Box 3**). Symptoms include stabbing or shooting pain in the C1 and C2 dermatomes, at times associated with dysesthesia or sensory loss in the same distribution. Examination discloses tenderness of the involved occipital nerve to palpation (**Fig. 1**).

Atypical facial pain (persistent idiopathic facial pain)

Atypical facial pain may be defined as chronic and nonspecific facial pain not fitting into other diagnostic categories and with no diagnostic features by examination or testing. Typically, a burning, continuous, unilateral pain, and often in place for years before diagnosis, may be severe and often associated with depression and anxiety. The patient has often undergone multiple evaluations by multiple specialists before presentation and is refractory to all treatments. The prognosis has been considered guarded to poor for recovery. Nonetheless, a multidisciplinary approach to diagnosis and management is suggested because newer interventional approaches may show benefit.[17,18]

Box 3
International Classification of Headache Disorders occipital neuralgia criteria

A. Unilateral or bilateral pain fulfilling criteria B–E

B. Pain is located in the distribution of the greater, lesser, and/or third occipital nerves

C. Pain has 2 of the following 3 characteristics:
 1. Recurring in paroxysmal attacks lasting from a few seconds to minutes
 2. Severe intensity
 3. Shooting, stabbing, or sharp in quality

D. Pain is associated with both of the following:
 1. Dysesthesia and/or allodynia apparent during innocuous stimulation of the scalp and/or hair
 2. Either or both of the following:
  a. Tenderness over the affected nerve branches
  b. Trigger points at the emergence of the greater occipital nerve or in the area of distribution of C2

E. Pain is eased temporarily by local anesthetic block of the affected nerve

Data from Olesen J. International classification of headache disorders. Lancet Neurol 2018;17(5):396–7.

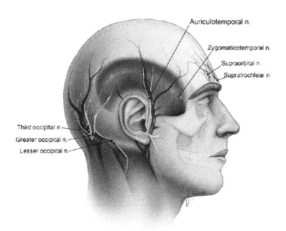

Fig. 1. Superficial nerves of the face and scalp. (*From* Gadient PM, Smith JH. The neuralgias: diagnosis and management. Curr Neurol Neurosci Rep 2014;14(7):459; with permission.)

New Daily Persistent Headache

This distinctive pattern of headache is currently classified as primary in origin and benign in nature. NDPH has only been described relatively recently, in 1986, by Vanast,[19] who resolved the pattern of a sudden onset of daily headache out of the background of his other chronic headache patients. The pattern has held up over time and has earned full status in the International Classification of Headache Disorders (ICHD) classification system. The essential feature of the diagnosis is a "distinct and clearly remembered onset, with pain becoming continuous and unremitting within 24 hours" and present for more than 3 months.[9]

Although NDPH may rarely remit or relapse, it is generally abrupt in onset and continuous, usually without any prior headache history or clear triggering features. Its unique temporal profile makes it instantly recognizable; often patients can specify the day and date of onset, if not the time of day and activity underway at the time. In perhaps 40%, it may be associated with a prior febrile illness at onset or prior noncranial surgery. NDPH typically persists, year after year, as a daily continuous pattern without aggravating, alleviating or modifying features. It has been postulated to represent persistent central nervous system (CNS) or systemic inflammation. The headache description itself may differ between individuals, looking more migrainelike in one, more tensionlike or clusterlike in another.[20]

The pathophysiology is unknown. Patients generally report no relief from medications; nonetheless, most patients at diagnosis continue their daily activities. Prevalence has been estimated at 0.1% to 13% of all patients presenting with chronic headache; chronic headaches in turn constitute 3% to 4% of all headache patients. Notwithstanding, NDPH has become a routine diagnosis in every headache center. Given the apparently benign nature of the pattern, little in the way of evaluation is usually performed. Other forms of headache may be considered, and the differential diagnosis is as listed in **Box 4**.

Case reports of response to treatment have been published and, early in the course, steroids may improve or even resolve symptoms (**Box 5** suggests a treatment paradigm). Otherwise, currently, treatment is often tailored to that of the phenomenology of the headache itself, that is, treating a cluster pattern as one would treat cluster.

Box 4
Differential diagnosis of new daily persistent headache

- Low-pressure headache
- Cerebral venous thrombosis
- Arterial dissection
- Giant cell arteritis
- CNS vasculitis
- Hemicrania continua
- Lymphocytic meningitis
- Recurrent herpes simplex virus meningitis (Mollaret)

Although the prognosis is considered guarded to poor, supportive management and medication trials are considered appropriate in most patients.

SELECTED SECONDARY HEADACHES
Vascular-Related Headache

Cervical artery dissection
Cervical artery dissection (CEAD) is a major cause of ischemic stroke in the young, typically occurring in the early 40s. CEAD presents with neck pain and headache, and as such, may be misdiagnosed as migraine or musculoskeletal pain initially.[21] However, most patients also present with focal neurologic signs. Dissection of the vertebral artery may result in cerebellar, brainstem (lateral medullary), or occipital lobe infarct, and dissection of the carotid artery may present with a partial Horner syndrome (ptosis and miosis) in addition to hemispheric strokes and dysautonomia. Patients with dissection are less likely to have traditional stroke factors in comparison to other causes of ischemic stroke.[22] Retrospective report of infection in the previous week, and report of minor cervical trauma in the last month, is relatively high, although subject to recall bias.[22] Fibromuscular and connective tissue disorders are risk factors, as is migraine. Given the high rates of migraine (more than one-third of patients with CEAD), it is important for the clinician to not be misled by this history when evaluating the patient with acute headache and neurologic complaints.[23] Pathognomonic radiodiagnostic findings include dissection flaps and "pearl-and-string" sign.

Box 5
New daily persistent headache treatment paradigm

- If recent onset:
  - Prednisone 60 to 80 mg/d, taper over 16 to 20 days
- If migrainous, treat with drugs for migraine: topiramate, beta-blockers, divalproex, tricyclics
- If neuralgic, use drugs for neuralgia: gabapentin, duloxetine, pregabalin
- Consider (based on case reports): doxycycline, naltrexone, naratriptan, prazosin, or mexiletine. Next consider onabotulinumtoxinA
- If response, maintain treatment for 6 months before tapering

Data from Joshi SG, Mathew PG, Markley HG. New daily persistent headache and potential new therapeutic agents. Curr Neurol Neurosci Rep 2014;14(2):425.

Treatment is typically antiplatelet therapy to prevent recurrence, because there does not appear to be increased benefit with anticoagulation.[24] Vascular surgery may be warranted in complicated cases.

Cerebral venous thrombosis

Cerebral venous thrombosis (CVT) is a rare cause of stroke that disproportionately affects women (74% of cases) and the young (mean age of presentation at 39 years).[25] Presentation may include headache (almost 90%), seizure (almost 40%), paresis, mental status change, aphasia, diplopia, papilledema, visual loss, and stupor/coma (**Fig. 2** provides a case and image encountered by one of the authors). Multiple venous sinuses are involved in almost half of the cases, with the superficial veins of the superior sagittal sinus and transverse sinus most commonly involved. Risk factors are similar to systemic venous thrombosis and include thrombophilia, malignancy, pregnancy/puerperium, infection, oral contraceptives, and dehydration. One potential severe consequence of infections of the face or sphenoid sinuses is a cavernous sinus thrombosis, which may present with palsy of cranial nerves passing through the cavernous sinus (abducens palsy being the most common). Treatment includes anticoagulation with intravenous heparin in most cases, including in cases of hemorrhagic infarct.[26] In severe cases, thrombectomy/thrombolysis may be considered. Mortality ranges from 6% to 20%, and as such, organized care in a stroke unit is recommended because it reduces mortality by 14%.[26]

Reversible cerebral vasoconstriction syndrome and posterior reversible encephalopathy syndrome

Reversible cerebral vasoconstriction syndrome (RCVS) is defined by the angiographic description of alternating segments of arterial constriction and dilatation, which present with recurring thunderclap headaches over the course of weeks, typically triggered by sexual activity, straining, or Valsalva maneuvers.[9] Although the disease is self-limiting, there is a high risk of neurologic sequelae from intracranial hemorrhage, infarction, or edema. Initial arterial imaging peaks 2 to 3 weeks after symptom onset,

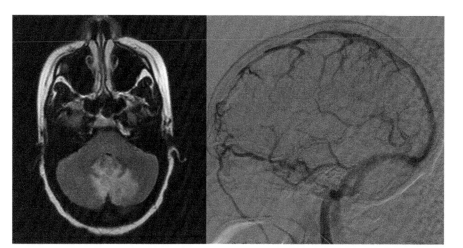

Fig. 2. A 35-year-old woman with an underlying hypercoagulable disorder (on anticoagulation) with subacute severe continuous headache with flashes of light and acute nausea, vomiting, bilateral papilledema, bilateral dysmetria, and ataxia. MR imaging revealed a straight sinus venous thrombosis causing bilateral cerebellar infarcts (*left*) with venous sinus thrombosis of the straight sinus identified on angiography (*right*).

and as such, normal imaging on presentation should be repeated.[27] Risk factors include postpartum state and vasoactive substances (including cocaine, marijuana, selective serotonin reuptake inhibitors, triptans, ergot derivatives, alpha-sympathomimetics). Treatment is typically supportive; however, medications that may prevent vasospasm (such as verapamil) are often used.[27]

Posterior reversible encephalopathy syndrome (PRES) may present with headache, altered consciousness, visual abnormalities, seizures, and most commonly, hypertension (in 60%–80% of patients). **Fig. 3** provides a case encountered by one of the authors. It has been proposed that the PRES and RCVS may share a common pathophysiologic mechanism secondary to several clinical and radiographic similarities. Imaging findings depict characteristic focal regions of symmetric hemispheric vasogenic edema, with a predilection in parieto-occipital regions, but may also depict infarcts and hemorrhages. Conditions that increase the risk of PRES include preeclampsia/eclampsia, infection, autoimmune disease, and immunosuppression. Vasogenic edema occurs from disruption of the blood-brain barrier in the more vulnerable regions of the posterior brain secondary to endothelial dysfunction, hypoperfusion, vasoconstriction, and hypertension.[28,29] Treatment targets the underlying illness or contributing factors. Up to one-third of patients may have marked functional impairment.[30]

Cerebrospinal Fluid Flow–Related Headache

Disorders of CSF fluid homeostasis often present with headache. An elevation of CSF pressure could be linked to factors that increase the contents of the fixed intracranial vault. These factors include pathologic conditions such as parenchymal edema, increased cerebral blood volume, increased CSF production and/or reduced reabsorption, or venous outflow obstruction.[31]

A reduction in CSF pressure could in theory be related to low CSF production but more often is considered to represent a loss of CSF due to leakage into surrounding tissues from a variety of pathologic conditions, natural and iatrogenic, which leads to a tear or rent in the dura.

Idiopathic intracranial hypertension

Idiopathic intracranial hypertension (IIH) is a condition characterized by increased intracranial pressure in the absence of identifiable intracranial pathologic condition capable of producing increased pressure. The current incidence of 1 to 2 cases per

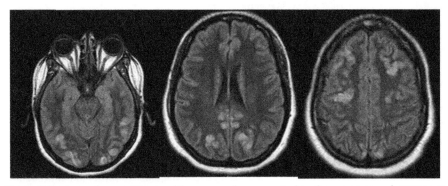

Fig. 3. MR images from a 28-year-old woman who presented to the emergency department on post-partum day 4 with a severe headache and blurry vision. Shortly thereafter, she had multiple convulsions. Her MRI (FLAIR images) showed bilateral cortical and subcortical edema throughout the brain, consistent with PRES.

100,000 may be increasing in proportion to the population incidence of obesity, and the incidence in obese women of childbearing age may be as high as 21 cases per 100,000.[31] The most common presenting symptom is often a nonspecific, subacute onset, progressive headache that may worsen with exertion. Associated features may include tinnitus, visual obscurations, and nausea. Bilateral papilledema, due to pressure effect on the optic nerves, is usually present on examination, although cases without this finding have been documented. Other visual findings may be present, and permanent visual loss can occur. Laboratory diagnosis rests on a CSF opening pressure on lumbar puncture of greater than 200 mm H_2O, although an upper limit of 250 mm H_2O may be considered in the obese patient. The CSF is otherwise normal. The pathophysiology is uncertain, but the condition is said to be self-limited in many patients. Besides an association with obesity, some possible etiologic factors have been associated, among them the use of tetracyclines and oral contraceptive medications. Treatment is aimed at symptom reduction and the prevention of visual complications. Repeat lumbar puncture for removal of CSF is performed less frequently than previously and is not recommended. Acetazolamide is considered first-line therapy for reducing CSF pressure, although topiramate could also be considered. Weight loss to reduce CSF pressure can also be effective. Surgical management with shunt placement or optic nerve sheath fenestration is performed only rarely in aggressive cases to prevent visual complications.

Low cerebrospinal fluid pressure headache/orthostatic headache

A reduction in intracranial CSF pressure/volume leads to loss of the cushioning effect or buoyancy of CSF on the brain, leading to excessive brain movement and traction on pain-sensitive dural structures. This traction results in an orthostatic headache pattern of headache, worse with the upright posture and better in recumbency. The most common cause is persistent CSF leakage after lumbar puncture, but multiple noniatrogenic, or spontaneous, causes have been described. The resulting headache is usually dull and generalized, ranging from mild to severe and relieved when the patient is flat. Associated features may include nausea, tinnitus, and imbalance.[32] Diagnostic evaluation usually begins with brain MRI. Characteristic MRI changes, including diffuse meningeal enhancement, subdural hematomas or hygromas, brain sagging or descent, venous engorgement, and pituitary enlargement, or some combination, are present in up to 80% of patients. An opening pressure of less than 60 mm H_2O on lumbar puncture is also indicative. MRI of the spine may show extra-arachnoid or extradural CSF fluid collections, which, with computed tomographic (CT) or MR myelography, may help localize the site of the leak. However, evaluation to determine the source of the leak is usually unrewarding unless the leak is especially large.

Many leaks will resolve spontaneously with bed rest, fluids, and supplemental caffeine administration. If not, an autologous lumbar blood patch may be curative, although at times more than one patch is required for resolution. To reduce the incidence of iatrogenic low-pressure headache related to lumbar puncture, use of a non-cutting or atraumatic LP needle has been advised.[33]

Inflammatory-Related Headache

Giant cell arteritis

Giant cell arteritis (GCA) is a common form of systemic vasculitis affecting medium and large arteries and presenting in adults over the age of 50. At highest risk are women of Northern European descent. There is a strong association with polymyalgia rheumatica, although the conditions are separate.[34]

Most of the symptoms of GCA relate to involvement of cranial and intracranial arteries and include new-onset headache, jaw claudication, diplopia, and transient and fixed visual loss. Constitutional symptoms include fever, anemia, weight loss, and fatigue. The headache may be nonspecific or may be a moderate-intensity, dull, temporal pain, at times associated with local temporal artery tenderness and nodularity. It is important to maintain a high index of clinical suspicion for this condition in anyone over the age of 50 presenting with any of the following: a new onset headache, jaw claudication, transient of permanent visual loss, or unexplained fever. The most serious complication, permanent visual loss, may arise suddenly and painlessly at any time before treatment and is rarely reversible. Involvement of vision on one side is commonly followed shortly by visual loss on the opposite side.

Because of the risk of sudden visual loss, the diagnosis of GCA constitutes a medical emergency, and treatment should be instituted as quickly as possible, often before the completion of the evaluation. Once the condition is treated, however, the risk of blindness falls to near zero. Initial evaluation includes the inflammatory markers: erythrocyte sedimentation rate and C-reactive protein. An outpatient temporal artery biopsy can confirm the diagnosis. Treatment is often initiated, before biopsy, with high-dose prednisone, and the patient is followed in rheumatology.[35]

REFERENCES

1. Nesbitt AD, Goadsby PJ. Cluster headache. BMJ 2012;344:e2407.
2. Weaver-Agostoni J. Cluster headache. Am Fam Physician 2013;88(2):122–8.
3. Rozen TD. Inhaled oxygen for cluster headache: efficacy, mechanism of action, utilization, and economics. Curr Pain Headache Rep 2012;16(2):175–9.
4. Lainez MJ, Pascual J, Pascual AM, et al. Topiramate in the prophylactic treatment of cluster headache. Headache 2003;43(7):784–9.
5. Gallagher RM, Mueller LL, Freitag FG. Divalproex sodium in the treatment of migraine and cluster headaches. J Am Osteopath Assoc 2002;102(2):92–4.
6. Silberstein SD, Mechtler LL, Kudrow DB, et al. Non-invasive vagus nerve stimulation for the acute treatment of cluster headache: findings from the randomized, double-blind, sham-controlled ACT1 study. Headache 2016;56(8):1317–32.
7. Pareja JA, Alvarez M, Montojo T. SUNCT and SUNA: recognition and treatment. Curr Treat Options Neurol 2013;15(1):28–39.
8. Baron R, Binder A, Wasner G. Neuropathic pain: diagnosis, pathophysiological mechanisms, and treatment. Lancet Neurol 2010;9(8):807–19.
9. Olesen J. International classification of headache disorders. Lancet Neurol 2018; 17(5):396–7.
10. Katusic S, Williams DB, Beard CM, et al. Epidemiology and clinical features of idiopathic trigeminal neuralgia and glossopharyngeal neuralgia: similarities and differences, Rochester, Minnesota, 1945-1984. Neuroepidemiology 1991; 10(5–6):276–81.
11. De Toledo IP, Conti Reus J, Fernandes M, et al. Prevalence of trigeminal neuralgia: a systematic review. J Am Dent Assoc 2016;147(7):570–6.e572.
12. Antonini G, Di Pasquale A, Cruccu G, et al. Magnetic resonance imaging contribution for diagnosing symptomatic neurovascular contact in classical trigeminal neuralgia: a blinded case-control study and meta-analysis. Pain 2014;155(8): 1464–71.
13. O'Connor AB, Schwid SR, Herrmann DN, et al. Pain associated with multiple sclerosis: systematic review and proposed classification. Pain 2008;137(1):96–111.

14. Cruccu G, Gronseth G, Alksne J, et al. AAN-EFNS guidelines on trigeminal neuralgia management. Eur J Neurol 2008;15(10):1013–28.
15. Zakrzewska JM, Linskey ME. Trigeminal neuralgia. BMJ 2015;350:h1238.
16. Obermann M. Treatment options in trigeminal neuralgia. Ther Adv Neurol Disord 2010;3(2):107–15.
17. Weiss AL, Ehrhardt KP, Tolba R. Atypical facial pain: a comprehensive, evidence-based review. Curr Pain Headache Rep 2017;21(2):8.
18. Zakrzewska JM. Chronic/persistent idiopathic facial pain. Neurosurg Clin N Am 2016;27(3):345–51.
19. Robbins MS, Vanast WJ, Allan Purdy R. New daily persistent headache: historical review and an interview with Dr. Walter Vanast. Headache 2017;57(6):926–34.
20. Rozen TD. New daily persistent headache: clinical perspective. Headache 2011; 51(4):641–9.
21. Arnold M, Cumurciuc R, Stapf C, et al. Pain as the only symptom of cervical artery dissection. J Neurol Neurosurg Psychiatry 2006;77(9):1021–4.
22. Debette S, Metso T, Pezzini A, et al. Association of vascular risk factors with cervical artery dissection and ischemic stroke in young adults. Circulation 2011; 123(14):1537–44.
23. Rist PM, Diener HC, Kurth T, et al. Migraine, migraine aura, and cervical artery dissection: a systematic review and meta-analysis. Cephalalgia 2011;31(8): 886–96.
24. Lyrer P, Engelter S. Antithrombotic drugs for carotid artery dissection. Cochrane Database Syst Rev 2010;(10):CD000255.
25. Ferro JM, Canhao P, Stam J, et al. Prognosis of cerebral vein and dural sinus thrombosis: results of the International Study on Cerebral Vein and Dural Sinus Thrombosis (ISCVT). Stroke 2004;35(3):664–70.
26. Saposnik G, Barinagarrementeria F, Brown RD Jr, et al. Diagnosis and management of cerebral venous thrombosis: a statement for healthcare professionals from the American Heart Association/American Stroke Association. Stroke 2011;42(4):1158–92.
27. Ducros A. Reversible cerebral vasoconstriction syndrome. Lancet Neurol 2012; 11(10):906–17.
28. Ay H, Buonanno FS, Schaefer PW, et al. Posterior leukoencephalopathy without severe hypertension: utility of diffusion-weighted MRI. Neurology 1998;51(5): 1369–76.
29. Fugate JE, Rabinstein AA. Posterior reversible encephalopathy syndrome: clinical and radiological manifestations, pathophysiology, and outstanding questions. Lancet Neurol 2015;14(9):914–25.
30. Legriel S, Schraub O, Azoulay E, et al. Determinants of recovery from severe posterior reversible encephalopathy syndrome. PLoS One 2012;7(9):e44534.
31. Skau M, Brennum J, Gjerris F, et al. What is new about idiopathic intracranial hypertension? An updated review of mechanism and treatment. Cephalalgia 2006; 26(4):384–99.
32. Hoffmann J, Goadsby PJ. Update on intracranial hypertension and hypotension. Curr Opin Neurol 2013;26(3):240–7.
33. Davis A, Dobson R, Kaninia S, et al. Change practice now! Using atraumatic needles to prevent post lumbar puncture headache. Eur J Neurol 2014;21(2): 305–11.
34. Caylor TL, Perkins A. Recognition and management of polymyalgia rheumatica and giant cell arteritis. Am Fam Physician 2013;88(10):676–84.

35. Ezeonyeji AN, Borg FA, Dasgupta B. Delays in recognition and management of giant cell arteritis: results from a retrospective audit. Clin Rheumatol 2011; 30(2):259–62.
36. Blumenfeld A, Nikolskaya G. Glossopharyngeal neuralgia. Curr Pain Headache Rep 2013;17(7):343.
37. Pareja JA, Lopez-Ruiz P, Mayo D, et al. Supratrochlear neuralgia: a prospective case series of 15 patients. Headache 2017;57(9):1433–42.

Concussion Evaluation and Management

William T. Jackson, MD, Amaal J. Starling, MD*

KEYWORDS

- Concussion • Postconcussion syndrome • Mild traumatic brain injury
- Traumatic brain injury • Posttraumatic headache

KEY POINTS

- Concussion is a public health crisis for which internists are on the front line of medical care.
- Rapid identification and appropriate diagnosis and management are essential components to concussion care.
- Multidomain symptoms require multidisciplinary, symptom-directed treatment.
- There are 2 primary goals in the management of concussion: (1) to provide symptomatic treatment and (2) to prevent reinjury while the brain is healing.
- A graduated return to learn/work and physical activity protocol, as well as controlled aerobic exercise, may be helpful for recovery from concussion.

INTRODUCTION

Concussion or mild traumatic brain injury (TBI) is a public health crisis, with the incidence approaching 4 million injuries per year.[1] A concussion is a TBI induced by biomechanical forces.[2] Although a concussion may have microstructural neuropathologic changes, acute symptoms and signs represent abnormal function of networks in the brain, rather than gross structural injury.[2] There is also increasing awareness of the short-term and potential long-term consequences of repetitive blows to the head on the national scale due to the extensive exposure to risk in professional sports and in the military.[3,4] One of the most significant consequences after a concussion is a recurrent concussion.[5] Individuals are at a higher risk of having a recurrent concussion within the first 7 to 10 days after the first concussion, likely due to both a physical vulnerability (poor balance, blurred vision, and so forth) and a physiologic neuronal

Disclosure Statement: Dr W.T. Jackson has nothing to disclose. Dr A.J. Starling receives research funding from the Migraine Research Foundation and Mayo Clinic. She serves as a consultant or on advisory boards for Alder, Amgen, Eli Lilly & Company, and eNeura.
Department of Neurology, Mayo Clinic College of Medicine, 13400 East Shea Boulevard, Scottsdale, AZ 85259, USA
* Corresponding author.
E-mail address: Starling.amaal@mayo.edu

Med Clin N Am 103 (2019) 251–261
https://doi.org/10.1016/j.mcna.2018.10.005
0025-7125/19/© 2018 Elsevier Inc. All rights reserved.
medical.theclinics.com

vulnerability.[6,7] Recurrent concussions demonstrate longer symptom resolution time, increased time out of play, and higher likelihood of loss of consciousness than the first concussion.[8] In addition, young brains seem to be at higher risk for injury due to immature neurologic, vascular, and musculoskeletal physiology.[9] This factor combined with less training experience can lead to increased forces of impact and a higher incidence of concussion.[10] Improving the rapid identification, diagnosis, and appropriate management of concussion is likely key to reducing the potential downstream negative consequences. This narrative review highlights the essentials for the in-office evaluation and management of concussion, including return to learn/work and return to physical activity recommendations.

Symptoms

Concussion can result in a range of symptoms that may vary greatly in quality, severity, and duration. They can often be very nonspecific in nature and overlap with preexisting medical conditions. In addition, they can have a delayed presentation. Some symptoms are present at the time of head impact; however, other symptoms may develop over the first several hours or even days after injury. All of these factors can make the symptomatic assessment of concussion challenging. The concussion symptom evaluation checklist from the Sports Concussion Assessment Tool, fifth edition (SCAT 5) is a thorough, easy-to-administer, helpful tool to capture many symptoms related to a concussion.[11] It has a list of 22 common symptoms in concussion assessed via a Likert scale from 0 to 6 to calculate not only the number of symptoms but also the symptom severity.

Symptoms of a concussion fall into multiple domains: physical, cognitive, emotional, and sleep (**Table 1**). The most commonly reported symptoms are in the physical and cognitive domains, including headache, dizziness, and difficulty with concentration; however, patients and families are often most concerned about the emotional and sleep symptoms. These symptoms can be overlooked during the evaluation, yet can be very debilitating and worrisome for the patient.

It has also been observed that depending on when the patient presents, the predominant symptoms can shift throughout the recovery course. The most common presenting symptoms, headache, dizziness, and difficulty with concentration, tend to become overshadowed at subsequent visits by sleep disturbances, frustration, forgetfulness, and fatigue.[12] There may be significant variability in symptom severity both at onset and throughout recovery, fortunately there is a consistent trend toward

Table 1
Symptoms of a concussion can be categorized into multiple domains: physical, cognitive, emotional, and sleep

Physical	Cognitive	Emotional	Sleep
Headache Sensitivity to light Sensitivity to sound Nausea/vomiting	Poor concentration	Irritability	Insomnia
Dizziness Lightheadedness Difficulty with balance	Difficulty with memory	Depressive symptoms or sadness	Hypersomnia
Blurred vision	Cognitive slowing	Anxiety or nervousness	Fatigue
Loss of energy	Inability to multitask	Mood swings	

symptom resolution seen in the most patients. However, a small population may have persistent symptoms over time.[13] It is hoped, with improved identification, diagnosis, and appropriate management, a greater percentage will make a more complete recovery.

Diagnostic Test/Imaging Study

Concussion remains a clinical diagnosis. At this time, there is no diagnostic test, clinical biomarker, or imaging study that can diagnose a concussion.[2] A clinical diagnosis is made based on symptoms from the clinical history and signs from the physical examination. There are several objective tools that can be used to aid the clinical diagnosis, including neuropsychological testing, vestibular and balance testing, oculomotor or eye tracking, and autonomic testing.

Clinical history and physical examination

The primary means of an in-office diagnosis of concussion revolve around the clinical history and physical examination. Although there are many objective screening tools, including brief computerized cognitive testing, in development and in practice to augment the evaluation, an expedited clinical history and physical examination are paramount. Concussed patients, specifically athletes, should be seen by a medical provider within 72 hours of injury to ensure appropriate management, to limit symptom exacerbation, and to prevent premature return to learn and play.

The specific nature of the initial injury should be discussed in great detail. This discussion should include the date of injury, a description of the mechanism of injury, location of impact, loss of consciousness, and the presence or absence of retrograde or anterograde amnesia. Immediate and delayed symptoms should also be noted with attention paid to the timing of symptom occurrence and progression. A systematic symptom screen can help in capturing the variety and severity of symptoms. The concussion symptom evaluation checklist includes a list of 22 common symptoms in concussion to identify and monitor the number of symptoms and symptom severity.[11] The symptom severity can be calculated at the initial postinjury visit and at subsequent visits to monitor recovery.

Headache is the most common symptom after a concussion.[14] In fact, there is a higher prevalence of headache after concussion or mild TBI compared with moderate to severe TBI.[14,15] A systematic approach to headache after a concussion starts with screening for headache red flag symptoms. These red flag symptoms may include focal neurologic symptoms, altered level of consciousness, postural or positional component to headache, progressively worsening headache, or intractable vomiting with headache. If red flags are present, neuroimaging is needed to evaluate for structural abnormalities that need to be addressed. A postural or headache exacerbated by being upright may indicate a low pressure headache due to cerebrospinal fluid (CSF) leak after injury.[16] An MRI Brain with and without contrast and MRI Spine without contrast would be appropriate in this situation to look for signs of a CSF leak, including pachymeningeal enhancement or spinal extradural fluid collections.[17]

After headache red flags have been ruled out, a detailed headache history will aid to determine the diagnosis and clinical features of the headache. The headache history should include the time of onset in relation to the head injury, frequency, duration, quality, severity, and location of headache attacks in addition to associated features, including sensory sensitivities, nausea or vomiting, exacerbation with movement, unilateral cranial autonomic features, and/or neck pain. As defined by the International Classification of Headache Disorder, third edition, a headache disorder that starts or a premorbid primary headache disorder that is significantly worsened within

7 days of a TBI is diagnosed as a secondary headache disorder called *headache attributed to traumatic injury to the head* or posttraumatic headache (PTH).[18] However, the definition of a PTH is devoid of clinical features.[18] In addition, there is a paucity of evidence-based treatment options specifically for PTH.[19] Thus, the treatment of PTH is based on the clinical features of the headache itself.[19] Most PTHs have clinical features consistent with migraine.[15,20] At this time, in the absence of evidence-based treatment of PTH, most patients with PTH are treated with evidence-based migraine treatment options. Treatment outcomes in PTH are not ideal, and it is hoped future research will improve the ability to treat these patients. Currently, there is an ongoing calcitonin gene-related peptide large-scale randomized controlled study in PTH (ClinicalTrials.gov Identifier: NCT03347188).

Other important historical components include medications, including over-the-counter pain medications for headache. There is a high risk of medication overuse headache (MOH) in this population due to limited access to care, lack of patient education, subpar treatment of PTH, and lack of evidence-based treatment of PTH.[21] The past medical history, developmental history, family history, social history, and level of education are also relevant to the evaluation of a concussed patient. There are multiple risk factors for prolonged recovery that can be elicited from this information, including personal history of migraine, mood disorders, and learning disabilities in addition to a family history of migraine or mood disorders.[9,22] In the past medical history, obtaining a detailed history of prior concussions is recommended. A history of prior concussion increases the risk of and prolongs the recovery for subsequent concussions.[9] Determine the number of prior concussions, mechanism of injury, and the length of recovery for each one. This information will also inform about the possibility of a reduced threshold, which means that less mechanical impact or force is causing more severe concussion symptoms and longer recovery.[23] A reduced threshold is concerning, and these athletes may be counseled to retire from contact sports.[23]

The physical examination in a concussion patient starts with orthostatic vitals due to the prevalence of autonomic dysfunction and postural tachycardia in patients with concussion.[24,25] Vitals should be followed by a detailed HEENT (head, eyes, ears, nose, and throat) examination looking for areas of ecchymosis or abrasions, tenderness to touch and palpation, otorrhea, rhinorrhea, impaired range of motion of the neck secondary to pain, or muscle spasms and identification of trigger points. Most importantly, a thorough neurologic examination should be performed, starting with a mental status examination. Many practitioners use the Standardized Assessment of Concussion (SAC), which is a validated sideline tool.[11] However, any in-office well-validated mental status examination can be used in this setting, including the mini-mental status examination, Kokmen short test of mental status, or Montreal Cognitive Assessment. Cranial nerves (CN) should be assessed in detail, including the presence/absence of anosmia (CN I), pupillary assessment (CN II and III), extraocular motor assessment (CN III, IV, and VI), facial sensory loss or allodynia (CN V), facial weakness (CN VII), hearing loss or vertigo (CN VIII), gag reflex/phonation/swallow (CN IX, X, XII), and shoulder elevation or head turning (CN XI). Special attention should be paid to the visual-vestibular assessment. Look for abnormalities such as nystagmus, saccadic intrusions during smooth pursuit, difficulty performing horizontal and vertical saccades, poor near point convergence and accommodation, and catch-up saccades during vestibulo-ocular reflex testing with the head impulse test.[26,27] Complete the neurologic examination with an assessment motor, including reflexes, sensory, coordination, and gait. During the gait examination, one should look for evidence of difficulties with balance and apply tests of dynamic balance. Timed tandem gait is often administered on the sideline as a part of the SCAT 5 and can easily be administered in the office during the initial visit and monitored at subsequent postinjury office visits.[11]

Objective tools used in concussion
One should also determine if any form of baseline or preseason testing had been performed for means of comparison during the postinjury in-office visit. Preseason assessments can play a role in the removal from play and return to play by aiding clinical judgment. Preseason assessments may include a baseline concussion symptom checklist, King-Devick Test (KDT),[27] and computerized neuropsychological testing.[2] Completion of brief computerized cognitive evaluation tools, when correctly completed and interpreted, can be helpful to determine baseline cognitive function and appropriate return to activity.

When counseling athletes, parents, or teams about sideline assessments, the most important factor to emphasize is to remove an athlete from play if a concussion is suspected until formally evaluated by a health care provider.[2] When in doubt, sit them out, and check them out by a health care provider. For any rapidly progressive symptoms, an emergency room evaluation is necessary to rule out intracranial injury, including hemorrhage. Athletic trainers are essential and can effectively serve as sideline health care providers. Sideline assessment tools are still in evolution, but currently the authors use the KDT[27] and the SCAT 5,[11] which include the concussion symptom checklist, a brief neuropsychological screen (SAC), and a measure of dynamic balance (timed tandem gait). The SCAT 5 must be completed by trained health care providers, including athletic trainers. The KDT is a rapid, number naming timed test with a high level of sensitivity and specificity as a screening tool for concussion.[28] The postinjury KDT time is compared with the baseline KDT time. If an athlete makes an error or is slower than the baseline, they should be removed from play until formally evaluated by a health care provider. The KDT can serve as a remove from play sideline screening tool.[29] At this time, no one test is 100% sensitive at screening for concussion; however, a combination of tools approaches that goal.[28] The combination of the SAC, KDT, and timed tandem gait appears to be the most sensitive and specific sideline protocol at this time.

At the initial and subsequent postinjury in-office visits, the KDT, SAC, timed tandem gait, and brief computerized cognitive evaluations can be completed to monitor recovery. In addition, gold-standard comprehensive neuropsychological testing may be needed for those who are experiencing slow recovery or significant cognitive symptoms that are interfering with return to learn or work.

Additional tools in the concussion toolbox include objective autonomic testing, vestibular testing, and neuroimaging. In regards to neuroimaging, computed tomographic scans are typically much less helpful than MRIs, which are capable of demonstrating microhemorrhages in susceptibility-weighted imaging, microstructural injuries in diffusion tensor imaging, metabolic changes in MR spectroscopy, and other abnormalities.[27]

Differential Diagnosis

The differential diagnosis of concussion is quite wide, due to the nonspecific nature of the symptoms and signs on examination, which can make the diagnosis very challenging.

Migraine and other primary headache disorders can exist on their own apart from the PTH or concussion. Vestibular migraine can mimic not only the head pain that can exist in migraine but also the visual-vestibular dysfunction and difficulties with balance.[30] A history of migraine, lack of physical trauma, and identification of triggers can be helpful in making these determinations. However, this should not sway the decision to keep players in games if concussion is suspected.

In certain areas of the country where high ambient temperatures and humidity are present, heat illness or exertional heat stroke can also be a concussion mimicker. However, a physical examination exhibiting progressing symptoms, and elevated core body temperature, and the absence of preceding trauma are most helpful in distinguishing between the 2 conditions.[31] Additional diagnoses to consider are hypoglycemia, dehydration, syncope, underlying psychiatric disorders such as anxiety, and malingering. Although it is good to keep all of these conditions in the differential diagnosis, a high index of suspicion for concussion should be maintained in order to prevent repeat injury or worsening of a TBI and premature return to play without a proper evaluation by a health care provider. When in doubt, sit them out.

Treatment

The treatment of concussion remains symptomatic therapy. There are targeted therapies for the most common symptoms experienced. The range of symptoms experienced by each patient will vary from person to person and cross multiple domains of medicine. Therefore, a multidisciplinary approach is quite important. The overarching goal in management of these patients is to provide symptomatic treatment, provide recommendations for return to mental and physical activity, and prevent reinjury while the brain is healing.

As mentioned earlier, headache is the most common and debilitating symptom after a concussion.[32] PTH results in pain and an inability to participate in rehabilitation. Patients with PTH can present with a myriad of associated clinical features that mimics a specific primary headache disorder, and specific therapies should be tailored to those clinical features. A migraine-like PTH is most common.[15,20]

There are no randomized, prospective, blinded trials for the treatment of PTH, but the current expert consensus is that early and aggressive treatment of PTH may prevent persistent headache and therefore should be aggressively pursued.[21,32] A systematic stepwise method of evaluating for and treating these headaches can be helpful. This evaluation should begin with the identification of red flag symptoms, the identification of the associated clinical feature to determine a headache phenotype, for example, migraine, and consideration of comorbidities, including a premorbid history of headache. Patients with a premorbid history of a primary headache disorder are more likely to develop PTH and are at a higher risk for persistence of PTH beyond 3 months after injury.[14]

Acute treatment of PTH should occur early in the course of management, within days. Symptomatic management can begin with nonspecific treatments, including aspirin, acetaminophen, naproxen, and ibuprofen. In PTH with a migraine phenotype, triptans can be trialed.[21] Acute headache treatment has the potential to cause MOH or rebound headache. Patients with PTH are at a high risk of developing MOH.[32] If acute treatment is needed more than 3 days per week and/or there are risk factors for PTH and prolonged recovery, consider a preventive medication within the first 1 to 2 months after injury.[21]

Preventative treatments, again, are chosen based on the PTH phenotype. Treatment options include many medications and supplements of varying mechanisms, including magnesium, riboflavin, coenzyme Q10, antidepressants, beta-blockers, anticonvulsants, and neuropathic pain medications.[19] Generally, the choice of preventative medication is made based on additional comorbidities, which may also be treated by the selected preventative medication, such as insomnia, depression, anxiety, autonomic instability or orthostatic tachycardia, and myofascial pain. Procedures including

CN blocks and onabotulinum toxin injections have also been tried in PTH with some success.[33] There is evidence supporting the use of these treatment options for primary headache disorders, but not specifically for PTH.[34,35] It is important to consider comorbidities when selecting medications to treat PTH. If a patient has orthostatic tachycardia, amitriptyline or venlafaxine may worsen tachycardia; if a patient is having cognitive impairment, topiramate may worsen concentration and word finding, and if a patient is having significant hypersomnia, sedating medications may not be ideal. Although considering comorbidities is relevant when selecting treatment options for any patient with headache, this is especially relevant for PTH in the setting of concussion recovery due to the multidomain symptoms present.

In addition to headache, the other symptoms should receive targeted therapies. For patients with neck pain, physical therapy, manual therapies, and trigger point injections can be helpful. Orthostatic or autonomic symptoms can sometimes respond to high-volume hydration, increased salt intake, compression stockings, exercise, and avoidance of triggers. Patients with vestibular or balance symptoms benefit from vestibular therapy. Patients with cognitive and/or emotional symptoms respond to biofeedback, cognitive behavioral therapy, psychotherapy, and cognitive rehabilitation.

Management

In addition to providing multidisciplinary symptomatic treatment for the multidomain symptoms, preventing recurrent head injury while the brain is healing is the cornerstone for concussion management. In the recent past, this was accomplished with rest. Rest reduces the risk of recurrent injury during a time of neurometabolic vulnerability, and immediate postinjury exercise seemed to prolong recovery.[36,37] In one study, strict cognitive and physical rest decreased symptoms and improved neurocognitive testing.[38] Based on these data, strict cognitive and physical rest with limited sensory stimulation and even removal from school was recommended to many.

More recent data have demonstrated that rest should not exceed 24 to 72 hours after injury. After the acute stage of the concussion, it is important to initiate symptom-limited cognitive and physical activity. One study demonstrated that concussed subjects assigned strict rest for 5 days regardless of symptoms had higher symptom severity scores and a slower symptom recovery compared with the cohort assigned 1 to 2 days of rest followed by symptom-limited return to school and physical activity.[39] The timing of initiating and intensity of active rehabilitation appears to be important for treatment outcomes and recovery. School reentry and light physical activity after injury had the best outcome in one study.[37]

Graduated return to cognitive activity

If the concussed athlete is in school, she or he will likely require academic accommodations in the learning environment to help with symptom exacerbation and to facilitate return to learning. Typically, adjustments are short term and do not require a 504 plan or Individualized Education Program.[40] The clinical barriers for returning to school include poorly treated PTH, visual-vestibular dysfunction, cognitive slowing, mood lability, and fatigue. Phenotype-specific treatment and reduction of sensory stimuli can help reduce the impact of PTH. Accommodations including low-light and low-sound environments may be helpful. Audiobooks and note-taking help are appropriate accommodations for difficulty reading present in visual-vestibular dysfunction. Decreased quantity and increased time to complete class and homework can help with slowed cognitive function without exacerbating frustration and mood lability. Frequent rest breaks and a shortened school day may also be necessary, especially in the first couple of weeks after injury. A 5-step graduated return to learn plan can provide the parent and school with a framework for the concussed student.[41] The plan can be adjusted for those who are trying to return to work. The key is to have a deliberate, graduated cognitive recovery plan.

Graduated return to physical activity

Consensus recommendations support the use of submaximal activity and controlled aerobic exercise to engage in active recovery. Symptom-limited return to physical activity can be used as a treatment approach. However, because recovery is sensitive to the timing and intensity of subthreshold exercise, postinjury physical activity recommendations must not be vague and must be prescriptive with regards to timing, duration, and intensity of exercise. However, several studies have suggested that a slow symptom-limited progression of physical activity and exercise is beneficial for recovery.[42–44] The Buffalo Concussion Treadmill Test, controlled aerobic exercise, has demonstrated symptomatic improvement[45] as well as faster normalization of cerebral blood flow abnormalities during a cognitive task.[46] Provide prescriptive instructions regarding exercise, increase intensity slowly under close monitoring, and ensure the absence of symptom exacerbation. Once the exertion protocol has been completed, initiate a sport-specific return to play protocol, and advance toward complete recovery.[47]

Full return to play

Returning to full game play is not only about symptom freedom. Having a systematic approach for returning an athlete to play reduces the risk of premature return to play after injury (**Box 1**). Once the concussed patient is symptom free at rest, is at school without accommodations, and has completed a full exertion protocol and sport-specific return to play protocol without symptom exacerbation, returning to full contact practice and game play can be considered.[9] Objective measures of rapid number naming and eye movements (KDT), vestibular function, and cognitive function must return to valid baseline scores or fall within normal limits in absence of preinjury baseline measurements before full-contact practice and game play. Returning an athlete to play is a clinical decision. Tools, such as brief computerized cognitive testing, should not dictate return to play. Before providing medical clearance and returning to contact sports, it is recommended to reestablish baseline measures of oculomotor, vestibular, and cognitive function and to counsel the patient and family that a prior history of concussion is a risk factor for future concussion and prolonged recovery.

Box 1
A systematic approach for making return to play decisions to reduce the risk of premature return to play postinjury

Return to play decision

1. Symptom free at rest

2. Return to learn without accommodation (or with preinjury accommodations)

3. Exertion protocol without symptom recurrence

4. Return to baseline or normalization of objective testing, if available

5. Sport-specific graduated return to play protocol

6. Consider return to full-contact practice and eventually game play

When to consider an outside referral
Comprehensive concussion programs can be an ideal resource for many patients with a complicated past medical history and/or a prolonged recovery after injury. Consider referral to a comprehensive concussion program if there is a high number and severity of symptoms because often several symptom-directed treatment approaches (physical, occupation, speech, cognitive therapies) exist under one roof and can be performed in a coordinated fashion. Consider referral if the PTH is impairing the patient's abilities to participate in active rehabilitation or return to school. Individuals who have premorbid risk factors for concussion, PTH, and prolonged recovery may also benefit from a comprehensive center.

SUMMARY

Physical activity and sports play a very positive role in all individuals, especially our youth, in the face of the digital world, metabolic syndrome, diabetes, and obesity. However, the potential dangers of concussion and brain injury, both short term and long term, must be recognized. Mismanagement can be devastating. We must educate those involved with the diagnosis and aftercare of concussion. The science of concussion is rapidly evolving. This narrative review is meant to serve as a summary of the currently recommended clinical care of patients with concussion. As new science and evidence emerge, the level of sophistication and confidence in the management of concussion will increase over time. Appropriate, specific, and timely management of concussion can make the difference between short-term symptoms with resolution and persistent symptoms with lifelong difficulties.

REFERENCES

1. McCrory P, Meeuwisse WH, Aubry M, et al. Consensus statement on concussion in sport: the 4th International Conference on Concussion in Sport held in Zurich, November 2012. Br J Sports Med 2013;47(5):250–8.
2. McCrory P, Meeuwisse W, Dvorak J, et al. Consensus statement on concussion in sport-the 5(th) international conference on concussion in sport held in Berlin, October 2016. Br J Sports Med 2017;51(11):838–47.
3. Strain J, Didehbani N, Cullum CM, et al. Depressive symptoms and white matter dysfunction in retired NFL players with concussion history. Neurology 2013;81(1): 25–32.
4. Plassman BL, Havlik RJ, Steffens DC, et al. Documented head injury in early adulthood and risk of Alzheimer's disease and other dementias. Neurology 2000;55(8):1158–66.
5. Guskiewicz KM, McCrea M, Marshall SW, et al. Cumulative effects associated with recurrent concussion in collegiate football players: the NCAA concussion study. JAMA 2003;290(19):2549–55.
6. McCrea M, Guskiewicz K, Randolph C, et al. Effects of a symptom-free waiting period on clinical outcome and risk of reinjury after sport-related concussion. Neurosurgery 2009;65(5):876–82 [discussion: 82–3].
7. Vagnozzi R, Signoretti S, Cristofori L, et al. Assessment of metabolic brain damage and recovery following mild traumatic brain injury: a multicentre, proton magnetic resonance spectroscopic study in concussed patients. Brain 2010;133(11): 3232–42.
8. Castile L, Collins CL, McIlvain NM, et al. The epidemiology of new versus recurrent sports concussions among high school athletes, 2005-2010. Br J Sports Med 2012;46(8):603–10.

9. Giza CC, Kutcher JS, Ashwal S, et al. Summary of evidence-based guideline update: evaluation and management of concussion in sports: report of the Guideline Development Subcommittee of the American Academy of Neurology. Neurology 2013;80(24):2250–7.

10. Daneshvar DH, Nowinski CJ, McKee AC, et al. The epidemiology of sport-related concussion. Clin Sports Med 2011;30(1):1–17, vii.

11. Echemendia RJ, Meeuwisse W, McCrory P, et al. The Sport Concussion Assessment Tool 5th Edition (SCAT5): background and rationale. Br J Sports Med 2017; 51(11):848–50.

12. Eisenberg MA, Meehan WP 3rd, Mannix R. Duration and course of post-concussive symptoms. Pediatrics 2014;133(6):999–1006.

13. Lovell MR, Iverson GL, Collins MW, et al. Measurement of symptoms following sports-related concussion: reliability and normative data for the post-concussion scale. Appl Neuropsychol 2006;13(3):166–74.

14. Lucas S, Hoffman JM, Bell KR, et al. A prospective study of prevalence and characterization of headache following mild traumatic brain injury. Cephalalgia 2014; 34(2):93–102.

15. Hoffman JM, Lucas S, Dikmen S, et al. Natural history of headache after traumatic brain injury. J Neurotrauma 2011;28(9):1719–25.

16. Mokri B. Spontaneous intracranial hypotension. Continuum (Minneap Minn) 2015; 21(4 Headache):1086–108.

17. Starling A, Hernandez F, Hoxworth JM, et al. Sensitivity of MRI of the spine compared with CT myelography in orthostatic headache with CSF leak. Neurology 2013;81(20):1789–92.

18. Headache Classification Committee of the International Headache Society (IHS) the international classification of headache disorders, 3rd edition. Cephalalgia 2018;38(1):1–211.

19. Seifert T. Post-traumatic headache therapy in the athlete. Curr Pain Headache Rep 2016;20(6):41.

20. Lucas S, Hoffman JM, Bell KR, et al. Characterization of headache after traumatic brain injury. Cephalalgia 2012;32(8):600–6.

21. Lucas S. Posttraumatic headache: clinical characterization and management. Curr Pain Headache Rep 2015;19(10):48.

22. Legarreta AD, Brett BL, Solomon GS, et al. The role of family and personal psychiatric history in postconcussion syndrome following sport-related concussion: a story of compounding risk. J Neurosurg Pediatr 2018;22(3):238–43.

23. Starling AJ, Choe MC, Giza CC. How many concussion are too many before an athlete should retire?. In: Valvovich McLeod TC, editor. Quick questions in sport-related concussion: expert advice in sports medicine. Thorofare (NJ): SLACK Inc; 2015. p. 113–8.

24. Goodman BP, Vargas B, Dodick D. Autonomic nervous system dysfunction in concussion. Neurology 2013;80(7 Supplement).

25. Miranda NA, Boris JR, Kouvel KM, et al. Activity and exercise intolerance after concussion: identification and management of postural orthostatic tachycardia syndrome. J Neurol Phys Ther 2018;42(3):163–71.

26. Ventura RE, Balcer LJ, Galetta SL. The neuro-ophthalmology of head trauma. Lancet Neurol 2014;13(10):1006–16.

27. Ventura RE, Balcer LJ, Galetta SL. The concussion toolbox: the role of vision in the assessment of concussion. Semin Neurol 2015;35(5):599–606.

28. Galetta KM, Morganroth J, Moehringer N, et al. Adding vision to concussion testing: a prospective study of sideline testing in youth and collegiate athletes. J Neuroophthalmol 2015;35(3):235–41.
29. Ventura RE, Balcer LJ, Galetta SL, et al. Ocular motor assessment in concussion: Current status and future directions. J Neurol Sci 2016;361:79–86.
30. Zaleski A, Bogle J, Starling A, et al. Vestibular evoked myogenic potentials in patients with vestibular migraine. Otol Neurotol 2015;36(2):295–302.
31. O'Connor FG, Heled Y, Deuster PA. Exertional heat stroke, the return to play decision, and the role of heat tolerance testing: a clinician's dilemma. Curr Sports Med Rep 2018;17(7):244–8.
32. Lucas S. Headache management in concussion and mild traumatic brain injury. PM R 2011;3(10 Suppl 2):S406–12.
33. Conidi FX. Interventional treatment for post-traumatic headache. Curr Pain Headache Rep 2016;20(6):40.
34. Holland S, Silberstein SD, Freitag F, et al. Evidence-based guideline update: NSAIDs and other complementary treatments for episodic migraine prevention in adults: report of the Quality Standards Subcommittee of the American Academy of Neurology and the American Headache Society. Neurology 2012; 78(17):1346–53.
35. Silberstein SD. Practice parameter: evidence-based guidelines for migraine headache (an evidence-based review): report of the Quality Standards Subcommittee of the American Academy of Neurology. Neurology 2000;55(6):754–62.
36. Crane AT, Fink KD, Smith JS. The effects of acute voluntary wheel running on recovery of function following medial frontal cortical contusions in rats. Restor Neurol Neurosci 2012;30(4):325–33.
37. Majerske CW, Mihalik JP, Ren D, et al. Concussion in sports: postconcussive activity levels, symptoms, and neurocognitive performance. J Athl Train 2008;43(3): 265–74.
38. Moser RS, Glatts C, Schatz P. Efficacy of immediate and delayed cognitive and physical rest for treatment of sports-related concussion. J Pediatr 2012;161(5):922–6.
39. Thomas DG, Apps JN, Hoffmann RG, et al. Benefits of strict rest after acute concussion: a randomized controlled trial. Pediatrics 2015;135(2):213–23.
40. Halstead ME, McAvoy K, Devore CD, et al. Returning to learning following a concussion. Pediatrics 2013;132(5):948–57.
41. DeMatteo C, Stazyk K, Giglia L, et al. A Balanced protocol for return to school for children and youth following concussive injury. Clin Pediatr (Phila) 2015;54(8):783–92.
42. Makdissi M, Cantu RC, Johnston KM, et al. The difficult concussion patient: what is the best approach to investigation and management of persistent (>10 days) postconcussive symptoms? Br J Sports Med 2013;47(5):308–13.
43. Leddy J, Hinds A, Sirica D, et al. The role of controlled exercise in concussion management. PM R 2016;8(3 Suppl):S91–100.
44. Leddy JJ, Baker JG, Willer B. Active rehabilitation of concussion and post-concussion syndrome. Phys Med Rehabil Clin N Am 2016;27(2):437–54.
45. Leddy JJ, Kozlowski K, Donnelly JP, et al. A preliminary study of subsymptom threshold exercise training for refractory post-concussion syndrome. Clin J Sport Med 2010;20(1):21–7.
46. Leddy JJ, Cox JL, Baker JG, et al. Exercise treatment for postconcussion syndrome: a pilot study of changes in functional magnetic resonance imaging activation, physiology, and symptoms. J Head Trauma Rehabil 2013;28(4):241–9.
47. May KH, Marshall DL, Burns TG, et al. Pediatric sports specific return to play guidelines following concussion. Int J Sports Phys Ther 2014;9(2):242–55.

The Alzheimer's Disease Clinical Spectrum
Diagnosis and Management

Alireza Atri, MD, PhD[a,b,c],*

KEYWORDS

- Alzheimer's disease • Mild cognitive impairment • Cognitive • Treatment
- Donepezil • Memantine • Neuroimaging • Review

KEY POINTS

- Evaluation of older individuals with cognitive or behavioral symptoms, or functional decline, should use structured history and multidomain symptom-function reviews from the patient and a care partner or informant; a focused examination including a standardized cognitive instrument; and multitiered tests (laboratory tests, neuroimaging). In vivo biomarkers of Alzheimer's disease (AD), such as cerebrospinal fluid and PET, are also now clinically available.
- Level of impairment (mild cognitive impairment, dementia) and delineation of cognitive-behavioral syndrome, along with test results (that help exclude confounders and include AD) inform etiologic diagnosis, management of symptoms, and care plans.
- AD management is multifactorial. A first step involves a thorough review of medications and supplements to eliminate redundancies and potentially deleterious substances.
- Anti-AD pharmacotherapies approved by the US Food and Drug Administration (the acetylcholinesterase inhibitors donepezil, galantamine, and rivastigmine; and the N-methyl-D-aspartate antagonist memantine) provide modest but meaningful benefits by mitigating symptoms, reducing clinical progression, and delaying disability.

Continued

Disclosure Statement: Dr. Atri has no equity, shares or salary from any pharma company and is not a member of any pharma speakers' bureau. He has received honoraria for consulting, educational lectures/programs/materials or advisory boards from AbbVie, Allergan, Alzheimer's Association, Biogen, Eisai, Grifols, Harvard Medical School Graduate Continuing Education, Lundbeck, Merck, Oxford University Press (medical book-related revenues), Sunovion, Suven, and Synexus. Dr. Atri's institution (Banner Health) has investigational observational study/trial related funding from Novartis. Dr. Atri's previous institution (California Pacific Medical Center) had contracts or received investigational clinical trial related funding from The American College of Radiology, AbbVie, Avid, Biogen, Lilly, Lundbeck, Merck, and vTV.
[a] Banner Sun Health Research Institute, Banner Health, 10515 W Santa Fe Drive, Sun City, AZ 85351, USA; [b] Department of Neurology, Brigham and Women's Hospital, 60 Fenwood Road, Boston, MA 02115, USA; [c] Harvard Medical School, 25 Shattuck Street, Boston, MA 02115, USA
* Banner Sun Health Research Institute, 10515 W Santa Fe Drive, Sun City, AZ 85351.
E-mail address: alireza.atri@bannerhealth.com

0025-7125/19/© 2018 The Author. Published by Elsevier Inc. This is an open access article under the CC BY-NC-ND license (http://creativecommons.org/licenses/by-nc-nd/4.0/).

Continued

- First-line treatment of behavioral problems is nonpharmacologic and involves identifying the trigger for the problem behavior. When identified, it is necessary to institute behavioral interventions, make environmental modifications, and to evaluate the impact of the interventions.

INTRODUCTION

Alzheimer's disease (AD) is the most common cause of cognitive impairment or dementia in individuals older than 65 years and, with rising longevity, a worldwide pandemic of mild cognitive impairment (MCI), AD, and AD-related dementia (ADRD) is anticipated.[1–5] AD is the sixth leading cause of death in the United States and the only top-10 cause still significantly increasing.[4] AD-related pathological changes often coexist with 1 or more other pathologies, particularly vascular-ischemic cerebral injury and diffuse Lewy body (DLB) disease.[1,6–9]

Timely detection, accurate diagnosis, and appropriate management of MCI, AD and ADRD are imperative.[4] Symptoms too often go undiagnosed, misattributed, or dismissed and ignored, which causes distressing, costly, and potentially harmful delays in receiving appropriate care.[1,4,5]

AD clinical (ADc) syndromes, Cognitive-Behavioral Syndromes (CBS) presumed to be due to AD, are heterogeneous, particularly in younger individuals (65 years of age or younger). MCI and dementia due to AD can be accurately diagnosed by a comprehensive evaluation that integrates pathologic AD biomarkers (cerebrospinal fluid [CSF] and amyloid PET). However, clinical use of AD CSF and PET biomarkers are not currently indicated in most symptomatic individuals to include or exclude AD pathology. These tests are reserved for atypical, rapidly progressive, or early-onset syndromes, or when comprehensive evaluation is inconclusive.[10,11] In relatively typical cases, an individualized approach to history, examination, and selected laboratory tests and neuroimaging (see later discussion) can provide a high-confidence diagnosis. No single biomarker, test, or score can provide the clinical diagnosis; this requires characterization of symptoms and level of impairment into a profile via a clinical evaluation.

Epidemiology, Risk Factors, Genetics, and Neuropathology

The prevalence of dementia, mostly attributed to AD or mixed AD, is increasing in the United States and globally.[4,5] By 2030, the number of Americans with dementia will increase by 35%[4,12] and will potentially triple by 2050.[13] **Table 1** shows the major risk factors for AD or dementia. AD or dementia prevalence approximately doubles every 5 years in individuals aged 65 to 85 years; from approximately 1% to 2% at 65 years, to more than 30% to 50% by age 85 years.[4] Of Americans of older than 60 years, 16% have MCI (6.7% prevalence for ages 60–64 years, 8.4% for 65–69 years, 10.1% for 70–74 years, 14.8% for 75–79 years, and 25.2% for 80–84 years), equating to 11.6 million individuals.

AD is a dual proteinopathy disease defined by a widespread but regionally specific pattern of intraparenchymal diffuse and neuritic ß-amyloid (Aß) plaques and intracytoplasmic (initially), then extracellular, neurofibrillary tangles with synaptic and neuronal loss and gliosis.[14–17] Neurofibrillary tangles consist of intracellular (then extracellular) deposits of hyperphosphorylated tau protein, a microtubule stabilizing protein. The AD pathway that leads to clinical stages of MCI or dementia starts decades before the

Table 1
Risk factors for Alzheimer's disease and dementia

Modifiable (in Early Life and Midlife Ages 45–65 y, or Later Life Ages >65 y)	Nonmodifiable
Vascular risks	Age
Diabetes (later life)	Gender (female more than male; ~1.5
Hypertension (midlife)	relative risk [RR][13,133])
Dyslipidemia (midlife)	Family history (first-degree or second-degree
Metabolic syndrome and obesity (midlife)	relative or multiple generations; RR 2–6)
Smoking tobacco (later life)	Race (African American and Hispanic
Low physical activity (later life)	individuals are at 1.5–2-fold RR compared
Cerebral hypoperfusion, cerebrovascular	with white individuals due to a
injury or stroke	combination of genetic, health disparity,
Depression (later life)	and socioeconomic factors[38])
Severe head trauma or traumatic brain injury	Down syndrome
Hearing loss (midlife)	Apolipoprotein (APOE)-ε4 allele carriers
Low cognitive reserve (early life and	(individuals who carry one or two APOE-ε4
potentially midlife). Cognitive reserve is	alleles of the APOE gene have a 3-fold and
"the brain's capacity to maintain cognitive	8–10-fold RR, respectively, compared to
function despite neurologic damage or	homozygous APOE-ε3 allele carriers)
disease"[1]. (Low Cognitive reserve, thought	Cerebral amyloidosis (positive biomarker of
to be due to low educational, professional	the AD pathologic process[a])
or social attainment, or low intelligence,	
carries ~1.5–2 RR)[132]	

[a] Is currently a nonmodifiable risk factor but primary and secondary prevention trials using amyloid-modifying drugs are in progress and early results support that cerebral amyloid plaque burden can be lowered; whether this would then translate to lowering risk of progression to MCI or dementia, potentially making this be a modifiable risk factor, is to be determined.

onset of symptoms.[2] The new AD biological framework and the model of pathologic AD biomarkers from Jack and colleagues[18] conceptualize a progressive sequence of measurable biochemical, neurophysiological, and neuroanatomical alterations that can be detected years before psychometrically and clinically noticeable deterioration in cognition, behavior, and function. Typical AD neuropathology starts and spreads in a consistent pattern. Pathologic tangle findings correlate best with symptoms. In the dementia stages of AD, many patients have cortical or cortico-subcortical microhemorrhages due to cerebral amyloid angiopathy-related vasculopathy and leakage[19]; hemosiderin microdeposition from microhemorrhages are seen on gradient-echo or susceptibility-weighted MRI sequences in 15% to 20% of patients.[20]

The genetics and cause of AD are complex and incompletely understood.[2,21] AD-risk attributable to genetic factors is estimated at 70%. Familial autosomal dominant AD is rare (<1%), usually manifests in early-onset AD (onset age <65 years; <4% of AD), and is caused by mutations in presenilin 1, amyloid precursor protein, or presenilin 2.[21] In the most common form of AD, sporadic late-onset AD, many genetic variations contribute to increase or lower risk; greater than 20 have been identified (AlzGene Database; www.alzgene.org).[22] The major risk or susceptibility gene in sporadic AD involves apolipoprotein-E (APOE). APOE-ε4 alleles are associated with accelerated Aß-deposition and earlier onset and higher risk of developing AD symptoms.[21,23]

The cause of AD remains controversial and is incompletely understood.[24–26] Prevailing models posit a central role of accumulation of synaptic neurotoxic forms of Aß to induce inflammatory and microglial cascades, broad ionic and neurotransmitter abnormalities, mitochondrial dysfunction, oxidative stress, and hyperphosphorylation of the microtubule stabilizing protein tau and formation of tangles.[26–31]

Tau-mediated processes cause further synaptic and neuronal dysfunction and destruction, leading to cortical dysfunction. Other models posit microvascular injury, tipping the balance in favor of toxic Aß accumulation.[25]

SYMPTOMS
Clinical Features

There can be large heterogeneity in ADc syndromes; particularly regarding development and progression of symptoms and clinical decline. Clinical criteria recognize atypical presentations, or atypical AD, as variants. The 2011 National Institute on Aging and Alzheimer's Association (NIA-AA) criteria for AD recognizes nonamnestic AD presentations that include language, visuospatial, and executive dysfunction features.[32]

At the MCI level of impairment, when daily function and behavior are not significantly affected, the most typical presentations of AD are amnestic (single or multidomain amnestic-MCI). Amnestic-MCI is greater than 90% associated with underlying AD pathology. MCI significantly increases risk of annual progression to dementia (relative risk [RR] 6–8). MCI with negative biomarkers versus 1 or more AD pathology biomarkers (ie, AD pattern in CSF, high amyloid load in amyloid PET) or biomarkers of neurodegeneration (eg, AD pattern on structural MRI or fluorodeoxyglucose [FDG]-PET; high CSF tau and phospho-tau levels) has a 2 to 3 relative risk of progression to dementia (8% vs 17%–22% per year[33]).

Clinical Characteristics of Alzheimer's Disease: Symptoms and Signs

Individuals with very mild or mild AD dementia manifest variable but significant changes and/or mild-to-moderate impairments in multiple cognitive, functional, and behavioral domains. Patterns of change may overlap but are not part of normal cognitive aging, as manifested by differential aging and AD effects on cognitive networks.[34] In normal aging, individuals typically retain longstanding personalities and interests, including their levels of initiative, motivation, sociability, empathy, affect, and behavior. AD changes are not synonymous with old age (**Box 1**).

In retrospect, some of the earliest symptoms manifest years before receiving a clinical diagnosis of dementia, including changes in mood, anxiety, and sleep. Heightened anxiety, depressive symptoms, apathy, and withdrawal are highly prevalent in preclinical or early stages of AD.[35–37] Progression to later-stage symptoms, such as impaired judgment, disorientation, and confusion; major behavioral changes, such as aggression and agitation; and neuropsychiatric symptoms, such as delusions and hallucinations, can go unrecognized and undertreated until diagnosis. Recognition of the 10 early warning symptoms or signs[38] (**Table 2**) and appropriate evaluation is the first step of effective care.

DIAGNOSIS

The first pillar in appropriate care is accurate and timely diagnosis. AD dementia remains a clinical diagnosis. Of individuals age 70 years or older, 20% to 40% without cognitive impairment have biomarker or autopsy evidence of AD pathology[2]; therefore, pathologic AD findings are not sufficient for symptoms.

The 3 major clinical criteria for the AD spectrum are the revised 2011 NIA-AA criteria,[32,39] the International Working Group (Dubois and colleagues[39,40]) 2010 revised new lexicon criteria, and the Diagnostic and Statistical Manual of Mental Disorders, 5th edition criteria.[41] The new 2018 NIA-AA research framework dissociates AD symptoms or phenotypes from the pathologic process. It defines AD, for research purposes, purely in terms of a biopathologic construct with the AD biomarkers of

---

Box 1
Cognitive changes across the lifespan: decline in fluid intelligence in early adulthood and preservation and increase in crystalized intelligence until late life

- Aspects of cognitive decline begin in early adulthood but there are large interindividual differences in rates of decline

- Cognitive domains decline differently

- Effects on fluid intelligence
  - Performance on measures of fluid intelligence, such as speed of mental processing; working memory; recall and retention of verbal and visual information (learning and memory), in particular visuospatial memory; and reasoning begin to decline in many individuals from age 20 to 30 years.[134,135]
  - These cognitive changes can affect creativity, abstract reasoning, and novel problem-solving abilities.
  - These changes can affect lower speed and efficiency in acquiring and remembering new information; translating into a lower learning rate and slower retrieval of information and memories.

- Effects on crystalized intelligence
  - With age, accumulation of greater experience and knowledge can allow for better performance on measures of crystallized intelligence.
  - Better crystalized intelligence can manifest in improved (compared with ages 20–30 years) or stable performance from age 50 to 70 years on tests of specific procedures (eg, acquired skills), semantic knowledge (eg, facts about the world), reading, and vocabulary.[134,135]

- These cognitive abilities still rely on successful retrieval of stored procedures and information; loss of information storage is not considered a normal part of cognitive aging.

---

amyloid, tau, and neurodegeneration (ATN) criteria, which aids in defining the disease stages.[2]

Box 2 shows the 2011 NIA-AA all-cause dementia definition; dementia-level impairment requires cognitive or behavioral symptoms "of sufficient magnitude to interfere with usual work or daily function." MCI diagnosis is a matter of "clinical judgment made by a skilled clinician" regarding the presence of cognitive impairment without "significant interference in the ability to function at work or in usual daily activities," and must be individualized to the patient in the context of the patient's particular circumstances and premorbid level of function and performance as appreciated through clinical interview with the patient and informant.[32]

Box 3 shows the 2011 NIA-AA criteria for AD dementia, categorized as

1. Probable AD dementia
2. Possible AD dementia
3. Probable or possible AD dementia with evidence of the AD pathophysiologic process.

The third category was intended for research purposes and is recently replaced by the new research framework, ATN classification, of the AD biopathologic spectrum.[2] A diagnosis of possible AD dementia is made if the individual has either an atypical course or an etiologically mixed presentation.

Evaluation of Alzheimer's Disease: History, Examination, Cognitive Assessment, and Tests

According to recent preliminarily announced multidisciplinary US national guidelines, the *Alzheimer's Association Best Clinical Practice Guidelines for the*

Table 2
Comparison of behaviors associated with normal aging and symptoms and behaviors that may be observed in cognitive-behavioral impairment in Alzheimer's disease

	Normal Aging (Occasional and Inconsistent Behaviors)	Behaviors and Symptoms in AD (Persistent and Progressively More Frequent Symptoms and Behaviors)
Memory	Minor lapses of information retrieval with later recall (eg, forgetting an appointment or names and remembering later) Recall slightly slower	Memory loss, especially for recently learned information Forgetting important dates and appointments Repetitive questioning for same answer in a short time frame Increasing reliance on memory aids for tasks that they used to do themselves
Planning or problem-solving	Develops a plan, follows recipes, occasional error when balancing checkbook, may find an error later	Difficulty with developing a plan Difficulty following a plan or using a familiar recipe Difficulty working with numbers or paying bills Difficulty starting, focusing, or completing on a project
Familiar task completion	Occasionally need help to record a television show or to use a device or application	Trouble using appliances and devices Confusion or trouble driving to a familiar location Trouble remembering rules of a favorite game Trouble managing a budget
Recognition of time or place	Occasionally confused about date but remember it later	Forget exact location, address, nearby streets, or the route taken to get there Often confused about dates, day of the week, or time; may confuse season in later stages Trouble processing future events; mostly only aware of immediate events Difficulty remembering or confusing the correct timeline of events; may up mix events and people
Comprehension of visual images and spatial relationships	Vision changes related to cataracts, myopia, less acuity; may affect driving at night and glare	Visual processing problems, such as difficulty reading, determining color or contrast, judging distance, recognizing familiar objects, or seeing full picture or surroundings May become disoriented; not knowing the location or how they arrived there Driving more difficult even in daylight due to lower ability to estimate distance and speed of oncoming traffic

(continued on next page)

Table 2
(continued)

	Normal Aging (Occasional and Inconsistent Behaviors)	Behaviors and Symptoms in AD (Persistent and Progressively More Frequent Symptoms and Behaviors)
Communication, use and recall of words and names during talking and writing	Occasional trouble finding word, name, or phrase	Difficulty joining or following a conversation Struggling with vocabulary; often puts words together to describe a word Forgetting meaning of some words Using the wrong or imprecise words Becoming less fluent, starting to stutter, getting stuck during speech or have broken speech.
Ability to retrace steps	May misplace an item but usually able to retrace steps to find the item	Frequently misplacing personal items May leave things in odd places and unable to retrace steps to find them
Judgment and interpersonal interactions	Making an occasional bad decision Being occasionally irritable or less interactive	Decline in sound judgment, may include money, finances, personal interactions and actions Engaging in more risky, inappropriate, or unusual behavior More vulnerable to being taken advantage of by unscrupulous telemarketers and fraud Less attention to grooming and hygiene
Work or social activities	Usually enjoy and participate in family and social events but sometimes need a break	May avoid social interactions because they sense a change in their behavior Attend and engage less or abandon or lose interest in previous hobbies, projects, sports, and social activities May not remember how to perform hobby or complete projects
Mood and personality	Experiencing mild anxiety or sadness in reaction to life events and stressors May prefer using a routine to do things	May become anxious, depressed, less motivated, fearful, suspicious, or having labile affect Can be easily upset when in out of comfort zone scenario Overreacting; often frustrated when cannot remember or do things or blaming others Becoming impulsive or insensitive through words or actions.

Data from Alzheimer's Association. 2013 Alzheimer's disease facts and figures. Alzheimers Dement 2013;9(2):208–45; and Schott JM. The neurology of aging: what is normal? Pract Neurol 2017;17(3):172–82.

Evaluation of Neurodegenerative Cognitive Behavioral Syndromes, Alzheimer's disease and Dementias in the United States,[42] the clinician's approach to the evaluation and disclosure process in suspected AD or ADRD should involve triggering an evaluation in individuals when there is a symptom or concern regarding cognitive, behavioral, or functional decline; involving the patient and a care partner or

---

Box 2
2011 National Institute on Aging and Alzheimer's Association core clinical criteria for all-cause dementia

Dementia: cognitive or behavioral (neuropsychiatric) symptoms are present that

1. Interfere with the ability to function at work or at usual activities
2. Represent a decline from previous levels of functioning and performing
3. Are not explained by delirium or major psychiatric disorder
4. Cognitive impairment is detected and diagnosed through a combination of
   a. History-taking from the patient and a knowledgeable informant
   b. An objective cognitive assessment, either a bedside mental status examination or neuropsychological testing (neuropsychological testing should be performed when the routine history and bedside mental status examination cannot provide a confident diagnosis)
5. The cognitive or behavioral impairment involves a minimum of 2 of the following domains
   a. Impaired ability to acquire and remember new information
      Symptoms include: repetitive questions or conversations, misplacing personal belongings, forgetting events or appointments, getting lost on a familiar route
   b. Impaired reasoning and handling of complex tasks, poor judgment
      Symptoms include: poor understanding of safety risks, inability to manage finances, poor decision-making ability, inability to plan complex or sequential activities
   c. Impaired visuospatial abilities
      Symptoms include: inability to recognize faces or common objects or to find objects in direct view despite good acuity, inability to operate simple implements or orient clothing to the body
   d. Impaired language functions (speaking, reading, writing)
      Symptoms include: difficulty thinking of common words while speaking, hesitations; speech, spelling, and writing errors
   e. Changes in personality, behavior, or comportment
      Symptoms include: uncharacteristic mood fluctuations, such as agitation, impaired motivation, initiative, apathy, loss of drive, social withdrawal, decreased interest in previous activities, loss of empathy, compulsive or obsessive behaviors, socially unacceptable behaviors

From McKhann GM, Knopman DS, Chertkow H, et al. The diagnosis of dementia due to Alzheimer's disease: recommendations from the National Institute on Aging-Alzheimer's Association workgroups on diagnostic guidelines for Alzheimer's disease. Alzheimers Dement 2011;7(3):265; with permission.

---

informant; and using a 3-step diagnostic formulation process. This process includes (1) identifying and classifying the overall level of impairment (eg, MCI, mild neurocognitive disorder, dementia, or major neurocognitive disorder); (2) defining the CBS; and (3) establishing likely cause or causes (diseases or conditions causing the CBS) using a multitiered, structured, and individualized testing approach (eg, assessments, laboratory tests and neuroimaging).

Diminished cognitive capacity can adversely affect the ability of patients to manage their medications and follow medical recommendations. Clinicians should retain a high index-of-suspicion for cognitive, functional, or behavioral changes and warning signs in older patients (see **Table 2**). Subclinical cognitive impairment or dementia should be considered as a cause or contributor in older patients with escalating decompensation of an otherwise well-managed and stable chronic medical condition (eg, diabetes, hypertension, congestive heart failure); new onset of confusion; delirium (in the context of medical illness, medications, or surgery);

Box 3
2011 National Institute on Aging and Alzheimer's Association core clinical criteria for probable Alzheimer's disease dementia

A diagnosis of probable AD dementia can be made when the patient
1. Meets criteria for dementia (see **Box 2**)
2. Has the following characteristics
    a. Insidious onset
        Symptoms have a gradual onset over months to years, not sudden over hours or days
    b. Clear-cut history of worsening of cognition by report or observation
    c. The initial and most prominent cognitive deficits are evident on history and examination in one of the following categories
        i. Amnestic presentation: most common syndromic presentation of AD dementia; deficits should include impairment in learning and recall of recently learned information; should also be evidence of cognitive dysfunction in at least 1 other cognitive domain (see article discussion)
        ii. Nonamnestic presentations
            1. Language presentation: the most prominent deficits are in word-finding; deficits in other cognitive domains should be present
            2. Visuospatial presentation: the most prominent deficits are in spatial cognition, including object agnosia, impaired face recognition, simultanagnosia, and alexia; deficits in other cognitive domains should be present
            3. Executive dysfunction: the most prominent deficits are impaired reasoning, judgment, and problem-solving; deficits in other cognitive domains should be present
3. The diagnosis of probable AD dementia should not be applied when there is evidence of
    a. Substantial concomitant cerebrovascular disease, defined by a history of a stroke temporally related to the onset or worsening of cognitive impairment; or the presence of multiple or extensive infarcts or severe white matter hyperintensity burden
    b. Core features of dementia with Lewy bodies other than dementia itself
    c. Prominent features of behavioral variant frontotemporal dementia
    d. Prominent features of semantic variant primary progressive aphasia or nonfluent or agrammatic variant primary progressive aphasia
    e. Evidence for another concurrent, active neurologic disease, or a nonneurological medical comorbidity or use of medication that could have a substantial effect on cognition

From McKhann GM, Knopman DS, Chertkow H, et al. The diagnosis of dementia due to Alzheimer's disease: recommendations from the National Institute on Aging-Alzheimer's Association workgroups on diagnostic guidelines for Alzheimer's disease. Alzheimers Dement 2011;7(3):265–6; with permission.

---

weight-loss; failure-to-thrive; anxiety; social withdrawal or apathy; depressive and behavioral symptoms (eg, agitation, personality changes, hoarding, delusions); symptoms of presyncope or syncope, transient ischemic attack, or chronic dizziness; and unsteadiness or falls of unclear cause or thought to be related to medications or dehydration.

The history should be obtained from the individual, as well as a knowledgeable care partner or informant. In addition to cognitive symptoms and warning signs (see **Table 2**), assessments of cognition, function, and behavior should be personalized and interpreted within the context of the individual's psychosocial background, level of education or intelligence, function and attainment, primary language, ethnicity, and culture. The AD-8 screening instrument provides a practical symptoms questionnaire for changes in thinking and memory that can be a red flag for ADc syndromes.[43]

History of Present Illness

Presenting symptoms, as well as the most salient symptoms, complaints, and problems, and how the patients has progressed, should be assessed. Helpful questions include

1. When was the last time the patient's thinking was normal?
2. In retrospect, what was the first major change that was noticed?
3. What is now the most prominent symptom or change?
4. What is the most bothersome symptom, problem, or behavior?
5. How have these symptoms progressed?

It is important to delineate both the course (eg, generally linear decline vs clearly stepwise decline) and the pace (eg, very slow initially but more rapid in the last 6 months) of the progression of symptoms or problems, including any major fluctuations or full or partial recovery.

Other important questions include whether there are any

1. Major fluctuations in symptoms on a day-to-day (or hour-to-hour) basis
2. Unusual associated features (eg, falls, weakness, tremor, parkinsonism, personality changes, or odd behaviors)
3. Temporal associations with symptoms onset or worsening (eg, a stepwise decline after a major illness or surgery; happening mostly at night or when the patient is tired).

For example, rapid onset and deterioration (hours and days) is most consistent with an overlying encephalopathy or delirium, whereas a more subacute onset and progression (over weeks and months) is a greater indication of an overlying indolent or chronic infection, metabolic disorder, mass lesion, medication side-effect, sequelae of vascular insults and infarcts, or hydrocephalus. Any of these may overlie and decompensate vulnerabilities in individuals with undetected CBS. AD or ADRD have insidious onset and slow progression over many months and years but can be unmasked in the context of delirium or other cognitive stressors.

Table 3 summarizes components of a comprehensive review of cognition, daily function, behavior, or neuropsychiatric symptoms; other pertinent neurologic and general reviews of systems; salient past medical history (focus on cerebrovascular and hypoxic-ischemic risk factors); medications and supplements (Beers criteria lists those avoided in older individuals, including anticholinergics and sedative-hypnotics[44]); educational, work, and social history; hobbies and health-related behaviors (particularly alcohol intake, sleep and exercise); and potential safety concerns.

Approach to Multitiered Testing: Laboratory Studies

Table 4 outlines a multitiered and individualized approach to testing. Studies help exclude common comorbid conditions in older individuals that can contribute to cognitive impairment in susceptible individuals and that can be treated. It is highly unlikely for a hormonal or vitamin deficiency, or a metabolic, infectious, autoimmune, toxic, neoplastic, or paraneoplastic condition, to mimic the clinical phenotype of typical late-onset AD dementia. Although many of these comorbid conditions can cause decompensation of cognitive-behavioral function in susceptible individuals with subclinical or unrecognized mild impairments or dementia, they are not a primary cause of dementing syndromes. A judicious and stepwise approach to tests that prioritizes more common and treatable conditions, and less invasive and more

Table 3
Elements of history and multidomain symptom-function reviews in evaluation of cognitive-behavioral syndrome due to Alzheimer's disease or Alzheimer's disease–related dementia

Review of cognitive, functional, and neuropsychiatric domains	Cognition	Changes or difficulty with memory, orientation, language, attention, executive functions, judgment, reasoning, problem-solving, visuospatial functions, insight
	Function or ADLs	Instrumental ADLs: keeping appointments and checkbook; making payments and managing finances; shopping; handling money; engaging in hobbies; driving, commuting, and traveling; preparing meals and cooking; using tools, electronics, and appliances; doing laundry, cleaning, and housekeeping; making household repairs; managing medications
		Basic ADLs: dressing, eating, bathing, grooming, feeding, mobility, toileting, continence
	Behavior and neuropsychiatric	Presence, frequency, and severity of personality changes; neuropsychiatric symptoms and problem behaviors; false beliefs and delusions; hallucinations; apathy and indifference; anxiety, irritability, and lability; dysphoria and depression; inappropriate elation or euphoria; agitation and aggression; disinhibition and impulsivity; aberrant or repetitive motor behaviors; disrupted sleep and aberrant nighttime behaviors; changes in eating habits and tastes; aberrant oral intake
Review of systems	Neurologic	New headaches, weakness, incoordination, numbness, dysesthesia
	Parkinsonism	Dysarthria, tremor, poverty of movements, imbalance, difficulty walking or shuffling gait, falls, abnormal movements, stiffness, weakness, dysphagia (choking or coughing with food or drink)
	General	Appetite, weight, continence, vision, hearing
	Sleep	Nature and quality of sleep, time to bed and awake, number of times awake or up and why, difficulty falling or staying asleep, early morning wakening, snoring, restlessness, kicking, acting out dreams, sleep walking, daytime somnolence or naps
Salient past medical history	Cardiovascular and cerebrovascular; hypoxic-ischemic	Transient ischemic attack, stroke, hypertension, dyslipidemia, diabetes, arrhythmias, coronary artery or vascular disease, myocardial infarction, congestive heart failure, cardiac or vascular procedures, smoking, obstructive sleep apnea, snoring, severe lung disease
	Neurologic	Seizures or epilepsy, concussion or traumatic brain injury (including duration of loss of consciousness and any sequelae), meningoencephalitis, delirium, encephalopathy
	Psychiatric, and mental health	Mood disorder, depression, anxiety, electroconvulsive therapy, alcohol or substance abuse
	Other general and medical	Hormonal disorders, thyroid disease or deficiency, vitamin deficiency (particularly vitamin B12 deficiency), immunosuppression, malignancy, exposure to environmental toxic substances
	Development and school	Prenatal and birth history, developmental milestones, learning, attentional or cognitive problems, school performance (need to repeat grade or receive extra academic support or special education programs)

(continued on next page)

Table 3
(continued)

Medications and supplements	Medications	With special attention to anticholinergic and sedative-hypnotic and narcotic medications; particularly avoid those on the updated Beers criteria in older individuals due to potential cognitive side-effects[44]
	Supplements	Ask for a full list and components
Educational, social and work history	Educational and work	Achievement, performance, and the nature of education and occupation to inform past level of function, cognitive reserve, and problem trends
	Social	Social history regarding interpersonal relationships and support networks
Hobbies, community activities and health-related habits	Hobbies	Nature, level, and changes in engagement, activity, and performance of hobbies
	Exercise	Nature or type, frequency, duration, and intensity of exercise; amount of daily activity
	Alcohol and substance intake	Past and current level of alcohol intake (quantify); history of problem drinking; use of other substances, past or current
Family history		Family members diagnosed or suspected to have AD, dementia, or senility; other neurologic and psychiatric diagnoses; age of onset, nature, and progression of symptoms; age at death; pathologic confirmation
Review of safety and well-being		Access, use, and monitoring of medications, driving (including changes, accidents, scrapes, tickets), power tools, firearms, stove, or cooking; wandering potential
Caregiver burden and distress		Assess level of stress, care burden, mood disorder, anxiety, burnout; can be formally quantified using structured instrument[136]

Table 4
Multitiered testing in cognitive-behavioral syndromes: a tiered approach to laboratory and ancillary studies in etiologic evaluation of mild cognitive impairment and dementia syndromes

Tier	Type	What	When or Who or How	Why or Comments
1	Serum	Thyroid stimulating hormone, vitamin B12, homocysteine, complete blood count with differential, complete metabolic panel (including calcium, magnesium, liver function tests), erythrocyte sedimentation rate, C-reactive protein	Always or almost always and routinely done as foundational dementia assessment laboratory tests and imaging All individuals All or almost all tests	Broad and relatively inexpensive tests for common conditions in older individuals that can contribute to cognitive and behavioral impairments
	Imaging	Brain MRI without gadolinium; if unavailable or contraindicated, obtain noncontrast head computed tomography (CT)		Brain MRI (or CT), assessing: atrophy patterns (hippocampal and cortical atrophy in temporal and lateral parietal lobes are consistent with AD); infarcts, leukoaraiosis, and microhemorrhages; nondegenerative conditions (eg, hydrocephalus, mass lesions)
2	Serum	ANA, HgbA1c, lipid profile, folate, ammonia, lead, Lyme antibody, RPR, HIV, SPEP, methylmalonic acid (MMA), PT, PTT	Sometimes Some individuals as-needed based on individual characteristics (epidemiology; clinical risk profile from history, examination, or laboratory tests or studies) Some or few tests	—
	Imaging	Chest plain film or radiograph		
	Other	Sleep study: for obstructive sleep apnea or REM sleep disorder		

(continued on next page)

Table 4
(continued)

Tier	Type	What	When or Who or How	Why or Comments
3–4	Serum, CSF, imaging, biopsy, genetics	Thyroid peroxidase antibodies (TPO), antithyroglobulin antibodies (TGA), AD CSF biomarker panel (AB_{42}, tau, phospho-tau) with calculation of amyloid-tau index; EEG; brain FDG-PET (or SPECT) scan, brain amyloid-PET scan, APOE-4 allele, testing for AD deterministic gene mutations	Very occasionally or rarely Very few individuals: some individuals with atypical clinical profiles, early-onset, or rapid progression Highly sparingly or very few tests	Most should be done by a specialist or in consultation with specialist[45] Assessment of early onset AD can include analysis of specific in vivo AD biomarkers such as CSF AD pattern and/or brain amyloid-PET, and, under special circumstances, testing for APOE-4 allele, and deterministic AD gene mutations[a]

Abbreviations: Ab, antibody; ANA, antinuclear antibody; EEG, electroencephalogram; HgbA1c, hemoglobin A1c; HIV, human immunodeficiency virus; PT, prothrombin time; PTT, partial thrombo-plastin time; REM, rapid eye movement; RPR, rapid plasma reagin; SPEP, serum protein electrophoresis.
[a] When there are 2 or more generational histories of AD or dementia syndrome suggestive of autosomal pattern or early-onset; testing for deterministic AD mutations should be done in consul-tation with genetic counseling.

cost-effective tests, is recommended in evaluating progressive profiles that are not atypical or rapidly progressive.

Tier-1 dementia assessment laboratory tests should be obtained in all or almost all patients evaluated for suspected CBS. Tier-1 laboratory tests are low cost, widely available, and relatively high-yield as a broad screen for common comorbid conditions that can contribute to symptoms or decompensate an underlying CBS in a susceptible individual. None of these conditions primarily cause dementia. For example, thyroid and vitamin B_{12} deficiencies are common in older adults and can cause neurologic or neuropsychiatric symptoms and decompensation. Hyperhomocysteinemia is asso-ciated with functional B_{12} deficiency, vascular damage, and cardiac or cerebrovascular risk. Other conditions informed by tier-1 laboratory tests include dehydration (eg, blood urea nitrogen-to-creatinine ratio >20:1), hyponatremia or hypernatremia, hypomagne-semia, hypercalcemia (and hypocalcemia), hypoglycemia or hyperglycemia, anemia, uremia, and hepatic dysfunction. Erythrocyte sedimentation rate and C-reactive pro-tein broadly screen for systemic indolent or insidious inflammatory or autoimmune in-fectious and neoplastic processes (eg, undetected lung, liver, or colon cancer).

Structural brain imaging, preferably with MRI, is a tier-1 test in suspected AD or ADRD (if unavailable or contraindicated, use a noncontrast head computed tomogra-phy [CT] scan). Hippocampal and cortical atrophy in temporal and parietal regions on MRI or CT support an AD-related neurodegenerative pattern; however, absence of this pattern does not exclude pathologic AD. MRI or CT can also provide evidence for leu-koaraiosis (white matter burden); vascular cognitive impairment (VCI) or dementia (injury); mixed AD or VCI; and, rarely, for conditions that are not neurodegenerative and are treatable that may cause the CBS (eg, a large frontal meningioma). It can also dictate a substantial change in management; for example, in individuals with copious microhemorrhages placed on blood thinners or those with a mass lesion.

Tier 2 tests can be ordered in some individuals with a low-threshold reason based on particular clinical and epidemiologic profiles, findings on examination, or other test results.

In individuals presenting with symptoms of early-onset, highly atypical, or rapidly progressive dementia, in which the cause remains in doubt by a dementia specialist, more comprehensive testing can be pursued (tier 3–4). This may include spinal fluid testing and/or amyloid brain PET for AD profile (ie, low CSF $A\beta_{42}$, high tau and phospho-tau with an amyloid-tau index of less than 1.0, excessive and widespread binding of an amyloid PET agent in the brain) and exclusion of other less common cognitive or behavior-impairing conditions.[3,45]

FDG-PET or single-photon emission CT (SPECT), and MRI or CT, do not directly measure AD-related pathology but suggest neurodegeneration and can support that AD is causative or contributory. Bilateral parietal and temporal hypometabolism on FDG-PET or SPECT is useful to distinguish AD versus *frontotemporal degeneration* in individuals with behavioral or dysexecutive CBS in whom cause is in doubt. Presence of pathologic AD does not exclude other pathologies causing or contributing to the patient's CBS; for example, 70% to 80% of individuals with DLB are also amyloid-positive on PET.[46] In 2016, Atri[47] reviewed neuroimaging in CBS, AD, or ADRD.

Office-Based Brief Cognitive Testing

Office-based brief cognitive testing should include administration of at least 1 standardized and validated brief instrument for detection of cognitive impairment or dementia, such as MoCA, GPCOG, Blessed Dementia Information-Memory-Concentration scale (BDS-IMC), MMSE, SLUMS, Mini-Cog, and MIS (these tests were compared by Cordell and colleagues[48]). Further tests should be individually adapted and performance should be interpreted in the context of the individual's symptoms, history, demographics, and expected level of performance. The MoCA is a good initial choice for detection; it takes approximately 8 to 12 minutes to administer, has good psychometric properties, acceptable sensitivity to detection of mild impairment, and is available in several forms and languages. The BDS-IMC is useful for tracking progression because it accommodates performance across a broad range of dementia stages, from mild to severe; in contrast, performance on the MoCA often reaches floor values in moderate to severe stages of AD dementia.

Formal Neuropsychological Evaluation

Formal neuropsychological evaluation is useful when higher confidence is needed regarding delineation of the level of impairment and characterization of the CBS; especially when the initial evaluation is borderline or has discrepancies, and when there are unusual clinical profiles, extremes of age or education, and English as a secondary language. It also assists in determining possible contribution of a mood disorder, the patient's capacity, differential diagnosis (DDx), individualized care planning, and recommendation of compensatory strategies to leverage cognitive strengths and avoid limitations.

DIFFERENTIAL DIAGNOSIS

Table 5 provides the DDx of ADc syndromes. Symptoms do not necessarily present or progress in a uniform pattern, and mixed AD syndromes and pathologies are common. Co-existent AD and vascular-ischemic pathology (causing the clinical spectrum of VCI, which includes dementia), and AD with DLB pathology (causing AD-DLB

Table 5
Differential diagnosis of Alzheimer's disease clinical syndromes and Parkinson's plus sensorimotor cognitive-behavioral syndromes

ADc Syndrome	ADc Syndrome Characteristic	DDx
Amnestic ADc	Difficulty with learning and remembering new information	AD and mixed AD (AD + VCI, AD + DLB > AD + VCI + DLB) >> Pure DLB, Hippocampal sclerosis dementia, Argyrophilic grain disease, pure VCI, TDP-43 Pathology and Primary Age-Related Tauopathy Of note: Korsakoff syndrome, TBI, sequelae of HSV encephalitis are readily distinguished by history
Language variant ADc (presenting as primary progressive aphasia (PPA) syndrome)	Variable difficulty with different aspects of language, such as word-finding or hesitancy, fluency, syntax or grammar, writing, reading, comprehension, word-meaning, and naming	Logopenic variant PPA (word-finding): AD > FTD (4R tau > 3R tau or Pick disease) Nonfluent or agrammatic variant PPA (pronunciation or syntax): FTD (4R tau > TDP-43) > AD Semantic variant PPA (word meaning and naming): FTD (TDP-43>>3R tau or Pick disease) >> AD
Visuospatial variant ADc (presenting as posterior cortical atrophy syndrome)	Difficulty with visuospatial cognition and visuoperception, including processing, integration, interpretation, identification	AD > DLB and mixed AD + DLB >> CJD
Behavioral or dysexecutive variant AD	Changes in behavior and personality and/or executive functions, judgment, reasoning, problem-solving	FTD (TDP-43 > Pick disease or 3R tau) >> AD, VCI, DLB, PDD, PSP, AD mixed pathologies, CTE
Mixed Cognitive-Behavioral Syndrome with motor or sensorimotor presentations; Parkinsons-Plus syndromes	Parkinsonism; and/or sensorimotor perception difficulties; and/or apraxia and neglect	Parkinsons-Plus Syndrome: DLB > AD/VCI mixed pathologies, PDD > PSP, MSA Corticobasal Syndrome: CBD > AD, PSP

Relative prevalence of pathology accounting for the observed Cognitive-Behavioral Syndrome: > denotes relatively more prevalent than; >> denotes relatively much more prevalent than.

ADc syndromes are defined by the nature of the cognitive-behavioral domain primarily, prominently, and progressively affected.

Abbreviations: CBD, corticobasal degeneration; CJD, Creutzfeldt-Jakob disease; CTE, chronic traumatic encephalopathy; DLB, dementia with Lewy bodies; FTD, frontotemporal dementia; MSA, multiple systems atrophy; PDD, Parkinson's disease dementia; PSP, progressive supranuclear palsy; TBI, traumatic brain injury.

variants), are prevalent in older individuals.[9,49,50] The DDx of atypical or variant ADc syndromes is broad and depends on the particular CBS characterized by the most prominent presenting domain of impairment. Prion diseases are very rare but Creutzfeldt-Jakob disease is on the DDx of atypical ADc syndromes when there is rapid onset and progression of symptoms (over weeks to months).

TREATMENT OF ALZHEIMER'S DISEASE

Management of AD requires shared goal setting and a triadic partnership between the clinician, patient, and care partners; it is also dynamic, multifactorial, and multidisciplinary. AD management involves (1) early recognition and diagnosis of symptoms, combined with a proactive customized care plan for the patient–caregiver dyad because without accurate diagnosis and appropriate disclosure no care can be provided; (2) nonpharmacologic interventions and behavioral approaches; (3) appropriate pharmacology; and (4) dynamic and pragmatic care plan adjustment according to changes in the patient–caregiver dyad's goals, capacity, condition, and resources, which facilitates continued therapeutic alliance, adherence, and patient and caregiver well-being and safety. Caregivers provide the glue for the therapeutic legs of the care plan.

The current AD treatment paradigm is multifaceted management of symptoms and reduction of long-term clinical decline. First and foremost, management should involve truthful and compassionate disclosure of the diagnosis, according to the patient–caregiver dyad's wants and capacities, along with tailored psychoeducation regarding the syndrome, level of impairment, the disease name and stage, expected course, management options and expectations, and life and care planning needs. Nonpharmacologic or behavioral approaches should be recommended based on the patient–caregiver dyad's priorities, strengths, limitations, resources, and environment. After this foundation is formed, a stage-appropriate pharmacologic treatment plan can be instituted. Long-term management of AD dementia requires proactive planning and flexibility to modify care plans according to changes in the condition and resources of the patient–caregiver dyad.

MANAGEMENT OF ALZHEIMER'S DISEASE DEMENTIA
Nonpharmacologic Management: Behavioral Interventions and Coping Strategies

Nonpharmacologic interventions and behavioral strategies should be used as the first-line option to ameliorate neuropsychiatric symptoms (eg, agitation, apathy, delusions, and disinhibition) and problem behaviors (eg, resistance to care, caregiver shadowing, hoarding, and obsessive-compulsive behaviors) in AD dementia.[51,52] Problem behaviors are distressing to patients and caregivers and, left untreated, exact a devastating toll and lead to poor outcomes.[53,54] During the course of their illness, as many as 85% to 90% of patients will experience neuropsychiatric symptoms or problem behaviors, such as noncognitive behavioral symptoms and behavioral and psychological symptoms of dementia (BPSD), which are associated with more rapid decline, earlier institutionalization, higher distress, worse quality of life, and greater health care utilization and costs.[53,54] Treatment of BPSD using pharmacology alone has low treatment benefit effect sizes (Cohen's $d \leq 0.2$) and, in some cases (eg, antipsychotics), is associated with substantial side-effects and short-term and long-term risks for morbidity and mortality.[55]

Early and ongoing BPSD screening, root-cause analysis, intervention, monitoring, and care plan modification are important components of comprehensive AD dementia care; they can facilitate prevention and treatment efficacy by eliminating triggers and directing treatments to the root cause, not just at the symptoms.

Psychoeducation should include caregiver education on the biopsychosocial substrates behind BPSD (eg, loss of behavioral and coping reserve, compromise of top-down control from fronto-striatal networks, regression to childhood capacities and behaviors in a progression-regression model of dementia), and strategies to avoid behavioral triggers and better communicate and care for the patient. It is important for caregivers to appreciate that overall poor and problem behaviors by the demented individual are not intentional (eg, to be mean, ornery, or vindictive) but are due to disease, brain injury or damage, and diminished capacities. This is nobody's fault; it is just part of the illness. Environmental modification, maintaining consistency, and simple routines can also be very helpful.[56,57]

Pharmacologic Management

Eliminating deleterious medications

The initial step in the pharmacologic management of AD consists of eliminating redundant and potentially deleterious medications. For example, diphenhydramine, often taken as an over-the-counter drug combination with acetaminophen for sleep and pain relief; other sedative-hypnotics; and medications for anxiety (eg, benzodiazepines) or urinary incontinence (antimuscarinic) are relatively contraindicated in elderly and cognitively vulnerable persons.[44,58]

Identification and treatment of comorbid conditions that decompensate dementia

Treating these conditions can affect better cognition, function, and behavior in patients with AD. In many, the symptoms and signs of decompensation can be subtle and chronic and do not manifest as acute delirium or encephalopathy. The delirium-dementia link has been reviewed in the literature.[59,60] Tier 1 to 2 CBS or dementia assessment laboratory tests or studies (see **Table 4**) can help identify common conditions that exacerbate symptoms, including dehydration, electrolyte and metabolic derangements, anemia, cardiac or cerebral ischemia, hypoxia, thyroid and vitamin deficiencies (eg, vitamin B_{12} deficiency), and infections (eg, urinary tract infections, pneumonia). Other conditions, such as pain from arthritis, constipation, hunger, thirst, or fatigue, are also common in AD, particularly in later stages when patients cannot appropriately recognize or communicate their symptoms. These can lead to BPSD, particularly anxiety, irritability, agitation, aggression, or sleep-wake disturbances.

Antipsychotics: use with extreme caution under strict specific circumstances

Antipsychotics carry a US Food and Drug Administration (FDA) black-box warning in dementia; they must be used with extreme caution, ongoing monitoring, and only when strict conditions are met.[55,56] Short-term and long-term antipsychotic use is associated with substantial risk of cognitive decline, morbidity (eg, parkinsonism, falls, pneumonia, or cardiovascular and cerebrovascular events), and mortality. Their use is reserved as a last resort for severe refractory behavioral disturbances without an identifiable and treatable cause (eg, severe aggression, agitation, or psychosis not due to delirium, pain, or infection) or when a serious risk of immediate harm or safety exists that cannot be otherwise ameliorated.[55,56] Risperidone is European Medicines Agency approved in Europe for short-term, 12-week, use in dementia when there is refractory severe agitation or psychosis. After a careful evaluation by a dementia specialist, cautious use of antipsychotics should be limited to the lowest effective dosages for short durations. Continued use requires ongoing monitoring, assessment of risk-benefit, and continued consent from the family or care providers regarding goals of treatment and trade-offs.

Approved anti-Alzheimer disease medications: cholinesterase inhibitors and memantine

Cholinesterase inhibitors (ChEls) (donepezil, galantamine, rivastigmine) and the N-methyl-D-aspartate (NMDA)-antagonist, memantine, are the only FDA-approved treatments for AD dementia and are recommended broadly in consensus guidelines and practice parameters.[1,52,61,62] ChEIs and memantine also have complementary mechanisms of action, potentially additive effects, and demonstrate acceptable tolerability and safety profiles.[63] A recent systematic review and meta-analysis by Tricco and colleagues[64] included 110 studies and 23,432 subjects supports efficacy, effectiveness, and safety. A pharmacologic foundation of anti-AD therapies, whether with a ChEI or memantine monotherapy, or, ultimately, combined together as add-on dual combination therapy, most often as memantine added on to stable background ChEI treatment, have demonstrated benefits in the short-term and long-term to reduce decline in cognition and function, retard the emergence and impact of neuropsychiatric symptoms, and to delay nursing home placement without prolongation of time to death.[64,65] Viewed from the social perspective, anti-AD pharmacotherapy (donepezil, memantine, galantamine, rivastigmine) can reduce the economic burden of the illness, even in later stages of illness.[66]

Short-term responses to anti-AD medications vary between individuals. Aggregate data suggest that during the initial 6 to 12 months of treatment, performance on measures of cognition, activities of dialing living (ADL), behavioral symptoms, or global clinical impression of change may significantly improve in a minority (10%–30%), plateau in nearly half (30%–50%), or continue to deteriorate in about a third (20%–40%) of treated patients. Discontinuation of ChEI treatment is, on aggregate, harmful. Patients taken off, or those inconsistently taking, anti-AD medications progress more rapidly than those who continue treatments, particularly ChEIs. Unless otherwise indicated, clinicians should avoid discontinuation trials of ChEIs to see if there is worsening. Even temporary discontinuation is associated with irreversible declines and greater risk of nursing home placement.[67–72]

Sustained treatments provide a modest expectation of short-term stabilization or improvement, and longer-term slowing of clinical decline. As the disease progresses, over several months to years, patients who may initially show improvement or stability, will eventually decline. It is important for clinicians to communicate practical issues associated with pharmacologic treatment, including rationale, need for monitoring, and expectations. In the long run, current treatments of AD dementia mitigate decline but do not prevent it. From a public health and economics perspective, therapies that minimize caregiver burden and delay nursing home entry translate into significant benefits related to worker productivity and health care savings.[66,73–75]

Cholinesterase inhibitors

ChEIs facilitate central cholinergic activity by reducing the physiologic breakdown of acetylcholine (ACh) by the enzyme acetylcholinesterase (AChE) in the synaptic cleft. No high-quality data support significant group-level efficacy differences between the 3 ChEIs generically available in the United States. Donepezil and rivastigmine are FDA-approved and labeled for mild, moderate, and severe AD dementia; galantamine has approval for mild and moderate AD.

Cholinesterase inhibitors safety and tolerability With slow titration in appropriate individuals, ChEIs are generally tolerated well and have an acceptable adverse effect profile.[64] The most common adverse effects, including nausea, vomiting, anorexia, flatulence, loose stools, diarrhea, salivation, and abdominal cramping, are related to peripheral cholinomimetic effects on the gastrointestinal (GI) tract. For the oral preparations, the adverse GI effects of ChEI can be minimized by administering the drug after a meal or in combination with memantine. Others can experience vivid dreams or mild insomnia; therefore, doses should ideally be given after a meal in the morning. The rivastigmine transdermal patch can also cause skin irritation, redness, or rash at the site of application. Overall, adverse effects may occur in 5% to 20% of patients starting on ChEIs but are usually mild and transient, and often related to the dosage and rate of dosage escalation. These medications may also decrease heart rate and increase the risk of syncope, particularly in susceptible individuals (eg, those with sick sinus syndrome or atrioventricular block) and with overdose. Use of these agents is contraindicated in patients with unstable or severe cardiac disease, uncontrolled epilepsy, unexplained syncope, and active peptic ulcer disease.

ChEIs efficacy and effectiveness In more than 40 short-term randomized controlled trials (RCTs) using placebos over 24 to 52 weeks investigating efficacy, and in meta-analyses of RCTs, all 3 ChEIs have demonstrated small to medium effect size treatment benefits at the sibject-group level in terms of improving, stabilizing, or delaying decline in cognition, ADL, and global status, and in ameliorating BPSD and caregiver burden.[35,65,70,71,76–87] Longer term benefits, from 2 to 4 or more years have been demonstrated in open-label extension[69,88–90] and long-term prospective observational clinical cohort studies.[91–95]

Level II or equivocal level I evidence suggest donepezil treatment may be beneficial in very mild stage AD or for subgroups with MCI due to AD (ie, carriers of APOE-ε4 allele,[96] those with depression or depressive symptoms[97]). Such off–FDA label pharmacotherapy is not sufficiently supported by level I evidence to warrant an unequivocal recommendation for all patients. However, efficacy or effectiveness, risk (tolerability and safety) and cost data, individual clinical circumstances, and patient–caregiver dyad preferences may warrant a discussion between clinicians, patients, and caregivers about this possibility.[96]

N-methyl-D-aspartate antagonists (memantine)

Memantine was the last FDA-approved treatment of AD dementia (2002) and remains the sole medication in its class. Memantine affects glutamatergic transmission; it is a renally cleared low-to-moderate affinity NMDA-receptor open-channel blocker.

Memantine safety and tolerability Titrated appropriately, memantine has a favorable safety and tolerability profile. Mild and transient treatment-emergent side effects include confusion, dizziness, constipation, headache, and somnolence. These may be encountered during, or soon after, titration to the maximum total daily dosage of 10 mg twice daily for immediate-release memantine (generically available in the United States) or 28 mg once daily for memantine XR. In patients with severe renal insufficiency (creatinine clearance <30 mL/min) a dosage-adjustment to 5 mg twice daily for immediate-release memantine and 14 mg daily for extended-release memantine is recommended.

Memantine efficacy and effectiveness Memantine is FDA-approved in moderate to severe AD dementia, as monotherapy or in combination with a ChEI (often added to an existing ChEI treatment). In moderate and severe AD, short-term efficacy of memantine monotherapy compared with placebo is reported in several RCTs of 12 to 50 weeks duration and supported by meta-analyses. Treatment benefits include improvement, stabilization, or reduced decline in the domains of cognition, function (ADLs), and global status; and by amelioration of BPSD and caregiver burden.[63,71,73,98–111] Short-term (6 months or less) memantine treatment effect sizes are small to medium in size and clinically significant at the moderate to severe stages of AD.[109,110,112,113] Longer-term prospective observational clinical patient cohort studies report reduced clinical decline in patients with AD treated at any stage.[114–119]

Add-on dual combination therapy with acetylcholinesterase inhibitors and memantine
Short-term (6–12 months) RCTs (level I evidence), longer-term (12–36 months) open-label extensions of RCTs (level II or III evidence), and long-term (2 to 5-plus years) observational prospective clinical cohort effectiveness studies (level II evidence) support the safety and benefits of anti-AD treatments in combination, most frequently as memantine added on to a stable regimen of background ChEI treatment.[114–121] Systematic reviews and meta-analysis also provide level II grade evidence for the benefits of ChEI and memantine add-on combination treatment in AD dementia.[63–65,79,80,122–124]

Safety and tolerability of cholinesterase inhibitor memantine add-on combination treatment Several studies have reported on safety and tolerability of combination therapy; overall, there is a good profile for both. Addition of memantine to stable dosages of a ChEI does not correspond to significant overall increases in adverse events.[63,64] The rates of discontinuation due to adverse events for ChEIs and memantine combination treatment are low, between 5% to 10%, and not generally significantly different from placebo.[100,120,121,125,126]

Vitamins, medical foods, and supplements
Other than vitamin E, large RCTs have failed to provide support from level III or IV epidemiologic association studies for potential benefits of vitamins or supplements at the AD dementia stage. Unless contraindicated due to bleeding diatheses, coronary artery disease, or another comorbidity, high-dose vitamin E (1000 IU twice daily was the regimen tested) may be considered based on results of 2 RCTs that supported approximately 20% lower rate of ADL decline over approximately 2 to 3 years; there were no concerning safely signals or increased mortality with high-dose vitamin E.[127,128] There is no compelling evidence that Souvenaid, a prescription nutritional supplement (ie, medical food) containing Fortasyn Connect provides additional benefits in patients with AD dementia treated with anti-AD medications.[129] Unfortunately, large RCTs have failed to support benefits from ginkgo biloba, high-dose vitamin B_{12} or folic acid combinations, omega-3 fatty acid or fish oil components or preparations, nonsteroidal anti-inflammatory drugs, and statin medications at the dementia stage of AD.[76,81]

Practical recommendations for implementation of pharmacotherapy
Unless contraindicated, ChEI therapy should be initiated and slowly titrated over months to a maximal clinical or tolerated dosage following diagnosis of AD dementia (**Table 6**). For patients with moderate to severe AD, memantine can be initiated (see **Table 6**) after patients have received stable ChEI therapy for several months without adverse effects. Memantine monotherapy can be initiated on-label in moderate or later stage AD. Conversely, a ChEI can be added after several months of stable memantine monotherapy. The latter is a useful strategy in patients who are very sensitive to or experience GI side effects with ChEIs. A very low and slow titration (eg, starting donepezil 2.5 mg daily after breakfast; increasing it to 5 mg daily if no side effects emerge within 6 weeks) may be helpful in patients who are very sensitive to cholinomimetic effects. In highly refractory situations, switching to another ChEI at a low-dosage can be tried. Persistence, higher dosage (in later dementia stages), and duration of treatment are associated with better outcomes, even in those with advanced dementia.[92,95,114,115,130]

Patients should have diligent management of their vascular risk factors, including lipids, blood pressure, and glucose. Managing vascular risk factors in patients with

Table 6
Recommended dosing for US Food and Drug Administration–approved anti–Alzheimer disease medications: cholinesterase inhibitors donepezil, rivastigmine, and galantamine; and the N-methyl-ᴅ-aspartate–antagonist, memantine

Drug	Dosage and Notes
Donepezil	Starting dosage: 5 mg/d; can be increased to 10 mg/d after 4–6 wk Before starting donepezil 23 mg/d, patients should be on donepezil 10 mg/d for at least 3 mo
Rivastigmine	Oral: starting dosage 1.5 mg twice daily; if well-tolerated, the dosage may be increased to 3 mg twice daily after 2 wk; subsequent increases to 4.5 and 6 mg twice daily should be attempted after 2-wk minimums at previous dosage; maximum dosage: 6 mg twice daily; oral rivastigmine can be difficult to tolerate Patch: starting dosage 1 4.6 mg patch once daily for a period of 24 h Maintenance dosage 1 9.5 mg or 13.3 mg patch once daily for a period of 24 h; before initiating a maintenance dosage, patients should undergo a minimum of 4 wk of treatment at the initial dosage (or at the lower patch dosage of 9.5 mg) with good tolerability
Galantamine	Extended-release: start at 8 mg once daily for 4 wk; increase to 16 mg once daily for 4 weeks; increase to 24 mg once daily Generic: start at 4 mg twice daily for 4 wk; increase to 8 mg twice daily for 4 wk; increase to 12 mg twice daily
Memantine	Immediate-release: starting dosage 5 mg once daily; increase dosage in 5-mg increments to a maximum of 20 mg daily (divided dosages taken twice daily) with a minimum of 1 week between dosage increases; in earlier stages may consider 10 mg daily dosage; the maximum recommended dosage in severe renal impairment is 5 mg twice daily Extended-release (XR): for patients new to memantine, the recommended starting dosage of memantine XR is 7 mg once daily, and the recommended target dosage is 28 mg once daily; the dosage should be increased in 7-mg increments every seventh day; the minimum recommended interval between dosage increases is 1 week, and only if the previous dosage has been well tolerated; the maximum recommended dosage in severe renal impairment is 14 mg once daily
Memantine XR or donepezil capsule (branded combo capsule)	Combination capsule consisting of 7–28 mg memantine or 10 mg donepezil given orally once daily; can be started in patients already on background stable donepezil 10 mg daily (with memantine dosage titration) or in patients already on combination treatment with each agent; maximum recommended dosage in severe renal impairment is 14 mg memantine XR or 10 mg donepezil once daily

AD is associated with slower cognitive decline (Deschaintre, Neurol 2009).[2] Anxiety and clinical depression should be monitored and treated (use a selective serotonin reuptake inhibitor with a low anticholinergic load and a favorable geriatric profile; eg, citalopram, escitalopram, sertraline). There should be proactive monitoring and optimization of sleep, stress level, hydration, and nutrition status; and any deficiencies (eg, thyroid, vitamin B_{12}) and systemic conditions that can decompensate mental functions should be treated (eg, urinary tract infection, dehydration, hyponatremia). Along with social and mental engagement, and stress management, daily exercise and physical activity should be an integral part of the care plan.

Potentially deleterious medications, including anticholinergics and benzodiazepines, should be weaned and avoided.[44] Off-label use of antipsychotics should be used with great caution, and only under specific circumstances when behavioral or environmental interventions have failed, and after careful consideration of risks, benefits, side-effects, and alternatives.[56] Stimulants are seldom indicated and may lower the threshold for irritability, agitation or aggression, and dysphoria.

When to start and stop anti-Alzheimer disease medications

Per FDA prescribing information, clinicians may start a ChEI in mild, moderate, or severe AD, and memantine in moderate or severe AD. In moderate stages, a ChEI or memantine can be started and, ultimately, the complementary agent can be added to achieve dual-combination therapy. Based on the patient–caregiver dyad preferences and clinician comfort and expertise, an individualized discussion can be prompted regarding the pros and cons, cost, and uncertainties of potential off-label prescription of anti-AD medications, such as ChEIs in MCI due to AD[96] and high-dose vitamin E.[127,128]

Box 4
Key elements of effective multifactorial management of Alzheimer's disease

Individualization of evaluation process, diagnosis, disclosure process, and care plan
- Early detection of symptoms, timely assessment and diagnosis, and appropriate disclosure
- Shared goal setting for diagnostic, disclosure, and management processes; sustained targeting and tailoring of a proactive care plan to patient and caregivers

Nonpharmacologic interventions and behavioral approaches to management
- Psychoeducation about AD; dementia in general; effects on cognition, function, and behaviors; dementia care; expectations; "the progression and regression model of aging and dementia"
- Behavioral approaches, both general and targeted to the patient–caregiver dyad; including simplification of environment; establishing routines; providing a safe, calm, and consistent care environment; using strategies such as interacting calmly, redirection to pleasurable activities and environment, reassurance, providing only necessary information in a manner that the patient can appreciate (ie, in simple language and small chunks) and at the appropriate time; benign therapeutic fibbing and never saying no (unless immediate safety is concerned) to allow the moment to pass
- Establishing and fostering support networks for the patient and caregivers
- Identifying and monitoring health and safety risks for patient and others, advance planning for medical, legal, and financial decision-making and needs (eg, stove, weapon, and driving safety; falling prey to fraud or poor work or financial decision-making)
- Caring for caregivers, including caregiver support and respite care

Pharmacologic treatment
- Elimination of redundant and inappropriate medications listed in Beers criteria.[44]
- Treating underlying medical and psychiatric conditions, and associated symptoms that can exacerbate cognitive-behavioral impairment or dementia (eg, dehydration, pain, constipation, infections, electrolyte and metabolic derangements, anxiety, depression, psychosis)
- Prescription of stage-appropriate FDA-approved anti-AD medications (ChEIs: donepezil, rivastigmine, galantamine; NMDA-antagonist: memantine) as monotherapy or add-on dual combination therapy (ChEI plus memantine)

Pragmatic modifications to sustain alliance, adherence, and well-being of patient–caregiver dyad
- Flexibility to modify care plan according to important changes in the patient–caregiver dyad
- Forging and sustaining a therapeutic alliance
- Promoting the safety, health, and well-being of the patient and her or his caregivers
- Adopting a pragmatic approach to ongoing care that includes establishing and simplifying care routines if possible; modifying the environment to suit the patient–caregiver dyad; and consideration of patient and caregiver preferences, capacity, environment, and resources in devising and implementing care plans

Anti-AD medications can be maintained in late-stages to support basic psychomotor processes, praxis, functional communication, the behavioral responses required to assist caregivers to deliver basic ADL care, and the elementary processes of movement and eating. The benefits may also extend to reducing antipsychotic use. In the end or terminal stages of AD, when personhood has disintegrated and when there is no meaningful communication or interaction, patients should only receive care (pharmacologic or otherwise) that is directed to provide palliation and comfort.[131]

SUMMARY OR FUTURE CONSIDERATIONS

Box 4 provides a summary of the evaluation, diagnosis, disclosure, and management process. Evaluation should use a structured history and multidomain symptom and function review from the patient and a care partner or informant, and a focused examination to assess the level of change or impairment and to characterize the CBS. Etiologic diagnosis is aided by a multitiered approach to tests, including laboratory tests and neuroimaging. The current AD treatment paradigm is to reduce progression of symptoms and disability. Despite ongoing efforts, a magic bullet or cure for AD in the dementia stages is unrealistic in the near future. By the time AD is in the dementia stages, neurodegeneration has wrought devastation in synapses, cells, and networks for a decade or more.

Nonpharmacologic management and pharmacologic therapies for AD dementia seek to minimize the disabling effects of cognitive and functional decline and emergence of problem BPSD. The FDA-approved anti-AD pharmacotherapies; the ChEIs donepezil, galantamine, and rivastigmine; and the NMDA antagonist memantine can reduce progression of clinical symptoms and disability.

Clinicians should establish a proactive and flexible individualized approach to compassionately care for individuals and caregivers. It is necessary to maintain a strong therapeutic alliance that is holistic, pragmatic, and involves psychoeducation, behavioral and environmental approaches to care, planning for current and future care needs, and promoting brain health and psychosocial well-being.

Intensive research efforts are underway to develop more accurate diagnostic tools (eg, using neuroimaging, blood, CSF, proteomic, and genomic biomarkers of AD) and better AD therapeutics. A myriad of ongoing phase1 to 3 human clinical trials for primary and secondary prevention, and symptomatic and disease-modifying treatment, are directed at diverse therapeutic targets in AD, including neurochemicals, amyloid and tau pathologic processes, mitochondria, inflammatory pathways, neuroglia, and multimodal lifestyle interventions.

REFERENCES

1. Livingston G, Sommerlad A, Orgeta V, et al. Dementia prevention, intervention, and care. Lancet 2017;390(10113):2673–734.
2. Deschaintre Y, Richard F, Fau-Leys D, et al. Treatment of vascular risk factors is associated with slower decline in Alzheimer's disease. Neurology 2009;73(9): 674–80.
3. Atri A. Alzheimer's disease and Alzheimer's dementia. In: Dickerson BC, Atri A, editors. Dementia: comprehensive principles and practices. 1st edition. New York: Oxford University Press; 2014. p. 360–432.
4. Alzheimer's Association. 2018 Alzheimer's disease facts and figures. Alzheimers Dement 2018;14(3):367–429.
5. Prince MJ, Wimo A, Guerchet MM, et al. World alzheimer report 2015 - the global impact of dementia: an analysis of prevalence, incidence, cost and trends. London: Alzheimer's Disease International (ADI); 2015.

6. Prince M, Prina M, Guerchet M. The world Alzheimer report 2013 'Journey of Caring: an analysis of long-term care for dementia'. Alzheimer's Disease International (ADI); 2013.
7. Wimo A, Prince M. The world Alzheimer report 2010 'The Global Impact of Dementia. Alzheimer's Disease International (ADI); 2010.
8. Saxena S. Dementia world report: a public health priority. World Health Organization (WHO); 2012.
9. Kapasi A, DeCarli C, Schneider JA. Impact of multiple pathologies on the threshold for clinically overt dementia. Acta Neuropathol 2017;134(2):171–86.
10. Johnson KA, Minoshima S, Bohnen NI, et al. Appropriate use criteria for amyloid PET: a report of the amyloid imaging task force, the Society of Nuclear Medicine and Molecular Imaging, and the Alzheimer's Association. Alzheimers Dement 2013;9(1):e-1-16.
11. Simonsen AH, Herukka SK, Andreasen N, et al. Recommendations for CSF AD biomarkers in the diagnostic evaluation of dementia. Alzheimers Dement 2017; 13(3):274–84.
12. Petersen RC, Lopez O, Armstrong MJ, et al. Practice guideline update summary: mild cognitive impairment: report of the guideline development, dissemination, and implementation subcommittee of the American Academy of Neurology. Neurology 2018;90(3):126–35.
13. Hebert LE, Weuve J, Scherr PA, et al. Alzheimer disease in the United States (2010-2050) estimated using the 2010 census. Neurology 2013;80(19):1778–83.
14. Braak H, Alafuzoff I, Arzberger T, et al. Staging of Alzheimer disease-associated neurofibrillary pathology using paraffin sections and immunocytochemistry. Acta Neuropathol 2006;112:389–404.
15. Jellinger KA, Bancher C. Neuropathology of Alzheimer's disease: a critical update. J Neural Transm 1998;54:77–95.
16. Parvizi J, Van Hoesen GW, Damasio A. The selective vulnerability of brainstem nuclei to Alzheimer's disease. Ann Neurol 2001;49:53–66.
17. Hyman BT, Phelps CH, Beach TG, et al. National Institute on Aging-Alzheimer's Association guidelines for the neuropathologic assessment of Alzheimer's disease. Alzheimers Dement 2012;8(1):1–13.
18. Jack C, Knopman D, Jagust W, et al. Hypothetical model of dynamic biomarkers of the Alzheimer's pathological cascade. Lancet 2010;9(1):119–28.
19. Attems J, Jellinger K, Thal DR, et al. Review: sporadic cerebral amyloid angiopathy. Neuropathol Appl Neurobiol 2011;37:75–93.
20. Atri A, Locascio JJ, Lin JM, et al. Prevalence and effects of lobar microhemorrhages in early-stage dementia. Neurodegener Dis 2005;2(6):305–12.
21. Loy CT, Schofield PR, Turner AM, et al. Genetics of dementia. Lancet 2014; 383(9919):828–40.
22. Bertram L, McQueen MB, Mullin K, et al. Systematic meta-analyses of Alzheimer disease genetic association studies: the AlzGene database. Nat Genet 2007; 39(1):17–23.
23. Corder EH, Saunders AM, Strittmatter WJ, et al. Gene dose of apolipoprotein E type 4 allele and the risk of Alzheimer's disease in late onset families. Science 1993;261(5123):921–3.
24. Davies P. A very incomplete comprehensive theory of Alzheimer's disease. Ann N Y Acad Sci 2000;924:8–16.
25. Zlokovic BV. Neurovascular pathways to neurodegeneration in Alzheimer's disease and other disorders. Nat Rev Neurosci 2011;12(12):723–38.

26. Hyman BT. Amyloid-dependent and amyloid-independent stages of Alzheimer disease. Arch Neurol 2011;68(8):1062–4.
27. Selkoe DJ, Abraham CR, Podlisny MB, et al. Isolation of low-molecular-weight proteins from amyloid plaque fibers in Alzheimer's disease. J Neurochem 1986;46(6):1820–34.
28. Haass C, Koo EH, Mellon A, et al. Targeting of cell-surface beta-amyloid precursor protein to lysosomes: alternative processing into amyloid-bearing fragments. Nature 1992;357(6378):500–3.
29. Selkoe DJ. Amyloid protein and Alzheimer's disease. Sci Am 1991;265(5): 68–71, 74–6, 78.
30. Hardy JA, Higgins GA. Alzheimer's disease: the amyloid cascade hypothesis. Science 1992;256(5054):184–5.
31. Hardy J, Selkoe DJ. The amyloid hypothesis of Alzheimer's disease: progress and problems on the road to therapeutics. Science 2002;297(5580):353–6.
32. McKhann GM, Knopman DS, Chertkow H, et al. The diagnosis of dementia due to Alzheimer's disease: recommendations from the National Institute on Aging-Alzheimer's Association workgroups on diagnostic guidelines for Alzheimer's disease. Alzheimers Dement 2011;7(3):263–9.
33. Petersen RC, Aisen P, Boeve BF, et al. Criteria for mild cognitive impairment due to Alzheimer's disease in the community. Ann Neurol 2013;74(2):199–208.
34. Chhatwal JP, Schultz AP, Johnson KA, et al. Preferential degradation of cognitive networks differentiates Alzheimer's disease from ageing. Brain 2018;141(5): 1486–500.
35. Farlow MR, Cummings JL. Effective pharmacologic management of Alzheimer's disease. Am J Med 2007;120(5):388–97.
36. Jost BC, Grossberg GT. The natural history of Alzheimer's disease: a brain bank study. J Am Geriatr Soc 1995;43(11):1248–55.
37. Jost BC, Grossberg GT. The evolution of psychiatric symptoms in Alzheimer's disease: a natural history study. J Am Geriatr Soc 1996;44(9):1078–81.
38. Alzheimer's-Association. 2013 Alzheimer's disease facts and figures. Alzheimers Dement 2013;9(2):208–45.
39. Dubois B, Feldman HH, Jacova C, et al. Revising the definition of Alzheimer's disease: a new lexicon. Lancet Neurol 2010;9(11):1118–27.
40. Dubois B, Feldman H, Jacova C, et al. Research criteria for the diagnosis of Alzheimer's disease: revising the NINCDS-ADRDA criteria. Lancet Neurol 2007; 6(8):734–46.
41. APA. Diagnostic and statistical manual of mental disorders - (DSM-V). 5th edition. Washington, DC: American Psychiatric Publishing; 2013.
42. Atri A, Norman M, Knopman D, et al. Alzheimer's association best clinical practice guidelines for the evaluation of neurodegenerative cognitive behavioral syndromes, Alzheimer's disease and dementias in the United States. Alzheimer's Association International Conference. Chicago, 22 July, 2018.
43. Galvin JE, Roe CM, Powlishta KK, et al. The AD8: a brief informant interview to detect dementia. Neurology 2005;65(4):559–64.
44. American Geriatrics Society 2012 Beers Criteria Update Expert Panel. American Geriatrics Society updated Beers Criteria for potentially inappropriate medication use in older adults. J Am Geriatr Soc 2012;60(4):616–31.
45. Rosenbloom MH, Atri A. The evaluation of rapidly progressive dementia. Neurologist 2011;17(2):67–74.
46. Gomperts SN, Rentz DM, Moran E, et al. Imaging amyloid deposition in Lewy body diseases. Neurology 2008;71(12):903–10.

47. Atri A. Imaging of neurodegenerative cognitive and behavioral disorders: practical considerations for dementia clinical practice. Handb Clin Neurol 2016;136: 971–84.
48. Cordell CB, Borson S, Boustani M, et al. Alzheimer's Association recommendations for operationalizing the detection of cognitive impairment during the Medicare Annual Wellness Visit in a primary care setting. Alzheimers Dement 2013; 9(2):141–50.
49. Jellinger KA, Attems J. Prevalence and impact of vascular and Alzheimer pathologies in Lewy body disease. Acta Neuropathol 2008;115(4):427–36.
50. Schneider JA, Arvanitakis Z, Bang W, et al. Mixed brain pathologies account for most dementia cases in community-dwelling older persons. Neurology 2007; 69(24):2197–204.
51. Bhalerao S, Seyfried LS, Kim HM, et al. Mortality risk with the use of atypical antipsychotics in later-life bipolar disorder. J Geriatr Psychiatry Neurol 2012;25(1): 29–36.
52. National Institute for Health and Care Excellence. Dementia: assessment, management and support for people living with dementia and their carers (NG97). NICE, UK, June 20, 2018.
53. Okura T, Plassman BL, Steffens DC, et al. Neuropsychiatric symptoms and the risk of institutionalization and death: the aging, demographics, and memory study. J Am Geriatr Soc 2012;59(3):473–81.
54. Kales HC, Chen P, Blow FC, et al. Rates of clinical depression diagnosis, functional impairment, and nursing home placement in coexisting dementia and depression. Am J Geriatr Psychiatry 2005;13(6):441–9.
55. Ballard C, Corbett A, Howard R. Prescription of antipsychotics in people with dementia. Br J Psychiatry 2014;205(1):4–5.
56. Kales HC, Gitlin LN, Lyketsos CG. Assessment and management of behavioral and psychological symptoms of dementia. BMJ 2015;350:h369.
57. Gitlin LN, Kales HC, Lyketsos CG. Nonpharmacologic management of behavioral symptoms in dementia. JAMA 2012;308(19):2020–9.
58. Rudolph JL, Salow MJ, Angelini MC, et al. The anticholinergic risk scale and anticholinergic adverse effects in older persons. Arch Intern Med 2008;168(5): 508–13.
59. Fong TG, Davis D, Growdon ME, et al. The interface between delirium and dementia in elderly adults. Lancet Neurol 2015;14(8):823–32.
60. Oh ES, Fong TG, Hshieh TT, et al. Delirium in older persons: advances in diagnosis and treatment. JAMA 2017;318(12):1161–74.
61. Schmidt R, Hofer E, Bouwman FH, et al. EFNS-ENS/EAN guideline on concomitant use of cholinesterase inhibitors and memantine in moderate to severe Alzheimer's disease. Eur J Neurol 2015;22(6):889–98.
62. Gauthier S, Patterson C, Chertkow H, et al. Recommendations of the 4th Canadian Consensus Conference on the Diagnosis and Treatment of Dementia (CCCDTD4). Can Geriatr J 2012;15(4):120–6.
63. Atri A, Molinuevo JL, Lemming O, et al. Memantine in patients with Alzheimer's disease receiving donepezil: new analyses of efficacy and safety for combination therapy. Alzheimers Res Ther 2013;5(1):6–16.
64. Tricco AC, Ashoor HM, Soobiah C, et al. Comparative effectiveness and safety of cognitive enhancers for treating alzheimer's disease: systematic review and network metaanalysis. J Am Geriatr Soc 2018;66(1):170–8.
65. Rountree SD, Atri A, Lopez OL, et al. Effectiveness of antidementia drugs in delaying Alzheimer disease progression. Alzheimers Dement 2013;9(3):338–45.

66. Cappell J, Herrmann N, Cornish S, et al. The pharmacoeconomics of cognitive enhancers in moderate to severe Alzheimer's disease. CNS Drugs 2010;24(11): 909–27.
67. Raskind MA, Peskind ER, Wessel T, et al. Galantamine in AD: a 6-month randomized, placebo-controlled trial with a 6-month extension. The Galantamine USA-1 study group. Neurology 2000;54:2261–8.
68. Courtney C, Farrell D, Gray R, et al. Long-term donepezil treatment in 565 patients with Alzheimer's disease (AD2000): randomised double-blind trial. Lancet 2004;363(9427):2105–15.
69. Doody R, Geldmacher D, Gordon B, et al. Open-label, multicenter, phase 3 extension study of the safety and efficacy of donepezil in patients with Alzheimer disease. Arch Neurol 2001;58(3):427–33.
70. Farlow M, Anand R, Messina J Jr, et al. A 52-week study of the efficacy of rivastigmine in patients with mild to moderately severe Alzheimer's disease. Eur Neurol 2000;44(4):236–41.
71. Howard R, McShane R, Lindesay J, et al. Donepezil and memantine for moderate-to-severe Alzheimer's disease. N Engl J Med 2012;366(10):893–903.
72. Howard R, McShane R, Lindesay J, et al. Nursing home placement in the Donepezil and Memantine in Moderate to Severe Alzheimer's Disease (DOMINO-AD) trial: secondary and post-hoc analyses. Lancet Neurol 2015;14(12):1171–81.
73. Weycker D, Taneja C, Edelsberg J, et al. Cost-effectiveness of memantine in moderate-to-severe Alzheimer's disease patients receiving donepezil. Curr Med Res Opin 2007;23(5):1187–97.
74. Getsios D, Blume S, Ishak KJ, et al. An economic evaluation of early assessment for Alzheimer's disease in the United Kingdom. Alzheimers Dement 2012;8(1): 22–30.
75. Getsios D, Blume S, Ishak KJ, et al. Cost effectiveness of donepezil in the treatment of mild to moderate Alzheimer's disease: a UK evaluation using discrete-event simulation. Pharmacoeconomics 2010;28(5):411–27.
76. Tayeb H, Yang H, Price B, et al. Pharmacotherapies for Alzheimer's disease: beyond cholinesterase inhibitors. Pharmacol Ther 2012;134:8–25.
77. Cummings JL. Alzheimer's disease. N Engl J Med 2004;351(1):56–67.
78. Cummings JL, Schneider L, Tariot PN, et al. Reduction of behavioral disturbances and caregiver distress by galantamine in patients with Alzheimer's disease. Am J Psychiatry 2004;161(3):532–8.
79. Raina P, Santaguida P, Ismaila A, et al. Effectiveness of cholinesterase inhibitors and memantine for treating dementia: evidence review for a clinical practice guideline. Ann Intern Med 2008;148(5):379–97.
80. Atri A, Rountree S, Lopez O, et al. Validity, significance, strengths, limitations, and evidentiary value of real-world clinical data for combination therapy in alzheimer's disease: comparison of efficacy and effectiveness studies. Neurodegener Dis 2012;10(1–4):170–4.
81. Ballard C, Gauthier S, Corbett A, et al. Alzheimer's disease. Lancet 2011; 377(9770):1019–31.
82. Birks J. Cholinesterase inhibitors for Alzheimer's disease. Cochrane Database Syst Rev 2006;(1):CD005593.
83. Greenberg SM, Tennis MK, Brown LB, et al. Donepezil therapy in clinical practice: a randomized crossover study. Arch Neurol 2000;57(1):94–9.
84. van de Glind EM, van Enst WA, van Munster BC, et al. Pharmacological treatment of dementia: a scoping review of systematic reviews. Dement Geriatr Cogn Disord 2013;36(3–4):211–28.

85. Rockwood K. Size of the treatment effect on cognition of cholinesterase inhibition in Alzheimer's disease. J Neurol Neurosurg Psychiatry 2004;75(5):677–85.

86. Mohs RC, Doody RS, Morris JC, et al. A 1-year, placebo-controlled preservation of function survival study of donepezil in AD patients. Neurology 2001;57(3): 481–8.

87. Cummings JL, McRae T, Zhang R. Effects of donepezil on neuropsychiatric symptoms in patients with dementia and severe behavioral disorders. Am J Geriatr Psychiatry 2006;14(7):605–12.

88. Burns A, Gauthier S, Perdomo C. Efficacy and safety of donepezil over 3 years: an open-label, multicentre study in patients with Alzheimer's disease. Int J Geriatr Psychiatry 2007;22(8):806–12.

89. Raskind MA, Peskind ER, Truyen L, et al. The cognitive benefits of galantamine are sustained for at least 36 months: a long-term extension trial. Arch Neurol 2004;61(2):252–6.

90. Doody RS, Dunn JK, Clark CM, et al. Chronic donepezil treatment is associated with slowed cognitive decline in Alzheimer's disease. Dement Geriatr Cogn Disord 2001;12(4):295–300.

91. Gillette-Guyonnet S, Andrieu S, Cortes F, et al. Outcome of Alzheimer's disease: potential impact of cholinesterase inhibitors. J Gerontol A Biol Sci Med Sci 2006; 61(5):516–20.

92. Wattmo C, Wallin A, Londos E, et al. Long-term outcome and prediction models of activities of daily living in Alzheimer disease with cholinesterase inhibitor treatment. Alzheimer Dis Assoc Disord 2011;25:63–72.

93. Wallin A, Andreasen N, Eriksson S, et al. Donepezil in Alzheimer's disease: what to expect after 3 years of treatment in a routine clinical setting. Dement Geriatr Cogn Disord 2007;23:150–60.

94. Wallin A, Gustafson L, Sjogren M, et al. Five-year outcome of cholinergic treatment of Alzheimer's disease: early response predicts prolonged time until nursing home placement, but does not alter life expectancy. Dement Geriatr Cogn Disord 2004;18(2):197–206.

95. Wallin A, Wattmo C, Minthon L. Galantamine treatment in Alzheimer's disease: response and long-term outcome in a routine clinical setting. Neuropsychiatr Dis Treat 2011;7:565–76.

96. Petersen RC, Thomas RG, Grundman M, et al. Vitamin E and donepezil for the treatment of mild cognitive impairment. N Engl J Med 2005;352(23):2379–88.

97. Lu PH, Edland SD, Teng E, et al. Donepezil delays progression to AD in MCI subjects with depressive symptoms. Neurology 2009;72(24):2115–21.

98. McShane R, Areosa Sastre A, Minakaran N. Memantine for dementia. Cochrane database Syst Rev 2006;(2):CD003154.

99. Winblad B, Poritis N. Memantine in severe dementia: results of the 9M-Best Study (Benefit and efficacy in severely demented patients during treatment with memantine). Int J Geriatr Psychiatry 1999;14(2):135–46.

100. Reisberg B, Doody R, Stoffler A, et al. Memantine in moderate-to-severe Alzheimer's disease. N Engl J Med 2003;348(14):1333–41.

101. Bullock R. Efficacy and safety of memantine in moderate-to-severe Alzheimer disease: the evidence to date. Alzheimer Dis Assoc Disord 2006;20(1):23–9.

102. Doody R, Wirth Y, Schmitt F, et al. Specific functional effects of memantine treatment in patients with moderate to severe Alzheimer's disease. Demenr Geriatr Cogn Disord 2004;18(2):227–32.

103. Grossberg GT, Pejovic V, Miller ML, et al. Memantine therapy of behavioral symptoms in community-dwelling patients with moderate to severe Alzheimer's disease. Dement Geriatr Cogn Disord 2009;27(2):164–72.

104. Schmitt F, van Dyck C, Wichems C, et al, Memantine MEM-MD-02 Study Group. Cognitive response to memantine in moderate to severe Alzheimer disease patients already receiving donepezil: an exploratory reanalysis. Alzheimer Dis Assoc Disord 2006;20:255–62.

105. van Dyck CH, Tariot PN, Meyers B, et al. A 24-week randomized, controlled trial of memantine in patients with moderate-to-severe Alzheimer disease. Alzheimer Dis Assoc Disord 2007;21(2):136–43.

106. Wilcock G, Ballard C, Cooper J, et al. Memantine for agitation/aggression and psychosis in moderately severe to severe Alzheimer's disease: a pooled analysis of 3 studies. J Clin Psychiatry 2008;69:341–8.

107. Wilkinson D, Andersen H. Analysis of the effect of memantine in reducing the worsening of clinical symptoms in patients with moderate to severe Alzheimer's disease. Dement Geriatr Cogn Disord 2007;24:138–45.

108. Wimo A, Winblad B, Stoffler A, et al. Resource utilisation and cost analysis of memantine in patients with moderate to severe Alzheimer's disease. Pharmacoeconomics 2003;21(5):327–40.

109. Winblad B, Jones R, Wirth Y, et al. Memantine in moderate to severe Alzheimer's disease: a meta-analysis of randomised clinical trials. Dement Geriatr Cogn Disord 2007;24:20–7.

110. Livingston G, Katona C. The place of memantine in the treatment of Alzheimer's disease: a number needed to treat analysis. Int J Geriatr Psychiatry 2004; 19(10):919–25.

111. Puangthong U, Hsiung GY. Critical appraisal of the long-term impact of memantine in treatment of moderate to severe Alzheimer's disease. Neuropsychiatr Dis Treat 2009;5:553–61.

112. Abbott BP, Abbott R, Adhikari R, et al. All-sky LIGO search for periodic gravitational waves in the early fifth-science-run data. Phys Rev Lett 2009;102(11): 111102.

113. Wilkinson D, Schindler R, Schwam E, et al. Effectiveness of donepezil in reducing clinical worsening in patients with mild-to-moderate Alzheimer's disease. Dement Geriatr Cogn Disord 2009;28:244–51.

114. Atri A, Shaughnessy L, Locascio J, et al. Long-term course and effectiveness of combination therapy in Alzheimer disease. Alzheimer Dis Assoc Disord 2008; 22:209–21.

115. Rountree S, Chan W, Pavlik V, et al. Persistent treatment with cholinesterase inhibitors and/or memantine slows clinical progression of Alzheimer disease. Alzheimers Res Ther 2009;1(2):7.

116. Chou YY, Lepore N, Avedissian C, et al. Mapping correlations between ventricular expansion and CSF amyloid and tau biomarkers in 240 subjects with Alzheimer's disease, mild cognitive impairment and elderly controls. Neuroimage 2009;46(2):394–410.

117. Lopez OL, Becker JT, Wahed AS, et al. Long-term effects of the concomitant use of memantine with cholinesterase inhibition in Alzheimer disease. J Neurol Neurosurg Psychiatry 2009;80(6):600–7.

118. Gillette-Guyonnet S, Andrieu S, Nourhashemi F, et al. Long-term progression of Alzheimer's disease in patients under antidementia drugs. Alzheimers Dement 2011;7(6):579–92.

119. Vellas B, Hausner L, Frolich L, et al. Progression of Alzheimer disease in Europe: data from the European ICTUS study. Curr Alzheimer Res 2012;9(8):902–12.
120. Tariot P, Farlow M, Grossberg G, et al. Memantine treatment in patients with moderate to severe Alzheimer disease already receiving donepezil: a randomized controlled trial. JAMA 2004;291:317–24.
121. Porsteinsson A, Grossberg G, Mintzer J, et al. Memantine treatment in patients with mild to moderate Alzheimer's disease already receiving a cholinesterase inhibitor: a randomized, double-blind, placebo-controlled trial. Curr Alzheimer Res 2008;5:83–9.
122. Patel L, Grossberg G. Combination therapy for Alzheimer's disease. Drugs & aging 2011;28:539–46.
123. Molinuevo JL. Memantine: the value of combined therapy. Rev Neurol 2011; 52(2):95–100 [in Spanish].
124. Gauthier S, Molinuevo JL. Benefits of combined cholinesterase inhibitor and memantine treatment in moderate-severe Alzheimer's disease. Alzheimers Dement 2013;9(3):326–31.
125. Choi SH, Park KW, Na DL, et al. Tolerability and efficacy of memantine add-on therapy to rivastigmine transdermal patches in mild to moderate Alzheimer's disease: a multicenter, randomized, open-label, parallel-group study. Curr Med Res Opin 2011;27(7):1375–83.
126. Grossberg GT, Manes F, Allegri RF, et al. The safety, tolerability, and efficacy of once-daily memantine (28 mg): a multinational, randomized, double-blind, placebo-controlled trial in patients with moderate-to-severe Alzheimer's disease taking cholinesterase inhibitors. CNS Drugs 2013;27(6):469–78.
127. Sano M, Ernesto C, Thomas RG, et al. A controlled trial of selegiline, alpha-tocopherol, or both as treatment for Alzheimer's disease. The Alzheimer's Disease Cooperative Study. N Engl J Med 1997;336(17):1216–22.
128. Dysken MW, Sano M, Asthana S, et al. Effect of vitamin E and memantine on functional decline in Alzheimer disease: the TEAM-AD VA cooperative randomized trial. JAMA 2014;311(1):33–44.
129. Shah RC, Kamphuis PJ, Leurgans S, et al. The S-Connect study: results from a randomized, controlled trial of Souvenaid in mild-to-moderate Alzheimer's disease. Alzheimers Res Ther 2013;5(6):59.
130. Wattmo C, Wallin AK, Londos E, et al. Predictors of long-term cognitive outcome in Alzheimer's disease. Alzheimers Res Ther 2011;3(4):23.
131. van der Steen JT, Radbruch L, Hertogh CM, et al. White paper defining optimal palliative care in older people with dementia: a Delphi study and recommendations from the European Association for Palliative Care. Palliat Med 2014;28(3):197–209.
132. Stern Y. Cognitive reserve. Neuropsychologia 2009;47:2015–28.
133. Seshadri S, Wolf PA, Beiser A, et al. Lifetime risk of dementia and Alzheimer's disease. The impact of mortality on risk estimates in the Framingham Study. Neurology 1997;49(6):1498–504.
134. Salthouse TA. When does age-related cognitive decline begin? Neurobiol Aging 2009;30(4):507–14.
135. Weintraub S, Dikmen SS, Heaton RK, et al. Cognition assessment using the NIH Toolbox. Neurology 2013;80(11 Suppl 3):S54–64.
136. Cummings JL, Mega M, Gray K, et al. The Neuropsychiatric Inventory: comprehensive assessment of psychopathology in dementia. Neurology 1994;44(12):2308–14.

Cerebrovascular Disease
Primary and Secondary Stroke Prevention

Fan Z. Caprio, MD*, Farzaneh A. Sorond, MD, PhD

KEYWORDS

- Stroke • Vascular risk factor • Primary stroke prevention
- Secondary stroke prevention • Stroke mechanism • Stroke etiology • Antiplatelets
- Anticoagulants

KEY POINTS

- Stroke, as the fourth leading cause of death and the number one cause of long-term disability in the United States, is a significant public health concern.
- Treatment of vascular risk factors is the most effective strategy for primary stroke prevention.
- Timely treatment of acute ischemic stroke with systemic thrombolysis and mechanical thrombectomy leads to improved functional outcomes.
- Prevention of stroke recurrence (secondary stroke prevention) as well as other associated vascular events should be tailored to specific stroke etiologies and patient risk factors.

INTRODUCTION

Over the past few decades, mortality due to cerebrovascular disease has decreased, likely due to earlier diagnosis and aggressive management of vascular risk factors with lifestyle modification and medical treatments. Despite these advances, stroke remains a leading cause of death and long-term disability worldwide, and disparities exist in stroke risk, rates of stroke, and treatment. Nonmodifiable risk factors of age, ethnicity, genetics, and family history contribute to significant stroke risk. Implementation of effective primary stroke prevention strategies for modifiable risk factors is of utmost importance to reduce the burden of stroke in an aging population.

Primary Prevention

In patients without a prior stroke or transient ischemic attack (TIA), treatments and interventions are considered primary stroke prevention. Potentially modifiable risk

Disclosures: No disclosures.
Division of Stroke and Neurocritical Care, Northwestern University Feinberg School of Medicine, 625 North Michigan Avenvue, Suite 1150, Chicago, IL 60611, USA
* Corresponding author.
E-mail address: Fan.Caprio@nm.org

Med Clin N Am 103 (2019) 295–308
https://doi.org/10.1016/j.mcna.2018.10.001
0025-7125/19/© 2018 Elsevier Inc. All rights reserved.

medical.theclinics.com

factors are associated with 90% of attributable risk for stroke worldwide; these include hypertension, smoking, obesity, diet, physical inactivity, diabetes, alcohol intake, psychosocial factors, cardiac disease, and apolipoprotein ratios.[1] Hypertension, hyperlipidemia, diabetes mellitus, obesity, and smoking are risk factors most closely linked to cardiovascular deaths, including those from cerebrovascular disease, ischemic heart disease, and systemic vascular disease.[2]

Therefore, the most effective strategy for preventing the first-ever stroke is through the control of identified modifiable risk factors. Specific risk factors and treatments are discussed in the next section.

HYPERTENSION

Hypertension is the single most important modifiable risk factor for stroke; more than half of all strokes worldwide are attributed to hypertension.[1,3] More than 90% to 95% of hypertension is of primary origin or due to genetic or general lifestyle factors.[4] The other 5% to 10% are considered secondary hypertension due to chronic or provoking disorders such as renal artery stenosis, endocrine tumors, or drug side effects. Primary hypertension is treated by ways of lifestyle modification and pharmacologic treatments. Recently revised recommendations aimed at individualizing risk assessment now define normal blood pressure as less than 120/80 mm Hg.[5] Lifestyle modifications including lowering dietary salt intake, avoiding excessive alcohol use, and effective weight control are recommended for those with blood pressure greater than 120/90 mm Hg and at low 10-year risk of a cardiovascular event (atherosclerotic cardiovascular disease risk, see later discussion). Patients with stage I hypertension as defined by blood pressure greater than 130/80 mm Hg with high 10-year risk of a cardiovascular event should be treated with antihypertensive medication in addition to lifestyle modifications. Several classes of antihypertensive medications are available, including beta-blockers, calcium channel blockers, diuretics, angiotensin-converting enzyme (ACE) inhibitors, and angiotensin II receptor blockers (ARB). Antihypertensive medication selection depends on individual comorbidities. For example, beta- or calcium channel blocker also provides heart rate control in patients with atrial fibrillation (AF); ACE inhibitors are renally protective in patients with diabetes. Otherwise, initial monotherapy for primary hypertension with a thiazide diuretic, ACE inhibitor, ARB, or dihydropyridine calcium channel blocker is reasonable.[5,6] Blood pressure control is more important than the medication choice. Many patients require combination treatment to achieve adequate blood pressure control. Despite multiple studies demonstrating the benefit of blood pressure lowering in older patients with hypertension,[7] patients older than 65 years have the lowest rates of adequate blood pressure control.[8] Although the same general principles should be followed in treating hypertension in older patients, one should bear in mind the physiologic changes that occur with aging and consider initial dose adjustments to avoid side effects such as dizziness.[8,9]

DIABETES MELLITUS

Diabetes mellitus (DM), a group of metabolic disorders that lead to elevated glucose levels in the vasculature, is known to cause microvascular (retinopathy, nephropathy, neuropathy) as well as macrovascular complications including stroke, cardiovascular, and peripheral vascular disease. The American Diabetes Association recommends assessment of fasting blood sugar, glucose tolerance, or A1C level in all at-risk patients and those older than 45 years for screening of prediabetes or diabetes.[10] Long-term glycemic control to A1C less than 7% in newly diagnosed type 2 DM patients is likely beneficial[11]; however, no randomized study has shown a clear beneficial effect of strict glycemic control on macrovascular outcomes in those with long-standing diabetes. Although strict glycemic control improves outcomes for microvascular disease in DM,[12] a multifaceted approach at glycemic control along with other vascular risk factor control, such as hypertension and dyslipidemia, is most beneficial for prevention of macrovascular (cerebral, cardiac, and peripheral vascular) disease.[13]

HYPERLIPIDEMIA

Most studies show that elevated total high cholesterol is a risk factor for stroke. Several prevention trials and meta-analyses have shown decreased vascular events and mortality rates in patients treated with statins for lipid (specifically LDL cholesterol) lowering.[14] The benefit of statins seems to be applicable across high-, moderate-, and low-risk groups.[15] Although weight management, healthy diet, and routine exercise should be encouraged in all patients with hyperlipidemia, determining when and in whom to start statin therapy is more controversial. Most guidelines recommend treatment for patients at higher levels of risk based on calculations of an estimated risk of a future cardiovascular event. For example, the AHA recommends treatment with moderate- or high-intensity statin in patients with an estimated 10-year cardiovascular disease risk of greater than 7.5%[16] (**Table 1**).

The only randomized trial of statins in stroke (SPARCL), evaluated the benefit of statin use in secondary stroke prevention, where patients with ischemic and hemorrhagic strokes were randomized to high-intensity statin (atorvastatin 80 mg daily) or placebo.[17] Patients in the statin arm had a significant stroke risk reduction. Although the relationship between lipid levels and initial stroke incidence is complex and studies of lipid lowering in primary stroke prevention are lacking, statins have become a mainstay in secondary stroke prevention, particularly in strokes related to large artery and small vessel atherosclerosis.

SMOKING

Smoking is a leading modifiable risk factor for cerebrovascular disease, with a dose-dependent increase in ischemic and hemorrhagic strokes.[18,19] Mechanisms linking

Table 1 Atherosclerotic cardiovascular disease risk factors	
ASCVD Risk Factor	Answer Units
Age	Years
Race	White/African American/Other
Sex	Male/Female
Systolic Blood Pressure	mm Hg
Total Cholesterol	mg/dL
High-Density Lipoprotein	mg/dL
Diabetes	Yes/No
HTN treatment	Yes/No
Smoking	Yes/No

These factors, along with prior history of vascular events, are taken into account when assessing and estimating an individual's 10-year risk of a cardiovascular (stroke or coronary) event.
Abbreviations: ASCVD, atherosclerotic cardiovascular disease; HTN, hypertension treatment.

smoking to vascular injury include endothelial damage, sympathetic activation, free radical generation, and inflammation.[20] Although there are no randomized studies for smoking cessation in primary or secondary stroke prevention, robust observational data show significant decrease in vascular risk after a few months of abstinence with elimination of risk after 5 years.[19,21–23] All cigarette smokers should be counseled to quit and abstain. Effective tobacco cessation strategies include behavioral therapy, nicotine replacement, other pharmacologic treatments, or a combination.

OTHER MODIFIABLE RISK FACTORS

Obesity, physical inactivity, and poor diet are also well-documented risk factors for stroke. Each is difficult to study in isolation due to the complex interaction and contributions to other cerebrovascular risk factors such as hypertension, diabetes, and dyslipidemia. Therapeutic lifestyle changes alone have a significant impact on these risk factors and can decrease the risk of cerebrovascular disease by up to 55%.[24]

Obesity, described as body mass index greater than 30 kg/m^2, affects up to 40% of the US population and its prevalence has multiplied at alarming rates in the past few decades, making it a top public health concern over the last decade. In patients with obesity, weight has a linear relationship with cardiovascular morbidity and mortality. Weight reduction leads to lower risk of stroke as well as myocardial infarction (MI), diabetes, and hypertension.[25] Treatment of obesity includes behavioral modification, diet, and exercise, although treatment selection depends on willingness and individual risk.

Physical inactivity has been linked to increased stroke incidence in observational studies. Exercise is protective against stroke risk, however, the relationship between intensity and type of exercise and stroke reduction is unclear. Adults are recommended to perform at least moderate-intensity aerobic activities for at least 40 minutes daily for 3 to 4 days weekly. Some of the benefit from exercise may be mediated by improvements in hypertension, diabetes, hyperlipidemia, and excess weight.[26]

Poor Diet: observational studies consistently show that people who eat healthily (rich in fruits, vegetables, fiber, omega-fatty acids, and monounsaturated fats such as in the Mediterranean diet) have lower rates of cardiovascular and cerebrovascular disease.[27] Lowering intake of sodium and increasing intake of potassium, along with a diet emphasizing fruits, vegetables, and low-fat dairy products is also recommended for lowering blood pressure and may decrease risk of stroke.[25]

ANTIPLATELETS IN PRIMARY CEREBROVASCULAR PREVENTION

Several randomized trials and meta-analyses have evaluated the efficacy and safety of aspirin (acetylsalicylic acid [ASA]) on cardiovascular disease. Overall, ASA provides a reduction in MI and all-cause mortality but no significant benefit in stroke prevention. Bleeding events offset the benefit of ASA in vascular prevention.[28–31] The USPSTF recommends low-dose ASA for men and women based on vascular risk and gastrointestinal hemorrhage.[32] Similarly, the AHA considers ASA to be reasonable for cardiovascular (including but not specific to stroke) prevention for those with a moderate-high 10-year risk.[25]

Primary prevention strategies for specific stroke mechanisms (AF, carotid stenosis) are reviewed in the next section in addition to secondary prevention.

In summary, primary stroke prevention in the general population is most successful when lifestyle modifications are made to lower multiple major risk factors.[33,34] Cerebrovascular risk factors are additive and possibly compounding. For example, having 5 vascular risk factors may pose a similar 10-year risk as that of person with a prior stroke or MI.[35] When recommending treatment, estimates of relative risk can be calculated based on number of traditional risk factors. Aggressive treatment of these risk factors is highly recommended for primary stroke prevention. In those with moderate to high risk of cardio- or cerebrovascular disease, the addition of statins and aspirin should be considered and tailored to the individual patient. Additional factors (such as renal disease or bleeding risk) should be considered when assessing individual patients. Unfortunately, there remains a gap between these evidence-based recommendations for lifestyle and medical interventions and their application in clinical practice and stroke prevention programs.

Acute Stroke Recognition and Treatments

In the acute setting of an ischemic stroke, timely treatment, even small reductions on the order of minutes, leads to significant increase in disability free life.[36,37] Intravenous tissue plasminogen activator (IV tPA) is an approved medication shown to improve functional outcomes when delivered within 3 hours of ischemic stroke onset and within 4.5 hours in select patients.[38] IV tPA seems to cause similar benefit in patients with different stroke subtypes (cardioembolic, large vessel, and small vessel disease)[39]; however, intracranial large vessel occlusions (LVO) are often refractory to IV tPA alone, which is then associated with poorer outcomes.[40] In 2014 to 2015, several large trials showed that direct, catheter-based endovascular treatments within 6 hours of stroke symptom onset in addition to IV tPA improved functional outcomes in patients with imaging-confirmed intracranial LVO.[41–45] DAWN and DEFUSE-3 further extended the treatment window for patients with LVO to up to 24 hours in those with small core infarction and significant salvageable penumbra as measured by CT or MR perfusion imaging.[46,47] Access to these extremely time-sensitive treatments requires rapid detection of acute stroke syndromes and complex coordination between emergency response teams, emergency room (including imaging and laboratory) staff, and neurology and interventional care providers.

Secondary Stroke Prevention

Secondary stroke prevention is about preventing recurrent stroke after an initial stroke or TIA. Most patients survive a first-time ischemic stroke but are at high risk for recurrent stroke as well as concomitant cardio- and peripheral vascular diseases. Patients are at highest risk of stroke in the first few days after TIA; therefore, rapid evaluation of stroke risk is of utmost importance. Secondary stroke prevention is targeted at mechanisms responsible for the index stroke. Generally speaking, a parallel goal is successful management of known vascular risk factors; this is likely as effective in secondary as it is in primary prevention. However, identifying stroke etiology for secondary prevention allows for more tailored medical treatments such as utilization of the appropriate antithrombotic regimen.

Mechanisms

In the United States, approximately 87% of strokes are ischemic and 13% are hemorrhagic, whereas worldwide, 68% of strokes are ischemic and 32% hemorrhagic.[48,49] This discussion here focuses on the ischemic type. Amongst ischemic strokes, cardioembolism, large vessel atherosclerosis, and small vessel disease account for 65% of cases; the remaining are due to other definite causes, 2 or more defined causes, or considered cryptogenic (**Fig. 1**).

Cardioembolism

Embolism from the heart accounts for approximately 25% of ischemic stroke cases. These can occur in setting of AF; cardiomyopathy; MI and left ventricular (LV)

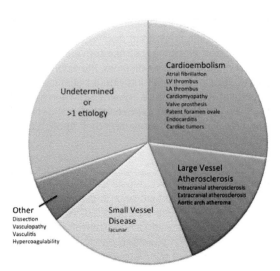

Fig. 1. More common causes of stroke can be categorized into several large subtypes of stroke, as classified by TOAST criteria. (*Data from* Adams HP Jr, Bendixen BH, Kappelle LJ, et al. Classification of subtype of acute ischemic stroke. Definitions for use in a multicenter clinical trial. TOAST. Trial of org 10172 in acute stroke treatment. Stroke 1993;24(1):35–41.)

thrombus; valve prostheses; patent foramen ovale (reviewed later); and other potential risk factors such as valvular disease, cardiac tumors, and paradoxic embolus.

AF accounts for 10% to 12% of all ischemic strokes and is typically detected on electrocardiograms or telemetry or on subsequent prolonged rhythm monitoring after stroke. Occult AF may be the underlying mechanism for up to one-third of cryptogenic strokes.[50] Oral anticoagulation with the vitamin K antagonist (VKA) warfarin or direct-acting oral anticoagulants (DOAC), such as thrombin inhibitor dabigatran or factor Xa inhibitor apixaban, is indicated for secondary prevention of stroke in patients with non-valvular AF.[25,51] Anticoagulation is also indicated for primary stroke prevention in AF with moderate-high risk of embolic events as calculated by the CHA2DS2-VASc score.[52] Selection of an oral anticoagulant should be individualized based on a patient's specific risk factors (ie, renal function), tolerability, and preference. Patients should be counseled on the increased risk of bleeding associated with systemic anticoagulation. Oral anticoagulants are generally underused for stroke prevention in AF[53]; however, the use of direct inhibitors may continue to increase after the recent approval for reversal agents.

Recent myocardial infarction and left ventricular thrombus
After large MI, wall motion abnormalities increase risk for mural thrombus formation and subsequent embolization. VKA anticoagulation for 3 months is indicated for secondary prevention after stroke due to LV thrombus. Concomitant use of dual antiplatelets (after cardiac stent placement) and anticoagulation (after embolic stroke)—so-called "triple therapy"—is controversial given the elevated bleeding risk, specifically hemorrhagic conversion after large cerebral infarction.

Cardiomyopathy
Patients with dilated cardiomyopathy are at increased stroke risk, likely due to turbulent or stagnant blood flow and occult thrombus formation. Additional risk factors include lower cardiac ejection fraction (EF) and prior stroke. Several randomized trials

evaluating antithrombotic options in patients with low EF in sinus rhythm show a reduction in ischemic stroke risk but an increase in major bleeding, including intracranial hemorrhages.[54] Barring finding of atrial or ventricular thrombi, the benefit of anticoagulation versus antiplatelets in patients with dilated or restrictive cardiomyopathy is unclear and the decision should be made on basis of the individual's risk. Mechanical LV assist devices are used in patients with advanced heart failure and carry a significant yearly stroke risk[55]; anticoagulation with warfarin is reasonable for secondary prevention barring major contraindications. Use of DOAC for stroke prevention in patients with cardiomyopathy has not been sufficiently studied. Atrial cardiopathy is an emerging mechanism for cardioembolic stroke and is under investigation.

Prosthetic heart valve

Patients with mechanical heart valves are at an increased risk for cerebral and systemic thromboembolic events, and VKA anticoagulation is recommended for secondary stroke prevention. The ideal international normalized ratio (INR) range depends on valve position and history of prior embolism. Increasing ASA dose and INR goals are considered reasonable approaches in patients with recurrent strokes despite initial anticoagulation.

Patients with bioprosthetic heart valves are at a lower risk for stroke than those with mechanical valves. Postsurgical occult AF may influence individual patient risk. Anticoagulation is typically used for 3 to 6 months after bioprosthetic valve placement, followed by long-term antiplatelet use.

Patent foramen ovale

About 25% of the general population has a patent foramen ovale (PFO).[56] When a PFO is detected (typically by echocardiography) during stroke workup for otherwise undetermined source, it is prudent to evaluate for visible thromboembolism (VTE) from the venous system causing paradoxic embolus. The presence of PFO alone is associated with cryptogenic stroke, particularly in younger patients (<55 years) with substantial right- to left-sided shunting and atrial septal aneurysm. Several earlier trials failed to show a clear benefit of PFO closure in secondary stroke prevention compared with medical management. Criticisms of these trials included usage of older closure devices, shorter follow-up timeframe, and patient selection. Since then, several additional studies, including a 5-year follow-up study of RESPECT, did show statistically significant reduction in stroke recurrence after PFO closure compared with medical treatment alone, with the greatest benefit in those with associated atrial septal aneurysm and more substantial shunts.[57,58] These patients were younger than 60 years and completed testing to rule out other potential causes of embolic stroke such as arterial stenosis and VTE. After a comprehensive search for stroke etiology, PFO closure may be considered for long-term secondary stroke prevention. Patients should be counseled on the increased risk of atrial fibrillation after PFO closure as seen in the recent studies and its potential implications.

Large vessel atherosclerosis

Cervical or extracranial carotid stenosis carries a high risk for recurrent strokes. Stroke can occur as a result of plaque rupture and artery-to-artery embolism or hemodynamic failure from critical stenosis. Treatment options for secondary stroke prevention are aimed at plaque stabilization and restoration of blood flow. Surgical and medical approaches are reviewed later.

Carotid endarterectomy Randomized studies including NASCET, ECST, and VACS have compared carotid endarterectomy (CEA) plus medical therapy with medical therapy alone and demonstrated superiority of the surgical group for prevention of recurrent stroke in patients with severe symptomatic stenosis (>70% stenosis). The benefit in moderate (50%–69%) stenosis was less pronounced favoring CEA, and there was no benefit of CEA for mild (<50%) stenosis for stroke prevention. Current recommendations are for patients with recent stroke due to ipsilateral severe carotid stenosis to undergo CEA for stroke prevention, if perioperative complications are less than 6%.[51] Similar recommendations are made for moderate-degree carotid stenosis in select patients with a favorable risk-benefit ratio considering age, sex, comorbidities, and perioperative risk.[51] To maximize benefit, CEA should ideally take place within 14 days of initial stroke barring contraindications including prohibitively large infarct burden.[59]

Carotid stenting and angioplasty Less invasive percutaneous treatments including carotid artery stenting (CAS) and angioplasty for symptomatic carotid stenosis have been studied in comparison with CEA in several randomized trials (CAVATAS, CREST, EVA3, SAPPHIRE, ICSS, SPACE) and meta-analyses.[60] Overall, older patients (>70 years) with favorable cervical anatomy had better outcomes from CEA compared with CAS, and similar periprocedural complications and future stroke risk were seen in younger patients in the 2 groups. Generally, CAS is a recommended alternative to CEA for patients with moderate-severe symptomatic carotid stenosis with reasonable low risk of perioperative complications.

Medical management Long-term secondary stroke prevention from symptomatic carotid stenosis includes an antiplatelet and statin regimen, as well as risk factor reduction for atherosclerotic disease. In the acute setting just after initial stroke, blood pressure should be judiciously monitored, and sudden relative hypotension should be avoided to preserve cerebral perfusion particularly in severe carotid stenosis.

For primary prevention of stroke in asymptomatic carotid atherosclerosis, intensive medical therapy should be mainstay of treatment. This includes risk reduction strategies of blood pressure control, lifestyle modification of smoking cessation, weight control, exercise regimen and healthy diet, as well as antiplatelet and statin therapy. Higher-risk features include progression in stenosis severity, presence of asymptomatic emboli (detected as silent infarcts on imaging or microembolic signal on transcranial doppler), ulcerated plaque or other morphologic abnormalities, and insufficient cerebrovascular reserve.[61] ACAS, ACST, and the VA study showed beneficial outcomes after CEA over medical treatments in asymptomatic carotid stenosis of 60% to 99%. Surgical revascularization may be considered for select patients who are medically stable, at particularly high risk of stroke from asymptomatic carotid stenosis, and in whom perioperative risk is acceptably low (<3%). Ultimately, routine CEA and CAS have not been sufficiently studied in comparison with modern medical therapies for purposes of primary stroke prevention; this is an area for further study given significant advancements in available medical treatments as well as surgical techniques.

Intracranial atherosclerotic disease

Intracranial atherosclerotic disease (ICAD) refers to atherosclerotic disease affecting the large intracranial vessels including internal carotid artery (ICA), middle cerebral artery (MCA), and basilar artery (BA); it carries a particularly high risk of recurrent stroke. ICAD is one of the most common causes of stroke worldwide and is more prevalent amongst blacks, Hispanics, and Asians in comparison with whites.[62,63] The SAMMPRIS trial showed significant benefit in stroke reduction in patients treated with short-term dual antiplatelets (DAPT) and aggressive medical management compared with those treated with angioplasty and stenting.[64] Intensive medical therapies are accepted as the initial strategy for secondary stroke prevention. Single antiplatelets and DAPT regimens have not been sufficiently compared in this population but short course of DAPT are generally considered safe. Angioplasty and stent placement may be considered in patients with recurrent strokes despite maximal medical therapies.

Arch atheroma

Atheromatous disease in the aortic arch is an important potential cause of large artery embolic stroke. Many studies have shown an association between aortic plaque disease and cerebrovascular events, including identification of larger (>4 mm) plaques as an independent risk factor for recurrent strokes.[65] Additional risk factors include atheroma morphology (large, complex), lack of calcification, and growth and mobile components. One randomized trial comparing DAPT with VKA anticoagulation for stroke prevention was stopped prematurely and did not detect a difference in preventing cerebral infarction.[66] Antiplatelet and statin treatments remain the mainstay of secondary stroke prevention in patients with arch atheromatous disease. Surgical resection is not indicated.

Small vessel disease

Also known as lacunar disease, stroke from small vessel disease (SVD) occurs as a result of pathologic changes such a lipohyalinosis, fibrinoid necrosis, or intimal hyperplasia. SVD accounts for up to 25% of all ischemic strokes. Classical clinical syndromes of lacunar stroke include pure motor hemiparesis, ataxia hemiparesis, dysarthria-clumsy hand, and pure sensory and mixed sensorimotor presentations. Secondary stroke prevention in small vessel pathology is generally through antiplatelet and statin therapy along with control of vascular risk factors. Multiple studies have compared different antithrombotic regimens in noncardioembolic stroke and ultimately any benefit of recurrent stroke reduction with anticoagulation and DAPT was countered by increased bleeding complications, although short-term DAPT use may be safe. The Chinese CHANCE study and a similar US study POINT compared short-term (21 and 90 days, respectively) DAPT with a single antiplatelet regimen in patients with minor stroke and high-risk TIA and showed a reduction in recurrent stroke in the DAPT group at 90 days.[67,68]

Other stroke etiologies

- Blood disorders
  - Antiphospholipid syndrome (APS) is an antibody-mediated syndrome associated with a hypercoagulable state, which predisposes to arterial and venous thromboembolism. Optimal antithrombotic regimen for secondary prevention of stroke in patients who fulfill criteria for APS has not been clearly established, although at least antiplatelet therapy is indicated, and anticoagulation is common.
  - Screening for inherited thrombophilia, such as protein C or S deficiency, antithrombin III deficiency, activated protein C resistance, factor V Leiden, and prothrombin gene mutation is, of unclear usefulness. These conditions are associated with a propensity for venous thromboses but not clearly associated with arterial thromboembolic events. Without evidence of VTE or recurrent strokes, either anticoagulation or antiplatelet therapy would be reasonable in these patients.
  - Sickle cell disease causes stroke via large vessel arteriopathy and possibly by hypercoagulability. Secondary stroke prevention entails reduction of

hemoglobin S (by transfusion or medication), antiplatelet treatment, and vascular risk factor reduction.

- Nonatherosclerotic arteriopathies include dissection, fibromuscular dysplasia, moyamoya disease, vasoconstriction disorders, and extracranial and intracranial vasculitides including Takayasu arteritis and primary arteritis of the central nervous system. Treatment of arteriopathies should be tailored to the specific stroke mechanism and might include revascularization therapies, immunosuppression, and antithrombotic treatment.
- Undetermined or cryptogenic stroke
  - As diagnostic tools have advanced, the original TOAST classification has been modified to include the likelihood of large artery, small artery atherosclerosis, cardioembolism, and other determined causes to be the likely stroke etiology. These are divided into categories of evident, probable, and possible levels of confidence.[69] A stroke of undetermined cause is further characterized as cryptogenic embolism (such as embolic stroke of undetermined source)[70]; other cryptogenic, incomplete evaluation; or unclassified wherein one probable cause cannot be established.

In conclusion, stroke is a heterogeneous disease with multiple additive risk factors and causes. Primary and secondary prevention of stroke should focus on reduction of known modifiable risk factors. Secondary prevention of recurrent strokes relies on the workup and a tailored treatment targeted at the mechanisms responsible for the incident stroke or TIA.

REFERENCES

1. O'Donnell MJ, Chin SL, Rangarajan S, et al. Global and regional effects of potentially modifiable risk factors associated with acute stroke in 32 countries (INTERSTROKE): a case-control study. Lancet 2016;388(10046):761–75.
2. Patel SA, Winkel M, Ali MK, et al. Cardiovascular mortality associated with 5 leading risk factors: national and state preventable fractions estimated from survey data. Ann Intern Med 2015;163(4):245–53.
3. Lawes CM, Vander Hoorn S, Rodgers A, et al. Global burden of blood-pressure-related disease, 2001. Lancet 2008;371(9623):1513–8.
4. Carretero OA, Oparil S. Essential hypertension. Part I: definition and etiology. Circulation 2000;101(3):329–35.
5. Whelton PK, Carey RM, Aronow WS, et al. 2017 ACC/AHA/AAPA/ABC/ACPM/AGS/APhA/ASH/ASPC/NMA/PCNA guideline for the prevention, detection, evaluation, and management of high blood pressure in adults: a report of the American College of Cardiology/American Heart Association task force on clinical practice guidelines. Hypertension 2018;71(6):e13–115.
6. Reboussin DM, Allen NB, Griswold ME, et al. Systematic review for the 2017 ACC/AHA/AAPA/ABC/ACPM/AGS/APhA/ASH/ASPC/NMA/PCNA guideline for the prevention, detection, evaluation, and management of high blood pressure in adults: a report of the American College of Cardiology/American Heart Association task force on clinical practice guidelines. Hypertension 2018;71(6):e116–35.
7. Lloyd-Jones DM, Evans JC, Levy D. Hypertension in adults across the age spectrum: current outcomes and control in the community. JAMA 2005;294(4):466–72.
8. Chobanian AV, Bakris GL, Black HR, et al. The seventh report of the joint national committee on prevention, detection, evaluation, and treatment of high blood pressure: the JNC 7 report. JAMA 2003;289(19):2560–72.

9. Pont L, Alhawassi T. Challenges in the management of hypertension in older populations. Adv Exp Med Biol 2017;956:167–80.
10. American Diabetes Association. Classification and diagnosis of diabetes: standards of medical care in diabetes-2018. Diabetes Care 2018;41(Suppl 1): S13–27.
11. Holman RR, Paul SK, Bethel MA, et al. 10-year follow-up of intensive glucose control in type 2 diabetes. N Engl J Med 2008;359(15):1577–89.
12. Hemmingsen B, Lund SS, Gluud C, et al. Targeting intensive glycaemic control versus targeting conventional glycaemic control for type 2 diabetes mellitus. Cochrane Database Syst Rev 2013;(11):CD008143.
13. Gaede P, Vedel P, Larsen N, et al. Multifactorial intervention and cardiovascular disease in patients with type 2 diabetes. N Engl J Med 2003;348(5):383–93.
14. Silverman MG, Ference BA, Im K, et al. Association between lowering LDL-C and cardiovascular risk reduction among different therapeutic interventions: a systematic review and meta-analysis. JAMA 2016;316(12):1289–97.
15. Cholesterol Treatment Trialists, Collaborators., Mihaylova B, Emberson J, Blackwell L, et al. The effects of lowering LDL cholesterol with statin therapy in people at low risk of vascular disease: meta-analysis of individual data from 27 randomised trials. Lancet 2012;380(9841):581–90.
16. Stone NJ, Robinson JG, Lichtenstein AH, et al. 2013 ACC/AHA guideline on the treatment of blood cholesterol to reduce atherosclerotic cardiovascular risk in adults: a report of the American College of Cardiology/American Heart Association task force on practice guidelines. Circulation 2014;129(25 Suppl 2):S1–45.
17. Amarenco P, Bogousslavsky J, Callahan A 3rd, et al. High-dose atorvastatin after stroke or transient ischemic attack. N Engl J Med 2006;355(6):549–59.
18. Ockene IS, Miller NH. Cigarette smoking, cardiovascular disease, and stroke: a statement for healthcare professionals from the American Heart Association. American Heart Association Task Force on Risk Reduction. Circulation 1997; 96(9):3243–7.
19. Wolf PA, D'Agostino RB, Kannel WB, et al. Cigarette smoking as a risk factor for stroke. The Framingham Study. JAMA 1988;259(7):1025–9.
20. Ambrose JA, Barua RS. The pathophysiology of cigarette smoking and cardiovascular disease: an update. J Am Coll Cardiol 2004;43(10):1731–7.
21. LaCroix AZ, Lang J, Scherr P, et al. Smoking and mortality among older men and women in three communities. N Engl J Med 1991;324(23):1619–25.
22. Kawachi I, Colditz GA, Stampfer MJ, et al. Smoking cessation and decreased risk of stroke in women. JAMA 1993;269(2):232–6.
23. Wannamethee SG, Shaper AG, Whincup PH, et al. Smoking cessation and the risk of stroke in middle-aged men. JAMA 1995;274(2):155–60.
24. Kurth T, Moore SC, Gaziano JM, et al. Healthy lifestyle and the risk of stroke in women. Arch Intern Med 2006;166(13):1403–9.
25. Meschia JF, Bushnell C, Boden-Albala B, et al. Guidelines for the primary prevention of stroke: a statement for healthcare professionals from the American Heart Association/American Stroke Association. Stroke 2014;45(12):3754–832.
26. Manson JE, Hu FB, Rich-Edwards JW, et al. A prospective study of walking as compared with vigorous exercise in the prevention of coronary heart disease in women. N Engl J Med 1999;341(9):650–8.
27. Sotos-Prieto M, Bhupathiraju SN, Mattei J, et al. Changes in diet quality scores and risk of cardiovascular disease among US men and women. Circulation 2015;132(23):2212–9.

28. Bartolucci AA, Tendera M, Howard G. Meta-analysis of multiple primary prevention trials of cardiovascular events using aspirin. Am J Cardiol 2011;107(12): 1796–801.

29. Raju N, Sobieraj-Teague M, Hirsh J, et al. Effect of aspirin on mortality in the primary prevention of cardiovascular disease. Am J Med 2011;124(7):621–9.

30. Antithrombotic Trialists, Collaboratuion, Baigent C, Blackwell L, Collins R, et al. Aspirin in the primary and secondary prevention of vascular disease: collaborative meta-analysis of individual participant data from randomised trials. Lancet 2009;373(9678):1849–60.

31. Guirguis-Blake JM, Evans CV, Senger CA, et al. Aspirin for the primary prevention of cardiovascular events: a systematic evidence review for the U.S. preventive services task force. Ann Intern Med 2016;164(12):804–13.

32. US Preventive Services Task Force. Aspirin for the prevention of cardiovascular disease: U.S. Preventive services task force recommendation statement. Ann Intern Med 2009;150(6):396–404.

33. Leening MJ, Berry JD, Allen NB. Lifetime perspectives on primary prevention of atherosclerotic cardiovascular disease. JAMA 2016;315(14):1449–50.

34. Chiuve SE, Rexrode KM, Spiegelman D, et al. Primary prevention of stroke by healthy lifestyle. Circulation 2008;118(9):947–54.

35. Jackson R, Lawes CM, Bennett DA, et al. Treatment with drugs to lower blood pressure and blood cholesterol based on an individual's absolute cardiovascular risk. Lancet 2005;365(9457):434–41.

36. Meretoja A, Keshtkaran M, Saver JL, et al. Stroke thrombolysis: save a minute, save a day. Stroke 2014;45(4):1053–8.

37. Meretoja A, Keshtkaran M, Tatlisumak T, et al. Endovascular therapy for ischemic stroke: Save a minute-save a week. Neurology 2017;88(22):2123–7.

38. Hacke W, Donnan G, Fieschi C, et al. Association of outcome with early stroke treatment: pooled analysis of ATLANTIS, ECASS, and NINDS rt-PA stroke trials. Lancet 2004;363(9411):768–74.

39. National Institute of Neurological Disorders and Stroke rt-PA Stroke Study Group. Tissue plasminogen activator for acute ischemic stroke. N Engl J Med 1995; 333(24):1581–7.

40. Rha JH, Saver JL. The impact of recanalization on ischemic stroke outcome: a meta-analysis. Stroke 2007;38(3):967–73.

41. Berkhemer OA, Fransen PS, Beumer D, et al. A randomized trial of intraarterial treatment for acute ischemic stroke. N Engl J Med 2015;372(1):11–20.

42. Goyal M, Demchuk AM, Menon BK, et al. Randomized assessment of rapid endovascular treatment of ischemic stroke. N Engl J Med 2015;372(11):1019–30.

43. Campbell BC, Mitchell PJ, EXTEND-IA Investigators. Endovascular therapy for ischemic stroke. N Engl J Med 2015;372(24):2365–6.

44. Jovin TG, Chamorro A, Cobo E, et al. Thrombectomy within 8 hours after symptom onset in ischemic stroke. N Engl J Med 2015;372(24):2296–306.

45. Saver JL, Goyal M, Bonafe A, et al. Stent-retriever thrombectomy after intravenous t-PA vs. t-PA alone in stroke. N Engl J Med 2015;372(24):2285–95.

46. Nogueira RG, Jadhav AP, Haussen DC, et al. Thrombectomy 6 to 24 hours after stroke with a mismatch between deficit and infarct. N Engl J Med 2018;378(1): 11–21.

47. Albers GW, Marks MP, Kemp S, et al. Thrombectomy for stroke at 6 to 16 hours with selection by perfusion imaging. N Engl J Med 2018;378(8):708–18.

48. Benjamin EJ, Blaha MJ, Chiuve SE, et al. Heart disease and stroke statistics-2017 update: a report from the American Heart Association. Circulation 2017;135(10): e146–603.

49. Krishnamurthi RV, Feigin VL, Forouzanfar MH, et al. Global and regional burden of first-ever ischaemic and haemorrhagic stroke during 1990-2010: findings from the global burden of disease study 2010. Lancet Glob Health 2013;1(5):e259–81.

50. Sanna T, Diener HC, Passman RS, et al. Cryptogenic stroke and underlying atrial fibrillation. N Engl J Med 2014;370(26):2478–86.

51. Kernan WN, Ovbiagele B, Black HR, et al. Guidelines for the prevention of stroke in patients with stroke and transient ischemic attack: a guideline for healthcare professionals from the American Heart Association/American Stroke Association. Stroke 2014;45(7):2160–236.

52. Lip GY, Nieuwlaat R, Pisters R, et al. Refining clinical risk stratification for predicting stroke and thromboembolism in atrial fibrillation using a novel risk factor-based approach: the euro heart survey on atrial fibrillation. Chest 2010;137(2): 263–72.

53. Hernandez I, Saba S, Zhang Y. Geographic variation in the use of oral anticoagulation therapy in stroke prevention in atrial fibrillation. Stroke 2017;48(8):2289–91.

54. Lee M, Saver JL, Hong KS, et al. Risk-benefit profile of warfarin versus aspirin in patients with heart failure and sinus rhythm: a meta-analysis. Circ Heart Fail 2013; 6(2):287–92.

55. Eckman PM, John R. Bleeding and thrombosis in patients with continuous-flow ventricular assist devices. Circulation 2012;125(24):3038–47.

56. Meissner I, Whisnant JP, Khandheria BK, et al. Prevalence of potential risk factors for stroke assessed by transesophageal echocardiography and carotid ultrasonography: the SPARC study. Stroke prevention: assessment of risk in a community. Mayo Clin Proc 1999;74(9):862–9.

57. Saver JL, Carroll JD, Thaler DE, et al. Long-term outcomes of patent foramen ovale closure or medical therapy after stroke. N Engl J Med 2017;377(11): 1022–32.

58. Abo-Salem E, Chaitman B, Helmy T, et al. Patent foramen ovale closure versus medical therapy in cases with cryptogenic stroke, meta-analysis of randomized controlled trials. J Neurol 2018;265(3):578–85.

59. Brott TG, Halperin JL, Abbara S, et al. 2011 ASA/ACCF/AHA/AANN/AANS/ACR/ ASNR/CNS/SAIP/SCAI/SIR/SNIS/SVM/SVS guideline on the management of patients with extracranial carotid and vertebral artery disease. Stroke 2011;42(8): e464–540.

60. Bonati LH, Lyrer P, Ederle J, et al. Percutaneous transluminal balloon angioplasty and stenting for carotid artery stenosis. Cochrane Database Syst Rev 2012;(9):CD000515.

61. Paraskevas KI, Spence JD, Veith FJ, et al. Identifying which patients with asymptomatic carotid stenosis could benefit from intervention. Stroke 2014;45(12): 3720–4.

62. Gorelick PB, Wong KS, Bae HJ, et al. Large artery intracranial occlusive disease: a large worldwide burden but a relatively neglected frontier. Stroke 2008;39(8): 2396–9.

63. Banerjee C, Chimowitz MI. Stroke caused by atherosclerosis of the major intracranial arteries. Circ Res 2017;120(3):502–13.

64. Chimowitz MI, Lynn MJ, Derdeyn CP, et al. Stenting versus aggressive medical therapy for intracranial arterial stenosis. N Engl J Med 2011;365(11):993–1003.

65. French Study of Aortic Plaques in Stroke Group, Amarenco P, Cohen A, Hommel M, et al. Atherosclerotic disease of the aortic arch as a risk factor for recurrent ischemic stroke. N Engl J Med 1996;334(19):1216–21.

66. Amarenco P, Davis S, Jones EF, et al. Clopidogrel plus aspirin versus warfarin in patients with stroke and aortic arch plaques. Stroke 2014;45(5):1248–57.

67. Wang Y, Wang Y, Zhao X, et al. Clopidogrel with aspirin in acute minor stroke or transient ischemic attack. N Engl J Med 2013;369(1):11–9.

68. Johnston SC, Easton JD, Farrant M, et al. Clopidogrel and aspirin in acute ischemic stroke and high-risk TIA. N Engl J Med 2018;379(3):215–25.

69. Ay H, Benner T, Arsava EM, et al. A computerized algorithm for etiologic classification of ischemic stroke: the causative classification of stroke system. Stroke 2007;38(11):2979–84.

70. Hart RG, Diener HC, Coutts SB, et al. Embolic strokes of undetermined source: the case for a new clinical construct. Lancet Neurol 2014;13(4):429–38.

Seizures and Epilepsy

Emily L. Johnson, MD

KEYWORDS

- Epilepsy • Seizure • Antiepileptic drugs • Epilepsy surgery • Women with epilepsy
- Epilepsy treatment • First seizure

KEY POINTS

- A seizure is a transient disruption of neurologic function caused by abnormal neuronal firing.
- Epilepsy is the condition of recurrent, unprovoked seizures.
- If epilepsy is refractory to two or more appropriately chosen antiepileptic drugs at therapeutic doses, patients should be referred to an epilepsy center.

INTRODUCTION
Symptoms and Definitions

An epileptic seizure is a "transient occurrence of signs and/or symptoms due to abnormal excessive or synchronous neuronal activity in the brain."[1] Depending on which areas of the brain are involved, epileptic seizures may consist of (among other symptoms) loss of awareness with body shaking, confusion, and difficulty responding; visual or other sensory symptoms; isolated posturing or jerking of a single limb; or brief loss of awareness. Seizures are provoked (eg, by hypoglycemia or alcohol withdrawal) or spontaneous, and spontaneous seizures may be caused by underlying epilepsy. Epilepsy is "a disorder of the brain characterized by an enduring predisposition to generate epileptic seizures."[1] Many patients with an isolated first seizure never have another seizure; however, after a second unprovoked seizure, the risk of recurrent seizures is high,[2] and individuals with two or more unprovoked seizures separated by at least 24 hours are diagnosed with epilepsy.[3] Similarly, individuals with a single seizure, but with a risk of future seizures of at least 60% (based on medical history or electroencephalogram [EEG]) are also considered to have epilepsy.[3]

Types of Seizures

The International League Against Epilepsy 2017 classification of seizure types emphasizes the origin of the seizure in the brain. Seizures may start in one location in the brain ("focal onset seizures"), or start in bilateral hemisphere networks simultaneously

Dr E.L. Johnson has no relevant financial disclosures.
Department of Neurology, Johns Hopkins School of Medicine, 600 North Wolfe Street, Baltimore, MD 21287, USA
E-mail address: ejohns92@jhmi.edu

Med Clin N Am 103 (2019) 309–324
https://doi.org/10.1016/j.mcna.2018.10.002
medical.theclinics.com
0025-7125/19/© 2018 Elsevier Inc. All rights reserved.

("generalized onset seizures").[4] Seizures are further classified depending on whether consciousness is retained or impaired (focal aware or focal impaired awareness seizures), and whether there is motor involvement. Specific symptoms and signs, such as automatisms, myoclonic jerks, or tonic-clonic activity, may be used to further classify the seizure.[4] The seizure origin, pattern of spread, and brain networks involved determine the signs and symptoms of a seizure. For example, a patient with a seizure starting in the left occipital region and spreading to both brain hemispheres may experience flashing lights and visual distortions in the right visual field, followed by bilateral tonic-clonic motor activity. Focal seizures with preserved awareness are also known as "simple partial" seizures or seizure auras, and focal seizures with impaired awareness are also known as "complex partial" seizures.

Seizures that lead to bilateral motor involvement often have a stiffening (tonic) phase, followed by a muscle jerking (clonic) phase, and are known as tonic-clonic seizures (also known as "grand mal" seizures).

One common type of seizure in children is the absence seizure, consisting of several seconds of staring and loss of awareness (occasionally with blinking or automatisms) followed by a quick return to consciousness, without confusion. These seizures are known colloquially as "petit mal" seizures.

The temporal lobe is the lobe most commonly involved in focal epilepsy. Temporal lobe seizures often consist of an aura of a gastric rising sensation followed by loss of awareness, frequently with oroalimentary automatisms and fumbling of the ipsilateral hand.

Types of Epilepsy

Depending on seizure origin in the brain, epilepsies are classified into generalized and focal epilepsies. Generalized epilepsies consist of abnormal brain activity involving both hemispheres at the onset, whereas focal epilepsies involve seizures with a localized origin (that may then spread).[5] Determining a patient's particular type of epilepsy is important, because antiepileptic drug (AED) choice is directed in part by epilepsy type.

Persons with a generalized epilepsy may have tonic-clonic seizures, absence seizures, myoclonic seizures, or atonic seizures. Persons with a focal epilepsy may have focal aware seizures, focal seizures with impaired awareness, or focal seizures that spread and become tonic-clonic seizures.[5]

EPIDEMIOLOGY

Each year, at least 170,000 individuals in the United States alone have a first seizure.[6,7] At least half do not go on to have further seizures; however, a proportion develop epilepsy.

Epilepsy affects at least 65 million people globally, most in underserved regions.[8] The rate in high-income countries is between 5 and 8/1000 persons affected.[8] The incidence and prevalence vary across the lifespan, with high rates in children younger than age 5, a low incidence of new cases in early adulthood, and an increase in new cases in adults older than 55.[9] The incidence continues to increase with age, and the rates of new-onset epilepsy in the elderly are higher than in any other age group. There is an estimated cumulative incidence of 4.4% by age 85.[10]

ETIOLOGIES

The most common etiologies of epilepsy vary across the lifespan. In children, genetic predisposition and congenital malformations or stroke are the most common causes.[10] Traumatic brain injury, infection, scarring, and tumors become significant causes in young adults. In older adults, stroke, neurodegenerative disease, and cerebrovascular disease are the most common causes.[10]

DIFFERENTIAL DIAGNOSIS

The differential diagnosis of an epileptic seizure must be considered when evaluating a person with a first seizure. In fact, one study of patients evaluated at a first seizure clinic found that 17% had had a "seizure mimic" rather than an epileptic seizure.[11] Syncope (particularly convulsive syncope)[12] is frequently mistaken for seizure. Other mimickers include transient ischemic attack; sleep disorders; panic disorders; other psychiatric conditions, such as dissociative disorders and psychogenic nonepileptic seizures[13]; complex migraine; medication intoxication or reaction; and transient global amnesia (**Box 1**). A careful history from the patient and from witnesses can help identify features, such as palpitations, tunnel vision, diaphoresis, and position changes, that are more suggestive of syncope,[14] and tongue biting (particularly of the lateral tongue)[15–18] or postictal confusion, which are more suggestive of seizure.

Some seizures are considered "provoked," if a toxic or metabolic cause within the previous 24 hours is identified. Hypoglycemia, severe hyponatremia, and other metabolic derangements are common causes of provoked seizures, as are alcohol withdrawal and exposure to certain illicit or prescribed drugs, such as cocaine or bupropion.

DIAGNOSTIC TESTS/IMAGING STUDIES

EEG and brain imaging are the mainstays of diagnostic testing for seizures and epilepsy; however, the EEG cannot "rule out" a seizure. A routine EEG consists of a 30-minute recording of brain activity as recorded by scalp electrodes. EEG after a first seizure shows an abnormality 12% to 73% of the time.[11,19] However, a normal EEG (**Fig. 1**) may be seen in up to 50% of people with epilepsy. After three EEGs, the likelihood of identifying an abnormality increases to 84%.[20] If the initial EEG did not capture sleep, it should be repeated: sleep-deprived EEGs, which capture drowsiness, have improved sensitivity over EEGs without state changes.[21] EEGs can detect focal sharp

Box 1
Differential diagnosis of epileptic seizures
Syncope and convulsive syncope
Medication intoxication or withdrawal
Migraine
Concussion
Transient ischemic attack
Dissociative episode
Psychogenic nonepileptic events
Panic attacks
Transient global amnesia
Sleep disorders

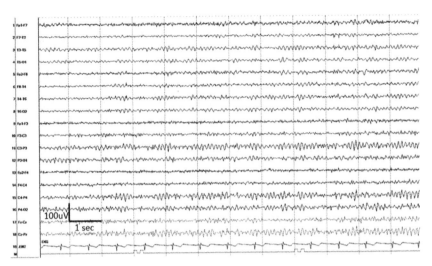

Fig. 1. A normal awake adult EEG.

waves or spikes characteristic of a focal epilepsy (**Fig. 2**), or bilateral (generalized) epileptiform activity characteristic of a generalized epilepsy (**Fig. 3**).

Brain imaging is important after a first seizure, to assess for serious conditions, such as hemorrhage, edema, or stroke,[22] and to identify possible causes of the seizure. MRI is preferred over computed tomography, because it is more sensitive for findings, such as hippocampal sclerosis and cortical dysplasias,[23] which may be the cause of seizures and epilepsy. In patients with chronic epilepsy and no known cause, repeat imaging with the more sensitive 3-T MRI now available may be indicated if the patient has had 1.5-T imaging in the past.[24,25]

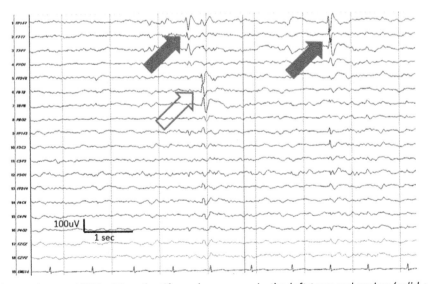

Fig. 2. Abnormal EEG with epileptiform sharp waves in the left temporal region (*solid arrows*) and right temporal region (*open arrow*).

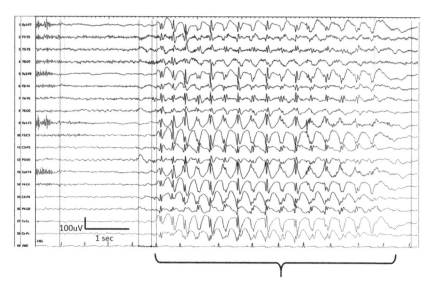

100uV
1 sec

Fig. 3. Abnormal EEG with generalized spike-and-slow-wave activity (bracket).

INITIAL TREATMENT

After a first seizure, the risks of future seizure recurrence must be weighed against the risks and benefits of starting an AED. Individuals with normal EEG, normal MRI, and normal neurologic examination have an approximately 35% risk of seizure recurrence by 5 years, after an unprovoked first seizure.[2] The risk is substantially higher in those with neurologic disorders or developmental delays,[2] abnormal EEG,[26] history of febrile seizures, or family history of epilepsy.[26] If there is a prior neurologic insult, such as stroke or traumatic brain injury, the seizure is considered "remote symptomatic" and the patient is also at an increased risk of future seizures, with recurrence rates of 26% by 1 year and 48% by 5 years.[27] Interestingly, patients with a first episode of status epilepticus and no prior seizures, or multiple seizures within 24 hours, have a similar risk of future seizures as those with an isolated first seizure.[28]

Once epilepsy is established (if the patient has had multiple unprovoked seizures, or through EEG with characteristic findings), AEDs are the first line of treatment. The ideal AED for a patient should be effective and well-tolerated. The choice of AED should be individualized keeping in mind the patient's medical and psychiatric comorbidities, and the risk of future seizures. Patients on multiple medications for other conditions, such as atrial fibrillation or HIV, may need to avoid enzyme-inducing AEDs, such as carbamazepine or phenobarbital, which can lead to significant drug-drug interactions. Patients with a history of depression or anxiety may wish to avoid levetiracetam as a first-line AED, because of the risk of exacerbating psychiatric symptoms. If the type of epilepsy (generalized or focal) is not known, clinicians should choose a broad-spectrum AED that is effective against both types of epilepsy. Well-tolerated AEDs include lamotrigine and levetiracetam (broad-spectrum), and oxcarbazepine (for focal epilepsy). **Table 1** lists commonly used AEDs, their spectrum of use, and common side effects.

MANAGEMENT

Clinicians should be aware of common side effects and counsel patients to monitor for these. If a patient's seizures respond to treatment but the patient has significant

Table 1
Commonly used antiepileptic drugs for focal and generalized epilepsies, and common side effects

	Focal Epilepsy		Broad Spectrum (Focal and Generalized Epilepsies)		Generalized Epilepsy	
Medication	Common Side Effects		Medication	Common Side Effects	Medication	Common Side Effects
Oxcarbazepine	Subclinical hyponatremia Dizziness Diplopia		Lamotrigine	Nausea Rash (minimize with slow up-titration)	Ethosuximide (absence seizures)	Cognitive effects Depression
Carbamazepine	Dizziness Sedation Ataxia Nausea Osteopenia (chronic use)		Levetiracetam	Irritability Aggressive behavior Depression		
Phenytoin	Sedation Dizziness Ataxia Cerebellar atrophy (chronic use) Peripheral neuropathy (chronic use) Osteopenia (chronic use)		Valproate	Teratogenicity in pregnancy Sedation Tremor Nausea Cognitive effects Weight gain Hair loss Osteopenia (chronic use)		

Drug	Side effects
Eslicarbazepine	Subclinical hyponatremia; Dizziness; Diplopia
Lacosamide	Dizziness; Nausea; Somnolence
Gabapentin	Sedation; Dizziness; Peripheral edema
Topiramate	Cognitive effects; Kidney stones; Weight loss; Paresthesias; Teratogenicity in pregnancy
Zonisamide	Sedation; Dizziness; Weight loss
Perampanel	Hostility; Aggressive behavior; Fatigue; Dizziness
Clobazam	Sedation; Increased salivation
Clonazepam	Sedation; Ataxia

adverse effects, the AED should be switched to a better-tolerated medication. Trials have shown that lamotrigine has significantly fewer adverse effects than carbamaze-pine or topiramate for focal epilepsy.[29] Lamotrigine, gabapentin, and levetiracetam seem to be well-tolerated in the elderly.[30,31] Lamotrigine is therefore often a good op-tion for patients with side effects on other AEDs; however, the need for long up-titration schedule and risk of rash must be taken into account, and it may not be optimal if a patient needs rapid protection against seizures.

If the first AED is not efficacious, the response rate (of seizure freedom) to the next AED chosen is 13% to 28%[32,33] and seems to be fairly similar across AEDs. Despite the many new AEDs introduced since 1990, the rates of seizure response to AEDs has been stable, and the proportion of patients who are seizure-free on medication re-mains around 60% to 70%.[32]

If a patient's seizures are not controlled after the first or second AED tried at thera-peutic doses, the likelihood of seizure control with the third or fourth medication dimin-ishes.[32,33] Patients whose seizures are not controlled after two appropriately chosen AEDs (which fail because of inefficacy, not because of side effects) are considered to have drug-resistant epilepsy,[34] and should be referred to an epilepsy specialist.

New AEDs are currently under development at all stages of clinical trials, and pa-tients with drug-resistant epilepsy may benefit from participating in a clinical trial. In recent years, there has been widespread public interest in the use of cannabis-derived cannabidiol for the treatment of refractory epilepsy. Cannabidiol has been shown to have efficacy in particularly severe types of childhood epilepsy (Dravet syn-drome and Lennox-Gastaut syndrome),[35] and is under study for other conditions.

Besides additional medications, patients with drug-resistant epilepsy may be eval-uated for treatment with surgery, neurostimulation, or dietary therapy.

SURGERY

Patients with focal epilepsy may be candidates for epilepsy surgery, if the seizure origin is in a part of the brain that can be safely resected. If a patient has not had seizure control after trials of two or more appropriately chosen AEDs at therapeutic doses, surgery may offer a higher chance of seizure freedom than do additional med-ications. Two randomized controlled trials found that epilepsy surgery provides a higher rate of seizure freedom than continued medical management in patients with temporal lobe epilepsy who qualified for surgery. The rate of seizure freedom in the surgery groups was 60% to 85%, compared with 0% to 8% seizure freedom in the continued medical management groups.[36,37] Social outcomes (quality of life, employ-ment status) were also improved in the surgery compared with medical management groups.

To determine whether a patient is a surgical candidate, extensive testing is needed. Epilepsy Monitoring Unit admission consists of prolonged video-EEG recording while the patient is hospitalized, to record several typical seizures. This recording helps determine the origin of the seizures, and whether there is more than one source of sei-zures. High-quality imaging with MRI helps clinicians select and counsel patients for surgery; patients with a lesion on MRI corresponding to the seizure onset zone have a higher rate of postoperative seizure-freedom than do patients with normal MRI.[38,39] If no lesion is found on MRI, PET can sometimes add to the surgical evalu-ation because approximately 40% of patients with epilepsy and normal MRI have localizing findings on PET.[40] Neuropsychology assessment before surgery is vital in determining the patient's presurgical verbal and nonverbal memory functioning. Be-tween 22% and 65% of patients who undergo dominant anterior temporal lobectomy have a postoperative decline in verbal memory. Patients with higher presurgical memory impairment may have less decline in memory after surgery, whereas those with normal memory may experience a larger decline.[41,42] Magnetoencephalogram is another noninvasive means of identifying the seizure source. Magnetoencephalogram uses the magnetic fields generated by interictal discharges to localize dipole sources. In one study, 78% of patients had a localizable interictal dipole source, and when that source was included in surgical resection, surgical outcomes were improved.[43]

In some cases, scalp EEG monitoring is insufficient to localize the seizure onset zone. Invasive monitoring with surgically implanted electrodes can improve localization and may allow some patients to become surgical candidates who otherwise would not be candidates.[44] Placement of intracranial electrodes may also allow for cortical mapping, in which low pulses of electric stimulation are given to the electrodes and the resulting function (eg, finger twitch, speech arrest, tingling of the tongue) recorded to accurately "map" the function of the precise area of cortex.[45]

In recent years, laser interstitial thermal ablation has become an alternative to open surgical resection for patients with certain types of focal epilepsy. In this procedure, the neurosurgeon uses MRI guidance to place a thermal probe targeting the seizure source (eg, the sclerotic hippocampus). Heat is then used to ablate the tissue.[46] The time needed to recover from this minimally invasive procedure is shorter than that from an open resection, and risk of cognitive decline may be lower compared with standard resection.[47] However, the rates of seizure freedom after thermal ablation for mesial temporal sclerosis are slightly lower than for standard temporal lobectomy, at 50% to 60%[46,48] compared with 80% to 90% in patients with unilateral mesial temporal sclerosis.[49]

NEUROSTIMULATION

Patients who are not surgical candidates because of seizure origin in eloquent cortex, such as primary language or primary motor areas, or multifocal or generalized seizures, may be candidates for treatment with neurostimulation.

Vagus nerve stimulation requires surgical placement of a subcutaneous stimulator in the chest, and placement of a stimulating wire in the neck attached to the vagus nerve. Intermittent stimulation of the vagus nerve helps reduce the frequency and perhaps severity of seizures over time in many of patients, with 31% to 38% of patients experiencing at least a 50% decrease in seizures. The seizure reduction improves over time.[50–52] However, reported rates of seizure freedom are low, especially compared with resective surgery.

Patients with focal or multifocal epilepsy who are not candidates for resection may have neurostimulation with the responsive neurostimulation device. Responsive neurostimulation is a closed-loop system using electrodes implanted at the sites of seizure onset in the brain, which detect the onset of seizure activity and deliver pulses of electrical stimulation designed to prevent the seizure from spreading and progressing.[53] After responsive neurostimulation placement, patients have a median 48% to 66% seizure reduction, and 16% are seizure free.[54] Similar to vagus nerve stimulation, seizure response is often delayed after therapy starts and improves over time, suggesting a neuromodulatory effect.

DIETARY TREATMENT

Dietary therapy has been used for epilepsy for nearly 100 years[55]; this type of treatment fell somewhat out of favor for some time after the introduction of phenytoin, but has experienced a resurgence in the past decades. Low-carbohydrate, high-fat diets are effective in the treatment of some medically refractory focal and generalized epilepsies, with 22% to 55% of patients experiencing at least a 50% reduction in seizures on the classical ketogenic diet (which requires that 90% of calories be from fat sources).[56,57] The less restrictive modified Atkins diet allows up to 20 g of carbohydrates per day, and 12% to 67% of patients experience at least a 50% seizure reduction on the modified Atkins diet.[58–60] Seizure response rates are comparable with and in many cases exceed responses to AEDs, with 33% of patients experiencing at least a 90% reduction in seizures in one study.[60] Other types of dietary therapy are available, including the medium-chain triglyceride diet[61] and low glycemic index diet.[62] Many patients report improved cognition and mood in addition to seizure control while on dietary therapies.[56,63–65]

The exact mechanisms underlying the efficacy of dietary treatment are unknown. Initially, ketone bodies were thought to control seizures. However, whether or not a patient achieves and maintains high levels of ketosis has not been shown to correlate with seizure response.[64,66] Other proposed mechanisms are through the action of decanoic acid (a component of medium-chain triglycerides), which inhibits the α-amino-3-hydroxy-5-methyl-4-isoxazolepropionic acid receptor, and via DNA methylation.[67]

SPECIAL CONSIDERATIONS: WOMEN

Women with epilepsy face unique challenges, particularly during the childbearing years. Treatment must be considered in the context of hormonal seizure exacerbations, contraception, and potential childbearing.

Up to one-third of women identify a seizure pattern related to the menstrual cycle,[68] termed "catamenial epilepsy." Seizures can be increased perimenstrually, around ovulation, or throughout the second half of an anovulatory menstrual cycle. An elevated estrogen to progesterone ratio is thought to cause these exacerbations.[68,69] Treatment may include an increase in baseline AEDs or additional AED around the projected days of seizure exacerbations, progesterone supplementation in rare cases with a strong catamenial pattern, or regulation of the menstrual cycle with exogenous hormones.

Enzyme-inducing AEDs, such as phenytoin, carbamazepine, and phenobarbital (among others; **Table 2**), can increase the metabolism of oral contraceptives, thereby reducing their effectiveness. Similarly, oral contraceptives can increase the metabolism of lamotrigine, reducing the serum level and requiring a dose increase. Alternative forms of contraception for women on enzyme-inducing medications include the intrauterine device,[70] barrier methods, tubal ligation if desired, and depot medroxyprogesterone.[71]

Epilepsy during pregnancy poses unique challenges. Generalized tonic-clonic seizures are harmful to mother and fetus during pregnancy, with earlier deliveries and lower birth weights in neonates born to mothers with tonic-clonic seizures,[72] and breakthrough seizures occur in 14% to 32% of women during pregnancy.[73] Although some AEDs (in particular, lamotrigine and levetiracetam) are thought to be safe in pregnancy and have minimally increased rates of major congenital malformations over those found in women on no medications,[74] other AEDs, such as valproic acid, phenobarbital, and topiramate have high rates of physical malformations and neurocognitive deficits.[74–76] Valproic acid especially should be avoided when at all possible in women of childbearing potential and substituted during pregnancy. Planning pregnancy and ensuring an AED regimen of preferred medications at the lowest effective doses (given the dose-dependent effects observed in some AEDs) is essential. There

Table 2
Interactions of common AEDs with estrogen-containing contraceptives

AED	Estrogen Reduced by AED
Carbamazepine	Yes
Clobazam	Yes
Clonazepam	No
Eslicarbazepine	Yes
Ethosuximide	No
Gabapentin	No
Lacosamide	No
Lamotrigine	No[a] (reduced by estrogen)
Levetiracetam	No
Oxcarbazepine	Yes
Perampanel	No[a]
Phenobarbital	Yes
Phenytoin	Yes
Topiramate	Yes[b]
Valproate	No
Zonisamide	No

[a] Reduces progesterone (perampanel at 12 mg).
[b] Dose-dependent.

is some evidence that higher doses of folic acid can reduce the risk of autism in children of women taking AEDs,[77] and folic acid supplementation should be encouraged in women with epilepsy even before pregnancy.

Lamotrigine and other medications have increased clearance in pregnancy,[78] and drug monitoring and dose adjustment is needed. However, dosages must be reduced back to baseline levels after delivery to avoid toxicity and side effects. Breastfeeding is generally thought to be safe and is encouraged for women with epilepsy taking AEDs,[79] because the dose of exposure in breastmilk does not exceed the dose of exposure in utero.

Women with epilepsy may also experience changes in seizure pattern around the time of menopause.[80–82] Women who have taken enzyme-inducing AEDs for years are at increased risk of osteoporosis,[9] and should have bone density monitoring and supplementation with calcium and vitamin D, or with other agents as appropriate.

FUTURE CONSIDERATIONS

Although the number of AEDs on the market has grown exponentially in the last 40 years, the percent of people with intractable seizures remains roughly similar.[32] New medications with novel mechanisms of action are under development, and are urgently needed. Similarly, although epilepsy surgery and the growing technique of laser interstitial ablation is an option for many patients with focal epilepsy, many patients are not candidates for these techniques because of multifocality, involvement of eloquent cortex (eg, primary motor or language areas), or widespread seizure onset regions. Increased understanding of the mechanisms of dietary therapy for epilepsy and the role of neurosteroid hormones in epilepsy exacerbations may open doors to new treatments. As new treatments become available, clinicians should continue to individualize treatment to a patient's needs, taking into account any psychiatric and medical comorbidities.

REFERENCES

1. Fisher RS, van Emde Boas W, Blume W, et al. Epileptic seizures and epilepsy: definitions proposed by the International League Against Epilepsy (ILAE) and the International Bureau for Epilepsy (IBE). Epilepsia 2005;46(4):470–2.
2. Kim LG, Johnson TL, Marson AG, et al. Prediction of risk of seizure recurrence after a single seizure and early epilepsy: further results from the MESS trial. Lancet Neurol 2006;5(4):317–22.
3. Fisher RS, Acevedo C, Arzimanoglou A, et al. ILAE official report: a practical clinical definition of epilepsy. Epilepsia 2014;55(4):475–82.
4. Fisher RS, Cross JH, French JA, et al. Operational classification of seizure types by the international league against epilepsy: position paper of the ILAE commission for classification and terminology. Epilepsia 2017;58(4):522–30.
5. Scheffer IE, Berkovic S, Capovilla G, et al. ILAE classification of the epilepsies: position paper of the ILAE Commission for Classification and Terminology. Epilepsia 2017;58(4):512–21.
6. Hauser WA, Beghi E. First seizure definitions and worldwide incidence and mortality. Epilepsia 2008;49(s1):8–12.
7. Krumholz A, Wiebe S, Gronseth GS, et al. Evidence-based guideline: management of an unprovoked first seizure in adults: report of the guideline development subcommittee of the American Academy of Neurology and the American Epilepsy Society. Neurology 2015;84(16):1705–13.
8. Moshe SL, Perucca E, Ryvlin P, et al. Epilepsy: new advances. Lancet 2015; 385(9971):884–98.
9. Cloyd J, Hauser W, Towne A, et al. Epidemiological and medical aspects of epilepsy in the elderly. Epilepsy Res 2006;68(Suppl 1):S39–48.
10. Hauser WA, Annegers JF, Kurland LT. Incidence of epilepsy and unprovoked seizures in Rochester, Minnesota: 1935-1984. Epilepsia 1993;34(3):453–68.
11. Jackson A, Teo L, Seneviratne U. Challenges in the first seizure clinic for adult patients with epilepsy. Epileptic Disord 2016;18(3):305–14.
12. Lempert T, Bauer M, Schmidt D. Syncope: a videometric analysis of 56 episodes of transient cerebral hypoxia. Ann Neurol 1994;36(2):233–7.
13. Chen DK, Sharma E, LaFrance WC. Psychogenic non-epileptic seizures. Curr Neurol Neurosci Rep 2017;17(9):71.
14. Sheldon R, Rose S, Ritchie D, et al. Historical criteria that distinguish syncope from seizures. J Am Coll Cardiol 2002;40(1):142–8.
15. Brigo F, Nardone R, Bongiovanni LG. Value of tongue biting in the differential diagnosis between epileptic seizures and syncope. Seizure 2012;21(8):568–72.
16. Brigo F, Bongiovanni LG, Nardone R. Lateral tongue biting versus biting at the tip of the tongue in differentiating between epileptic seizures and syncope. Seizure 2013;22(9):801.
17. Akor F, Liu N, Besag F, et al. Value of tongue biting in differentiating between epileptic seizures and syncope. Seizure 2013;22(4):328.
18. Oliva M, Pattison C, Carino J, et al. The diagnostic value of oral lacerations and incontinence during convulsive "seizures". Epilepsia 2008;49(6):962–7.
19. Krumholz A, Wiebe S, Gronseth G, et al. Practice parameter: evaluating an apparent unprovoked first seizure in adults (an evidence-based review): report

of the Quality Standards Subcommittee of the American Academy of Neurology and the American Epilepsy Society. Neurology 2007;69(21):1996–2007.

20. Salinsky M, Kanter R, Dasheiff RM. Effectiveness of multiple EEGs in supporting the diagnosis of epilepsy: an operational curve. Epilepsia 1987;28(4):331–4. Available at: http://www.ncbi.nlm.nih.gov/pubmed/3622408. Accessed October 8, 2017.

21. Schreiner A, Pohlmann-Eden B. Value of the early electroencephalogram after a first unprovoked seizure. Clin Electroencephalogr 2003;34(3):140–4. Available at: http://www.ncbi.nlm.nih.gov/pubmed/14521275. Accessed September 22, 2017.

22. Kotisaari K, Virtanen P, Forss N, et al. Emergency computed tomography in patients with first seizure. Seizure 2017;48:89–93.

23. Radue EW, Scollo-Lavizzari G. Computed tomography and magnetic resonance imaging in epileptic seizures. Eur Neurol 1994;34(Suppl 1):55–7. Available at: http://www.ncbi.nlm.nih.gov/pubmed/8001611. Accessed October 8, 2017.

24. Ladino LD, Balaguera P, Rascovsky S, et al. Clinical benefit of 3 Tesla magnetic resonance imaging rescanning in patients with focal epilepsy and negative 1.5 Tesla magnetic resonance imaging. Rev Invest Clin 2016;68(3):112–8. Available at: http://www.ncbi.nlm.nih.gov/pubmed/27408997. Accessed May 9, 2018.

25. Knake S, Triantafyllou C, Wald LL, et al. 3T phased array MRI improves the presurgical evaluation in focal epilepsies: a prospective study. Neurology 2005; 65(7):1026–31.

26. Hauser WA, Rich SS, Annegers JF, et al. Seizure recurrence after a 1st unprovoked seizure: an extended follow-up. Neurology 1990;40(8):1163–70.

27. Hauser WA, Anderson VE, Loewenson RB, et al. Seizure recurrence after a first unprovoked seizure. N Engl J Med 1982;307(9):522–8.

28. Kho LK, Lawn ND, Dunne JW, et al. First seizure presentation: do multiple seizures within 24 hours predict recurrence? Neurology 2006;67(6):1047–9.

29. Marson AG, Al-Kharusi AM, Alwaidh M, et al. The SANAD study of effectiveness of carbamazepine, gabapentin, lamotrigine, oxcarbazepine, or topiramate for treatment of partial epilepsy: an unblinded randomised controlled trial. Lancet 2007;369(9566):1000–15.

30. Werhahn KJ, Trinka E, Dobesberger J, et al. A randomized, double-blind comparison of antiepileptic drug treatment in the elderly with new-onset focal epilepsy. Epilepsia 2015;56(3):450–9.

31. Rowan AJ, Ramsay RE, Collins JF, et al. New onset geriatric epilepsy: a randomized study of gabapentin, lamotrigine, and carbamazepine. Neurology 2005; 64(11):1868–73.

32. Chen Z, Brodie MJ, Liew D, et al. Treatment outcomes in patients with newly diagnosed epilepsy treated with established and new antiepileptic drugs a 30-year longitudinal cohort study. JAMA Neurol 2018;75(3):279–86.

33. Kwan P, Brodie MJ. Early identification of refractory epilepsy. N Engl J Med 2000; 342(5):314–9.

34. Kwan P, Arzimanoglou A, Berg AT, et al. Definition of drug resistant epilepsy: consensus proposal by the ad hoc Task Force of the ILAE Commission on Therapeutic Strategies. Epilepsia 2010;51(6):1069–77.

35. Devinsky O, Cross JH, Laux L, et al. Trial of cannabidiol for drug-resistant seizures in the Dravet syndrome. N Engl J Med 2017;376(21):2011–20.

36. Engel J. Early surgical therapy for drug-resistant temporal lobe epilepsy. JAMA 2012;307(9):922.

37. Wiebe S, Blume WT, Girvin JP, et al. A randomized, controlled trial of surgery for temporal-lobe epilepsy. N Engl J Med 2001;345(5):311–8.

38. Berkovic SF, McIntosh AM, Kalnins RM, et al. Preoperative MRI predicts outcome of temporal lobectomy: an actuarial analysis. Neurology 1995;45(7):1358–63. Available at: http://www.ncbi.nlm.nih.gov/pubmed/7617198. Accessed May 11, 2018.
39. Ferrier CH, Engelsman J, Alarcón G, et al. Prognostic factors in presurgical assessment of frontal lobe epilepsy. J Neurol Neurosurg Psychiatry 1999;66(3): 350–6.
40. Menon RN, Radhakrishnan A, Parameswaran R, et al. Does F-18 FDG-PET substantially alter the surgical decision-making in drug-resistant partial epilepsy? Epilepsy Behav 2015;51:133–9.
41. Dulay MF, Busch RM. Prediction of neuropsychological outcome after resection of temporal and extratemporal seizure foci. Neurosurg Focus 2012;32(3):E4.
42. Chelune GJ, Naugle RI, Lüders H, et al. Prediction of cognitive change as a function of preoperative ability status among temporal lobectomy patients seen at 6-month follow-up. Neurology 1991;41(3):399–404. Available at: http://www.ncbi.nlm.nih.gov/pubmed/2006008. Accessed May 11, 2018.
43. Englot DJ, Nagarajan SS, Imber BS, et al. Epileptogenic zone localization using magnetoencephalography predicts seizure freedom in epilepsy surgery. Epilepsia 2015;56:949–58.
44. Weinand ME, Wyler AR, Richey ET, et al. Long-term ictal monitoring with subdural strip electrodes: prognostic factors for selecting temporal lobectomy candidates. J Neurosurg 1992;77:20–8.
45. So EL, Alwaki A. A guide for cortical electrical stimulation mapping. J Clin Neurophysiol 2018;35(2):98–105.
46. Willie JT, Laxpati NG, Drane DL, et al. Real-time magnetic resonance-guided stereotactic laser amygdalohippocampotomy for mesial temporal lobe epilepsy. Neurosurgery 2014;74(6):569–84.
47. Drane DL, Loring DW, Voets NL, et al. Better object recognition and naming outcome with MRI-guided stereotactic laser amygdalohippocampotomy for temporal lobe epilepsy. Epilepsia 2015;56(1):101–13.
48. Kang JY, Wu C, Tracy J, et al. Laser interstitial thermal therapy for medically intractable mesial temporal lobe epilepsy. Epilepsia 2016;57(2):325–34.
49. Cascino GD. Surgical treatment for epilepsy. Epilepsy Res 2004;60(2–3 SPEC. ISS.):179–86.
50. Handforth A, DeGiorgio CM, Schachter SC, et al. Vagus nerve stimulation therapy for partial-onset seizures: a randomized active-control trial. Neurology 1998; 51(1):48–55. Available at: http://www.ncbi.nlm.nih.gov/pubmed/9674777. Accessed May 11, 2018.
51. DeGiorgio CM, Schachter SC, Handforth A, et al. Prospective long-term study of vagus nerve stimulation for the treatment of refractory seizures. Epilepsia 2000; 41(9):1195–200. Available at: http://www.ncbi.nlm.nih.gov/pubmed/10999559. Accessed May 11, 2018.
52. The Vagus Nerve Stimulation Study Group. A randomized controlled trial of chronic vagus nerve stimulation for treatment of medically intractable seizures. Neurology 1995;45(2):224–30. Available at: http://www.ncbi.nlm.nih.gov/pubmed/7854516. Accessed May 11, 2018.
53. Ben-Menachem E, Krauss GL. Responsive neurostimulation: modulating the epileptic brain. Nat Rev Neurol 2014;10(5):247–8.
54. Bergey GK, Morrell MJ, Mizrahi EM, et al. Long-term treatment with responsive brain stimulation in adults with refractory partial seizures. Neurology 2015; 84(8):810–7.

55. Barborka J. Ketogenic dietary therapy of epilepsy in adults. JAMA 1928;91:73–8.
56. Sirven J, Whedon B, Caplan D, et al. The ketogenic diet for intractable epilepsy in adults: preliminary results. Epilepsia 1999;40(12):1721–6.
57. Schoeler NE, Wood S, Aldridge V, et al. Ketogenic dietary therapies for adults with epilepsy: feasibility and classification of response. Epilepsy Behav 2014; 37:77–81.
58. Smith M, Politzer N, MacGarvie D, et al. Efficacy and tolerability of the modified Atkins diet in adults with pharmacoresistant epilepsy: a prospective observational study. Epilepsia 2011;52(4):775–80.
59. Kossoff EH, Krauss GL, McGrogan JR, et al. Efficacy of the Atkins diet as therapy for intractable epilepsy. Neurology 2003;61(12):1789–91.
60. Kossoff EH, Henry BJ, Cervenka MC. Efficacy of dietary therapy for juvenile myoclonic epilepsy. Epilepsy Behav 2013;26(2):162–4.
61. Liu YC. Medium-chain triglyceride (MCT) ketogenic therapy. Epilepsia 2008;49: 33–6.
62. Pfeifer HH, Thiele EA. Low-glycemic-index treatment: a liberalized ketogenic diet for treatment of intractable epilepsy. Neurology 2005;65(11):1810–2.
63. Coppola G, Veggiotti P, Cusmai R, et al. The ketogenic diet in children, adolescents and young adults with refractory epilepsy: an Italian multicentric experience. Epilepsy Res 2002;48(3):221–7.
64. Mosek A, Natour H, Neufeld MY, et al. Ketogenic diet treatment in adults with refractory epilepsy: a prospective pilot study. Seizure 2009;18(1):30–3.
65. Lambrechts DAJE, Wielders LHP, Aldenkamp AP, et al. The ketogenic diet as a treatment option in adults with chronic refractory epilepsy: efficacy and tolerability in clinical practice. Epilepsy Behav 2012;23(3):310–4.
66. Kossoff EH, Turner Z, Bluml RM, et al. A randomized, crossover comparison of daily carbohydrate limits using the modified Atkins diet. Epilepsy Behav 2007; 10(3):432–6.
67. Boison D. New insights into the mechanisms of the ketogenic diet. Curr Opin Neurol 2017;30(2):187–92.
68. Herzog AG. Catamenial epilepsy: update on prevalence, pathophysiology and treatment from the findings of the NIH Progesterone Treatment Trial. Seizure 2015;28:18–25.
69. Logothetis J, Harner R, Morrell F, et al. The role of estrogens in catamenial exacerbation of epilepsy. Neurology 1959;9(5):352–60. Available at: http://www.ncbi. nlm.nih.gov/pubmed/13657294. Accessed November 4, 2016.
70. Espinera AR, Gavvala J, Bellinski I, et al. Counseling by epileptologists affects contraceptive choices of women with epilepsy. Epilepsy Behav 2016;65:1–6.
71. O'Brien MD, Guillebaud J. Contraception for women with epilepsy. Epilepsia 2006;47(9):1419–22.
72. Rauchenzauner M, Ehrensberger M, Prieschl M, et al. Generalized tonic–clonic seizures and antiepileptic drugs during pregnancy: a matter of importance for the baby? J Neurol 2013;260(2):484–8.
73. Harden CL, Hopp J, Ting TY, et al. Practice parameter update: management issues for women with epilepsy; focus on pregnancy, obstetrical complications and change in seizure frequency. Neurology 2009;73:126–32.
74. Hernandez-Diaz S, Smith CR, Shen A, et al. Comparative safety of antiepileptic drugs during pregnancy. Neurology 2012;78(21):1692–9.
75. Meador KJ, Baker GA, Browning N, et al. Fetal antiepileptic drug exposure and cognitive outcomes at age 6 years (NEAD study): a prospective observational study. Lancet Neurol 2013;12(3):244–52.

76. Hernández-Díaz S, Mittendorf R, Smith CR, et al. Association between topiramate and zonisamide use during pregnancy and low birth weight. Obstet Gynecol 2014;123(1):21–8.

77. Bjørk M, Riedel B, Spigset O, et al. Association of folic acid supplementation during pregnancy with the risk of autistic traits in children exposed to antiepileptic drugs in utero. JAMA Neurol 2018;75(2):160–8.

78. Pennell PB, Newport DJ, Stowe ZN, et al. The impact of pregnancy and childbirth on the metabolism of lamotrigine. Neurology 2004;62(2):292–5.

79. Meador KJ, Baker GA, Browning N, et al. Breastfeeding in children of women taking antiepileptic drugs: cognitive outcomes at age 6 years. JAMA Pediatr 2014; 168(8):729.

80. Abbasi F, Krumholz A, Kittner SJ, et al. Effects of menopause on seizures in women with epilepsy. Epilepsia 1999;40(2):205–10.

81. Harden CL, Koppel BS, Herzog AG, et al. Seizure frequency is associated with age at menopause in women with epilepsy. Neurology 2003;61(4):451–5. Available at: http://www.ncbi.nlm.nih.gov/pubmed/12939416. Accessed September 11, 2016.

82. Harden CL, Herzog AG, Nikolov BG, et al. Hormone replacement therapy in women with epilepsy: a randomized, double-blind, placebo-controlled study. Epilepsia 2006;47(9):1447–51.

Multiple Sclerosis and Autoimmune Neurology of the Central Nervous System

Kristin M. Galetta, MD[a,b], Shamik Bhattacharyya, MD, MS[a,*]

KEYWORDS

- Autoimmune neurology • Multiple sclerosis • Neuromyelitis optica
- Acute disseminated encephalomyelitis • Autoimmune encephalitis • Sarcoidosis

KEY POINTS

- Multiple sclerosis is the most common autoimmune disease of the central nervous system and is characterized by recurrent disease activity affecting different parts of the central nervous system.
- Neuromyelitis optica is associated with antibody to aquaporin-4 and is characterized by severe episodes of optic neuritis, myelitis, or brainstem/cerebral attacks.
- Acute disseminated encephalomyelitis is primarily a pediatric disease and generally includes encephalopathy and focal neurologic deficits.
- Autoimmune encephalitis is a broad category of disease with different causes characterized by subacute onset of memory disorder, psychiatric symptoms, or confusion generally with evidence of inflammation on imaging or in cerebrospinal fluid.
- Most patients with neurosarcoidosis will have evidence of systemic sarcoidosis even if the systemic involvement is clinically silent.

INTRODUCTION

Although the central nervous system was once thought of as an immune-privileged site hidden behind the blood brain barrier, we now know that there is active and continuous immunologic surveillance in the central nervous system. This was brought to the forefront in the human immunodeficiency virus epidemic when immunosuppression was accompanied by opportunistic infections affecting the brain, suggesting that immunity is active in the central nervous system. Although generally protective,

Disclosure Statement: The authors do not have any relevant disclosures.
[a] Department of Neurology, Brigham and Women's Hospital, Harvard Medical School, 75 Francis Street, Boston, MA 02115, USA; [b] Department of Neurology, Massachusetts General Hospital, 55 Fruit Street, Boston, MA 02114, USA
* Corresponding author.
E-mail address: sbhattacharyya3@partners.org

Med Clin N Am 103 (2019) 325–336
https://doi.org/10.1016/j.mcna.2018.10.004
0025-7125/19/© 2018 Elsevier Inc. All rights reserved.

medical.theclinics.com

inflammation in the central nervous system can be injurious when not properly regulated. This aberrant inflammation (or autoimmunity) can be triggered by a variety of mechanisms including granulomatous disease, cell-mediated processes, and autoantibodies targeting neuronal antigens. The authors review here some of the more common autoimmune syndromes of the central nervous system.

MULTIPLE SCLEROSIS

Multiple sclerosis (MS) is a chronic immune-mediated disease of the central nervous system. Although MS most often presents in women between 20 to 40 years of age, the disease affects both genders and can occur in children and the elderly. Clinically, MS most frequently presents as *relapsing-remitting* disease. Relapses can affect any part of the central nervous system. Some common syndromes include optic nerve dysfunction, diplopia, dizziness, and weakness or numbness of an extremity. These relapses typically evolve over the course of hours to days (in contrast to symptoms lasting minutes associated with migraine or seizure or transient ischemic attack). The severity is variable ranging from mild symptoms ignored by the patient to severe deficits presenting to the emergency room. In untreated patients, the symptoms spontaneously improve over the course of days to weeks.

MS can also present with slow progressive symptoms instead of discrete relapses. These progressive symptoms include gait disorder, bladder/bowel dysfunction, blindness, or lack of dexterity in a hand. This form of the disease is called progressive MS. Progressive disease can be present from the onset (called primary progressive MS). More commonly, patients who initially had relapsing-remitting disease evolve to have slow progression of neurologic deficits (called secondary progressive MS) as they age.

The cause of MS is unknown. MS incidence varies significantly by continent but is most commonly identified in Canada, Europe, the United States, New Zealand, and Southern Australia and less commonly in the Asia and the tropics.[1] Both genetic and environmental factors affect the development of the disease. Environmental associations include vitamin D levels, cigarette smoking, and exposure to Epstein–Barr virus.[2] The incidence of MS correlates with the distance from the equator in the Southern hemisphere in a latitudinal gradient. Risk of MS also increases with relatedness of individuals with monozygotic twins of patients with MS having more than 100x higher risk of developing the disease than the general population.

Pathologically, dysregulation of the blood-brain barrier and simultaneously cytokine and chemokine release occurs early. It is hypothesized that myelin antigens are presented by macrophages, microglia, and astrocytes to T cells leading to immune attack on myelin-oligodendrocyte complex.[3] These inflammatory changes result in destruction of myelin, axons, and neurons. The role of B cells (antibody producing cells) in MS is increasingly recognized but the exact mechanism of their involvement remains unclear. One of the cardinal features of MS is excess antibody synthesis within the central nervous system detectable clinically as elevated oligoclonal bands and immunoglobulin G (IgG) index in cerebrospinal fluid (CSF).

When suspected clinically, the diagnosis of MS is based on the dissemination of neurologic events in time and space (affecting different parts of central nervous system).[4] Classically, the diagnosis was made when 2 discrete clinical attacks occurred. For example, a patient might present with optic neuritis and then myelitis a year later. At present, evidence on MRI of typical demyelinating lesions can substitute for a clinical event and enables earlier diagnosis and treatment (**Fig. 1**). Lesion enhancement with intravenous gadolinium contrast indicates current disease activity (**Fig. 2**). Computed tomography of the brain does not provide sufficient information to

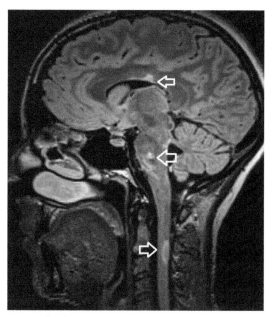

Fig. 1. Sagittal brain MRI fluid attenuation inversion recovery sequence shows typical MS hyperintense lesions in the corpus callosum (*top arrow*), brainstem (*middle arrow*), and spinal cord (*bottom arrow*).

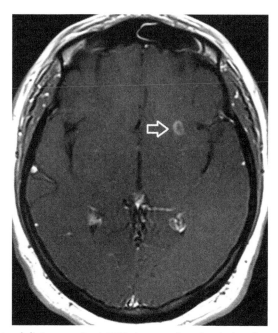

Fig. 2. Axial postgadolinium contrast MRI shows enhancing lesion (*arrow*) that indicates active inflammatory lesion in multiple sclerosis.

diagnose MS. CSF analysis is used as ancillary testing when the diagnosis is ambiguous or early in the disease when few or nonspecific lesions are present on imaging. The presence of oligoclonal bands (which indicates antibody synthesis within the central nervous system) increases the probability of MS. Ultimately, short of pathology, there is no "gold standard" test for the disease. Alternate causes of recurrent neurologic dysfunction including strokes, infections, and other inflammatory processes must be excluded before diagnosing MS.

In the current era of easily accessible imaging, many patients without symptoms can have imaging findings that suggest MS forming the entity *radiologically isolated syndrome*. Nonetheless, two-thirds of these patients will develop new findings on follow-up MRI scans and one-third will develop new neurologic symptoms within 5 years.[5] Male sex, younger age (<37 years), and spinal cord lesions are the most significant predictors of symptom development.

Most medical treatment for MS has been focused on immunomodulation and reducing relapses of the disease. MS flares are typically treated with high-dose intravenous (IV) methylprednisolone (such as 1000 mg) for 3 to 5 days. This short course has been shown to improve symptoms and immediate disability; however, there is no clear evidence that corticosteroids improve long-term disability.[6] There is emerging evidence that oral courses of corticosteroids such as with high-dose prednisone may have the same benefit as IV therapy and avoids visits to infusion centers.[7] Although beneficial for symptoms, corticosteroids have multiple negative side effects such as hypertension, hyperglycemia, insomnia, and irritability. Thus, steroids should be used sparingly and only when an acute event is suspected.

Over the last 3 decades many medications to prevent relapses have been developed. With the number of therapies, the choice can initially seem overwhelming. Broadly speaking, therapies can be subdivided into injectables, oral medications, and infusions. In terms of efficacy, the infusions generally are most efficacious followed by the oral agents and finally by the injectables. On the other hand, the infusion medications suppress the immune system (hence predisposing to adverse effects) most significantly followed by oral agents and then the injectables. As of yet, there is no clear way to match individual therapy to individual patients. There is wide variability in choice of therapy regionally and between institutions. There are 2 general paradigms. The "step up" approach starts with the safest but least efficacious agents such as the injectables and then therapy is escalated if the patient has disease breakthrough. The other approach is to start with more efficacious therapy early (such as an infusion) to protect the nervous system from injury early that may become manifest years later. The optimum strategy is unclear. Finally, most therapies were developed to address relapsing-remitting forms of MS. Only ocrelizumab has been shown in a trial to have modest effect on primary progressive MS.[8]

Among injectables, interferon-β (INF-β) and glatiramer acetate were the earliest disease-modifying therapies approved for use in MS in the 1990s and are still among the most widely used agents. Interferon-β is estimated to reduce the annual rate of relapse by about 30% compared with placebo. The mechanism by which INFs work remains unclear. It has both pro- and antiinflammatory effects but treatment is thought to potentially reduce trafficking of inflammatory cells across the blood-brain barrier.[9] The main side effects are flulike symptoms and liver enzyme elevations. Glatiramer acetate also decreases relapse rates compared with the natural history of MS and likely has similar efficacy compared with INF-β.[10] The most common side effects related to glatiramer acetate are injection site reaction and more infrequently immediate postinjection reaction, which includes vasodilatation, chest pain, tachycardia, and shortness of breath.

There are 3 main oral agents for treatment of MS: fingolimod, dimethyl fumarate, and teriflunomide. Fingolimod was the first Food and Drug Administration (FDA)-approved oral agent and is superior to IFN-1βa and placebo at preventing relapses.[11] It works by binding to sphingosine receptors on lymphocytes preventing them from exiting lymphatic tissue. Its use is limited by its risk of causing arrhythmia, macular edema, and immunosuppression resulting in infection. Teriflunomide also reduces clinical and radiographic relapse. It may result in leukopenia and can produce serious hepatotoxicity. The mechanism of dimethyl fumarate is unclear but likely involves dual roles of immunosuppression and neuroprotection. Dimethyl fumarate has been shown to reduce relapse rate and radiographic disease progression. Fingolimod and dimethyl fumarate have both been associated with opportunistic infections including progressive multifocal leukoencephalopathy (PML).

Infusion therapies for MS generally consist of monoclonal antibodies. Natalizumab is a monoclonal antibody that impairs the ability of leukocytes to adhere to the lining of cerebral vascular walls and then to enter through the blood-brain barrier. It has been shown to reduce the relapse rate by 68% as compared with placebo.[12] The most concerning side effect is PML. Risk for PML increases amongst those who are with positive anti-JCV antibody status, who have prolonged duration of natalizumab treatment extending over 2 years, and who use prior immunosuppressants. Monoclonal B-cell depleting anti-CD20 agents are increasingly being used for the treatment of both relapsing-remitting MS and primary progressive MS. Included in this group of rituximab are ocrelizumab (FDA approved for MS), and ofatumumab. These therapies potently lower rates of clinical and radiographic relapse activity as compared with other disease modifying agents. Infusion reactions and infections are common. Alemtuzumab is a monoclonal antibody that targets CD52 antigen in lymphocytes and results in complement-dependent and antibody-mediated cytolysis and apoptosis. This very potent therapy has prolonged effects lasting years even after one infusion cycle. Infusion side effects include immune thrombocytopenia purpura, infections (herpes), and thyroid-related disease.

In contrast to the disease-modifying agents discussed earlier, most patients with MS are also treated with supplemental vitamin D, which has been associated with a lower risk of MS. Observational studies from longitudinal cohorts indicate that there might be a disease-modifying effect.[13] This remains to be substantiated in a randomized clinical trial. However, moderate doses (such as 2000 IU of cholecalciferol) are tolerated and often recommended in the treatment of MS.

NEUROMYELITIS OPTICA

Neuromyelitis optica (NMO) is an inflammatory disorder of the central nervous system associated with autoantibody to aquaporin-4 (AQP4). As heralded by its name, NMO typically clinically manifests with episodes of inflammation of the optic nerves and spinal cord. In contrast to MS, recovery from optic neuritis or myelitis in NMO is more incomplete with significant residual deficits. NMO is most common in young adults and particularly in women. For many years, NMO was believed to be a monophasic illness, but studies have shown that most patients will relapse if untreated.[14] NMO spectrum disorder is a more recent term that describes the ongoing discovery of range of diseases presenting with a positive AQP4 antibody including brainstem and cerebral syndromes.

In patients with suggestive clinical syndrome such as unexplained optic neuritis or myelitis, the AQP4 antibody should be tested for. The modern test by cell-binding assay is highly specific (>90%) and moderately sensitive (>70%).[15] To make the diagnosis of NMO amongst patients with a positive AQP4 antibody, clinical lesions in 1 of 6 characteristic locations are required: optic nerve, spinal cord, area postrema (located in the medulla and clinically presenting with intractable hiccups and vomiting), brainstem, diencephalon, or cerebrum.[16] For those without anti-AQP4 antibody, more strict criteria must be met. These individuals must have 2 or more clinical attacks at 1 of the 6 locations mentioned earlier with at least one manifesting as optic neuritis, myelitis, or as an area postrema syndrome.

The diagnosis of NMO cannot be made amongst those patients with a positive AQP4-IG but without a clinical attack. As compared with MS, NMO typically has more inflammatory CSF (commonly more than 50 nucleated cells in the CSF). Unlike MS, CSF in NMO usually does not have oligoclonal bands. On imaging, NMO has more longitudinally extensive spinal cord lesions (**Fig. 3**). Further the brain MRI of NMO does not typically meet criteria for MS based on location of lesions.

Amongst those patients who are negative for the NMO antibody, a certain proportion will be positive for the newly discovered antibody against myelin oligodendrocyte glycoprotein (MOG). Debate currently exists whether these individuals should be included within the NMOSD disease entity or if it should be categorized as its own entity given different suggested pathology. These diseases will likely become distinct entities in the future because of the different targets of the antibodies. The AQP4-IgG targets astrocytes in the aquaporin water channels, whereas those with anti-MOG do not show astrocyte destruction.[17]

Steroids are typically first-line treatment for NMO attacks. In those without improvement or in those with particularly severe clinical syndrome, plasmapheresis is used either after steroids or concurrently with steroids.[18] Because NMO is a relapsing disease, preventive therapy is generally recommended. More studies are needed for

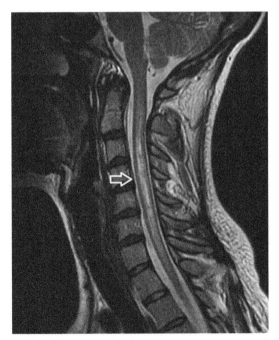

Fig. 3. Sagittal cervical spine MRI in patient with neuromyelitis optica shows longitudinally extensive hyperintense lesion (*arrow*).

immunosuppressive treatment strategies; however, the most common treatments used are typically azathioprine, mycophenolate mofetil, and rituximab. Selection amongst these options is based on comorbidities and patient preference. Treatments more classically used to treat MS, such as INFs, fingolimod, or natalizumab, should be avoided because they are ineffective or may even worsen the course of disease.

ACUTE DISSEMINATED ENCEPHALOMYELITIS

Acute disseminated encephalomyelitis (ADEM) is an immune-mediated disease primarily of children that causes widespread central nervous system demyelination.[19] In about two-third of cases, a preceding infection or vaccination can be identified. The course is typically monophasic although recurrent forms have been infrequently described. Clinically, patients usually have nonspecific flulike prodromal symptoms followed by neurologic symptoms, most typically a combination of encephalopathy and focal neurologic deficits. The most commonly reported focal deficits are weakness, ataxia, cranial nerve palsies, sensory abnormalities, and speech impairment.[20] Seizures may also occur in severe forms.

When suspected clinically, MRI often shows new white-matter lesions that are large and multifocal (**Fig. 4**). These lesions especially involve the deep structures of the brain such as the basal ganglia and thalamus. A single lesion is less common but does occur. CSF typically shows a lymphocytic pleocytosis and/or elevated protein. Unlike MS there are typically no oligoclonal bands present. Nonetheless, up to 30% of patients with ADEM may go on to be diagnosed with MS.[21] Anti-MOG antibodies have been found in a large fraction of children with ADEM. These levels become

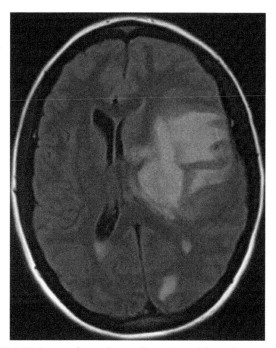

Fig. 4. Axial FLAIR MRI image shows large disseminated hyperintense lesions typical of ADEM.

undetectable in those children who have monophasic courses, whereas those with re-lapsing disease more commonly continued to have elevated anti-MOG levels.

Treatment of ADEM typically consists of high-dose steroids followed by a prolonged oral taper over weeks.[21] In patients who progress despite steroids, IVIG, and plasma-pheresis are considered second-line treatment. There are multiple reports for use of other agents including cyclophosphamide. In follow-up, vigilance should be main-tained for relapses, which often signal the diagnosis of MS.

AUTOIMMUNE ENCEPHALITIS

Autoimmune encephalitis refers to immune-mediated inflammatory brain disorder causing encephalopathy. The syndrome of autoimmune encephalitis can be caused by many factors some of which are known (such as particular antineuronal antibodies), whereas others are still being investigated. Clinically, autoimmune encephalitis should be suspected when there is otherwise unexplained subacute onset over weeks of memory disorder, psychiatric symptoms, or confusion.[22] There can be accompanying seizures or focal findings on neurologic examination. Inflammation is typically shown by pleocytosis in CSF or by MRI of brain showing evidence of inflammatory injury.

Within this broad category of patients with likely autoimmune encephalitis are more discrete syndromes. Perhaps the most important initial distinction is adverse event (AE) associated with cancer (paraneoplastic) and those that are not associated with cancer. The paraneoplastic AE disorders classically consist of progressive cerebellar degeneration, limbic encephalitis (combination of memory deficit, seizures, and neuropsychiatric symptoms), opsoclonus-myoclonus, or encephalomyelitis.[23] Neuro-logic symptoms can precede the detection of the cancer itself, and patients present-ing with one of these syndromes should be screened for presence of occult tumor with appropriate imaging. Paraneoplastic AE are associated with onconeural autoanti-bodies that target intracellular neuronal targets (such as anti-Hu or anti-Yo antibodies) although paraneoplastic syndromes certainly can occur without an identifiable auto-antibody in the serum. In paraneoplastic AE, the autoantibodies themselves are not thought to be pathogenic but rather a marker of the disease. Most patients with para-neoplastic AE have an abnormal CSF profile consisting of elevated cell count, elevated protein, or presence of oligoclonal bands (>90% sensitivity).[24] Paraneoplastic AE syn-dromes are poorly responsive to immunomodulatory therapy unless the underlying cancer has been adequately treated.

In contrast to paraneoplastic AE are syndromes mediated by autoantibodies that target antigens on neuronal surface. These neuronal cell surface antibodies are thought to be directly pathogenic. The spectrum of disease associated with these an-tibodies is expanding rapidly as more antibodies and associated syndromes are char-acterized. Some of the more common clinical syndromes encountered are those associated with anti-N-methyl-D aspartate receptor (anti-NMDAR) and anti-leucine-rich glioma-inactivated 1 (anti-LGI1) antibodies.[25]

Anti-NMDAR encephalitis was first described in 2007 in a small cohort of young fe-male patients most of whom had ovarian teratomas.[26] Anti-NDMAR encephalitis typi-cally starts with a systemic sense of unwellness with headache and fever that progresses over the course of days to weeks to neuropsychiatric changes including psychosis, catatonia, and delusions. Many patients are diagnosed with primary psy-chiatric disorders at this stage. However, patients with anti-NMDAR encephalitis develop progressively more symptoms including memory disorder, seizures, fluctu-ating consciousness, dyskinesias, and autonomic instability (fluctuations of blood pressure, heart rate, and respiratory rate).[26] Majority have abnormal CSF studies including lymphocytic pleocytosis, sometimes elevated protein or oligoclonal bands. MRI of the brain can show signal abnormalities although there is no characteristic abnormality.

The disease is caused by IgG antibodies against the GluN1 subunit of the NMDA receptor. The presence of the autoantibody causes receptor dysfunction and the progressive neuropsychiatric effects. In young women, anti-NMDAR encephalitis is associated with the presence of ovarian teratoma—about 45% of the female patients will have an ovarian teratoma.[27] The teratoma is thought to provoke autoimmunity by displaying neuronal antigens within the tumor.

Immunotherapy along with tumor removal (if applicable) results in improvement in more than 80% of individuals at 2 years. First-line therapy is considered steroids, IVIG, or plasmapheresis individually or combined.[28] Recovery typically starts within the first month of treatment. For those who continue to do poorly there is evidence that second-line therapy with rituximab or cyclophosphamide improves outcomes. Even after recovery, patients with anti-NMDAR encephalitis are at risk of relapse in the future with a similar stereotypic course.

The most common autoimmune cause of isolated limbic encephalitis (the combination of neuropsychiatric changes, seizure, and memory difficulty) is anti-LGI1 encephalitis. In contrast to other autoimmune disease, older men are predominantly affected by anti-LGI1 encephalitis.[29] This disease can evolve more slowly over weeks with a combination of psychiatric and cognitive changes. Behavioral changes typically consist of apathy and disinhibition, whereas cognitive changes generally at least involve memory deficits.[29] When seizures develop, a particular form called faciobrachial dystonic seizure is characteristic. This seizure is characterized by brief unilateral contraction of the face and arm occurring many times a day. Patients can have other neurologic symptoms including sleep disturbance, generalized seizures, and dysautonomia.

Clinical suspicion is key to diagnosing anti-LGI1 encephalitis. Majority has normal CSF, and MRI can be normal initially and only later show abnormalities in the temporal lobes (**Fig. 5**). A helpful laboratory clue is hyponatremia, which is associated with anti-LGI1 encephalitis. Treatment of anti-LGI1 encephalitis is based on observational series and generally consists of prolonged courses of corticosteroids.[30] For patients with persistent symptoms, additional agents including IVIg, rituximab, and oral immunosuppressants have been used. Although patients generally improve, many are left with some cognitive and psychiatric deficits.

SYSTEMIC AUTOIMMUNE DISEASE AND SARCOIDOSIS

The central nervous system can be affected by systemic autoimmune diseases. Examples include systemic lupus erythematosus, vasculitis, Sjögren syndrome, Behçet's disease, and sarcoidosis. As an example of these diseases, the authors discuss sarcoidosis, which is a granulomatous disorder that can affect almost every organ system but most commonly causes pulmonary disease. Neurosarcoidosis occurs in 5% to 15% of patients with systemic sarcoidosis; isolated sarcoidosis of the central nervous system is much rarer, estimated at around 1% of those with sarcoidosis.[31] Consequently, most patients who present with neurosarcoidosis as their initial clinical symptom have disease elsewhere even if not clinically apparent. The most common manifestation is cranial neuropathy, and among the cranial nerves, facial nerve, optic nerve, or trigeminal nerve is frequently affected.[32] Sarcoidosis has a predilection for the meninges and for the skull base region. Hence, in addition to cranial neuropathy, hypothalamic and pituitary dysfunction can occur. More infrequently, sarcoidosis can also present as isolated myelopathy or masslike lesion of the brain.

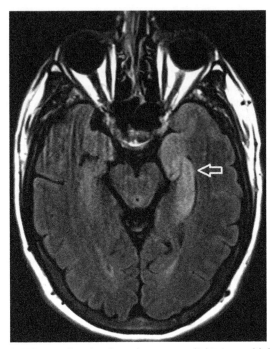

Fig. 5. Axial FLAIR MRI image showing hyperintense medial temporal lobe (*arrow*) in a patient with anti-LGI1 encephalitis.

Most patients with neurosarcoidosis have a specific phenotype of disease (such as cranial neuropathy or myelopathy or pituitary dysfunction), and relapses of the disease tend to follow the same phenotype.

A diagnosis of definite neurosarcoidosis can only be made with nervous system histology in the appropriate clinical context without any other cause. Probable neurosarcoidosis can be diagnosed with evidence of systemic sarcoidosis and involvement of central nervous system shown by imaging and laboratories such as inflammatory CSF. Possible neurosarcoid is a clinical presentation that suggests without an alternative diagnosis.[33] MRI is sensitive for disease involvement in sarcoidosis and frequently shows gadolinium-enhancing lesions involving both the parenchyma and meninges.[34] CSF is generally inflammatory but is nonspecific. Angiotensin-converting enzyme (ACE) is an insensitive and nonspecific marker of granulomatous disease and can be elevated in sarcoidosis. Estimates of ACE sensitivity in neurosarcoidosis vary widely among series but should not rely on to diagnose or exclude the disease.

Treatment for neurosarcoidosis is based on observational series. High-dose steroids with prolonged taper are generally the first-line therapy. For those who remain unresponsive to steroids or cannot tolerate prolonged courses, other agents such as methotrexate are used. More recently, there is compelling evidence that neurosarcoidosis responds well to anti-TNF therapy.[35] Duration of how long to treat is unclear but many patients have remissions during which therapy can be tapered down.

FUTURE CONSIDERATIONS

Autoimmune neurology is one of the more rapidly expanding subspecialties within neurology, and knowledge about novel mechanisms of injury to the central nervous system is emerging rapidly. The growing sophistication of imaging, laboratory testing, and treatment can be daunting to the internist. Clinical algorithms for when to suspect autoimmune disease and how to treat possible central nervous system autoimmunity are being developed and need to be simple and applicable.

REFERENCES

1. Koch-Henriksen N, Sørensen PS. The changing demographic pattern of multiple sclerosis epidemiology. Lancet Neurol 2010;9(5):520–32.
2. Ascherio A, Munger KL. Epidemiology of multiple sclerosis: from risk factors to prevention-an update. Semin Neurol 2016;36(2):103–14.
3. Hemmer B, Kerschensteiner M, Korn T. Role of the innate and adaptive immune responses in the course of multiple sclerosis. Lancet Neurol 2015;14(4):406–19.
4. Thompson AJ, Banwell BL, Barkhof F, et al. Diagnosis of multiple sclerosis: 2017 revisions of the McDonald criteria. Lancet Neurol 2018;17(2):162–73.
5. Yamout B, Al Khawajah M. Radiologically isolated syndrome and multiple sclerosis. Mult Scler Relat Disord 2017;17:234–7.
6. Ciccone A, Beretta S, Brusaferri F, et al. Corticosteroids for the long-term treatment in multiple sclerosis. Cochrane Database Syst Rev 2008;(1):CD006264.
7. Le Page E, Veillard D, Laplaud DA, et al. Oral versus intravenous high-dose methylprednisolone for treatment of relapses in patients with multiple sclerosis (COPOUSEP): a randomised, controlled, double-blind, non-inferiority trial. Lancet 2015;386(9997):974–81.
8. Montalban X, Hauser SL, Kappos L, et al. Ocrelizumab versus placebo in primary progressive multiple sclerosis. N Engl J Med 2017;376(3):209–20.
9. Kieseier BC. The mechanism of action of interferon-β in relapsing multiple sclerosis. CNS Drugs 2011;25(6):491–502.
10. O'Connor P, Filippi M, Arnason B, et al. 250 microg or 500 microg interferon beta-1b versus 20 mg glatiramer acetate in relapsing-remitting multiple sclerosis: a prospective, randomised, multicentre study. Lancet Neurol 2009;8(10):889–97.
11. Cohen JA, Barkhof F, Comi G, et al. Oral fingolimod or intramuscular interferon for relapsing multiple sclerosis. N Engl J Med 2010;362(5):402–15.
12. Polman CH, O'Connor PW, Havrdova E, et al. A randomized, placebo-controlled trial of natalizumab for relapsing multiple sclerosis. N Engl J Med 2006;354(9):899–910.
13. Rotstein DL, Healy BC, Malik MT, et al. Effect of vitamin D on MS activity by disease-modifying therapy class. Neurol Neuroimmunol Neuroinflamm 2015;2(6):e167.
14. Wingerchuk DM, Hogancamp WF, O'Brien PC, et al. The clinical course of neuromyelitis optica (Devic's syndrome). Neurology 1999;53(5):1107–14.
15. Jarius S, Wildemann B. Aquaporin-4 antibodies (NMO-IgG) as a serological marker of neuromyelitis optica: a critical review of the literature. Brain Pathol 2013;23(6):661–83.
16. Wingerchuk DM, Banwell B, Bennett JL, et al. International consensus diagnostic criteria for neuromyelitis optica spectrum disorders. Neurology 2015;85(2):177–89.
17. Pache F, Zimmermann H, Mikolajczak J, et al. MOG-IgG in NMO and related disorders: a multicenter study of 50 patients. Part 4: afferent visual system damage after optic neuritis in MOG-IgG-seropositive versus AQP4-IgG-seropositive patients. J Neuroinflammation 2016;13(1):282.

18. Kimbrough DJ, Fujihara K, Jacob A, et al. Treatment of neuromyelitis optica: review and recommendations. Mult Scler Relat Disord 2012;1(4):180–7.
19. Koelman DLH, Mateen FJ. Acute disseminated encephalomyelitis: current controversies in diagnosis and outcome. J Neurol 2015;262(9):2013–24.
20. Tenembaum S, Chitnis T, Ness J, et al, International Pediatric MS Study Group. Acute disseminated encephalomyelitis. Neurology 2007;68(16 Suppl 2):S23–36.
21. Pohl D, Tenembaum S. Treatment of acute disseminated encephalomyelitis. Curr Treat Options Neurol 2012;14(3):264–75.
22. Graus F, Titulaer MJ, Balu R, et al. A clinical approach to diagnosis of autoimmune encephalitis. Lancet Neurol 2016;15(4):391–404.
23. Dalmau J, Rosenfeld MR. Paraneoplastic syndromes of the CNS. Lancet Neurol 2008;7(4):327–40.
24. Psimaras D, Carpentier AF, Rossi C, et al. Cerebrospinal fluid study in paraneoplastic syndromes. J Neurol Neurosurg Psychiatry 2010;81(1):42–5.
25. Dalmau J, Graus F. Antibody-mediated encephalitis. N Engl J Med 2018. https://doi.org/10.1056/NEJMra1708712.
26. Dalmau J, Gleichman AJ, Hughes EG, et al. Anti-NMDA-receptor encephalitis: case series and analysis of the effects of antibodies. Lancet Neurol 2008;7(12):1091–8.
27. Ramanathan S, Mohammad SS, Brilot F, et al. Autoimmune encephalitis: recent updates and emerging challenges. J Clin Neurosci 2014;21(5):722–30.
28. Titulaer MJ, McCracken L, Gabilondo I, et al. Treatment and prognostic factors for long-term outcome in patients with anti-NMDA receptor encephalitis: an observational cohort study. Lancet Neurol 2013;12(2):157–65.
29. Bastiaansen AEM, van Sonderen A, Titulaer MJ. Autoimmune encephalitis with anti-leucine-rich glioma-inactivated 1 or anti-contactin-associated protein-like 2 antibodies (formerly called voltage-gated potassium channel-complex antibodies). Curr Opin Neurol 2017;30(3):302–9.
30. Ariño H, Armangué T, Petit-Pedrol M, et al. Anti-LGI1–associated cognitive impairment. Neurology 2016;87(8):759–65.
31. Segal BM. Neurosarcoidosis: diagnostic approaches and therapeutic strategies. Curr Opin Neurol 2013;26(3):307–13.
32. Krumholz A, Stern BJ. Neurologic manifestations of sarcoidosis. Handb Clin Neurol 2014;119:305–33.
33. Zajicek JP, Scolding NJ, Foster O, et al. Central nervous system sarcoidosis—diagnosis and management. QJM 1999;92(2):103–17.
34. Flanagan EP, Kaufmann TJ, Krecke KN, et al. Discriminating long myelitis of neuromyelitis optica from sarcoidosis. Ann Neurol 2015. https://doi.org/10.1002/ana.24582.
35. Gelfand JM, Bradshaw MJ, Stern BJ, et al. Infliximab for the treatment of CNS sarcoidosis: a multi-institutional series. Neurology 2017;89(20):2092–100.

Parkinson's Disease

Stephen G. Reich, MD*, Joseph M. Savitt, MD, PhD

KEYWORDS

- Parkinsonism • Parkinson's disease • Tremor • Levodopa • Dyskinesias
- REM sleep behavioral disorder

KEY POINTS

- The diagnosis of Parkinson's disease (PD) is based on the presence of bradykinesia and either resting tremor or rigidity and the absence of features from the history or examination suggesting an alternative cause of parkinsonism.
- Alternative causes of parkinsonism include drug-induced parkinsonism and parkinsonian syndromes such as multiple system atrophy or progressive supranuclear palsy.
- Although PD is usually considered a purely motor disorder, there is a long list of nonmotor manifestations that are equally, if not more, disabling and significantly affect quality of life. Many of them precede the onset of motor symptoms, such as hyposmia and a rapid eye movement sleep behavioral disorder.
- Levodopa remains the mainstay of treatment for PD.
- For patients with PD with drug-resistant tremor or problematic motor fluctuations including dyskinesias, which cannot be medically managed, deep brain stimulation should be considered.

INTRODUCTION

Parkinson's disease (PD) is the second most common neurodegenerative disorder after Alzheimer disease. Although most patients are managed by neurologists, PD presents initially to the primary care physician who should be able to make the diagnosis, which is based on the history and physical examination. The term "parkinsonism" refers to a clinical syndrome, including bradykinesia, cogwheel rigidity, resting tremor, a slow shuffling gait, and imbalance. The most common cause of parkinsonism is PD but there is a lengthy differential diagnosis and the challenge is to determine if the patient has PD or another cause of parkinsonism such as drug-induced or a parkinsonian syndrome, such as multiple system atrophy (MSA, formerly Shy–Drager syndrome). In addition to the cardinal motor signs of PD, there is a broad array of nonmotor features,

Disclosure: None.
Department of Neurology, University of Maryland School of Medicine, 110 South Paca Street, 3rd Floor, Baltimore, MD 21201, USA
* Corresponding author.
E-mail address: sreich@som.umaryland.edu

Med Clin N Am 103 (2019) 337–350
https://doi.org/10.1016/j.mcna.2018.10.014
0025-7125/19/© 2018 Elsevier Inc. All rights reserved.

medical.theclinics.com

which for many patients are equally if not more disabling, such as orthostatic hypotension, dream enactment (a rapid eye movement (REM) sleep behavioral disorder [RBD]), or hallucinations. Because of space limitations, the nonmotor features will not be covered in detail. The diagnosis of PD and the available medical and nonmedical therapies to treat the motor features are reviewed in this article.

Parkinsonism

PD was described by James Parkinson's, a general practitioner in London, just over 2 centuries ago, in 1817. His succinct description is still applicable:

> Involuntary tremulous motion, with lessened muscular power, in parts not in action and even when supported; with a propensity to bend the trunk forwards, and to pass from a walking to a running pace.[1]

There have been tremendous advances in our understanding of PD since 1817,[2] more than can be covered here, and the authors focus instead on practical clinical aspects of diagnosis and management. In brief, PD is characterized pathologically by degeneration of dopaminergic neurons in the substantia nigra of the midbrain, leading to pathophysiologic changes in the circuitry of the downstream basal ganglia.[3] The Lewy body is the cytologic hallmark of PD and contains misfolded α-synuclein, the same protein that also accumulates in related disorders including multiple system atrophy and dementia with Lewy bodies, collectively referred to as "synucleinopathies."[4] Although a small percentage of patients with PD have a monogenetic cause, either dominant or recessively inherited (such as the genes LRRK2 or *parkin*, among others) most cases are sporadic and of unknown cause.[5]

Consider the following patient:

> A 60-year-old man complains of tremor of the dominant right hand for the past 6 months. All fine motor tasks with his right hand are more difficult such as brushing his teeth, turning pages, and texting. His handwriting has become smaller. He tends to scuff the right foot and has trouble sliding the right foot into a loafer. His wife has noticed that he does not swing the right arm while walking and that his voice is softer. Although not appreciated until asked, he acknowledges that his sense of smell has diminished. There is a history of constipation. When asked about sleep, his wife reports that for the past 10 years he has occasionally acted out a dream, appearing to be fighting, and during one episode he struck her during his sleep. Although he always was mildly anxious, this worsened recently with irritability and insomnia. On examination, there is decreased facial expression and his voice is mildly soft with diminished volume. There is a tremor at rest of the right hand. He has no difficulty arising from the chair. He walks a little slowly; the right arm does not swing, and the right shoe scuffs the floor, which can be both seen and heard. His posture is mildly flexed. He does not lose his balance when given a sudden pull backwards. His handwriting starts off normally but gets smaller toward the end of a sentence. Rapid repetitive movements of the right limbs are mildly slow but normal on the left. Strength is normal as are reflexes. When the right arm is passively moved, there is mild rigidity. Shoulder shrug is slower on the right.

Does this patient have PD? To answer this question, it is appropriate to evaluate this case using the diagnostic criteria for PD proposed by the Movement Disorder Society (MDS) (please refer to the criteria for a complete discussion).[6] There are 4 steps in the diagnosis of PD (**Box 1**); the first is to ensure the patient actually has parkinsonism. This is defined by the presence of bradykinesia and either a resting tremor or rigidity

---

Box 1
Four-step approach to the diagnosis of Parkinson's disease

Step 1: Establish the presence of parkinsonism
- Bradykinesia plus
- Rest tremor OR
- Rigidity

Step 2: Identify features supporting the diagnosis of PD
- Unequivocal and dramatic response to levodopa
- Presence of resting tremor
- Olfactory loss
- Other

Step 3: There should be no absolute exclusion criteria
- Cerebellar signs
- Supranuclear vertical ophthalmoplegia
- Treatment of dopamine receptor blocker or depletor within the past year
- Cortical sensory signs (agraphesthesia, astereognosis)
- Normal functional imaging of the presynaptic dopamine receptor
- Other

Step 4: Search for red flags that cast doubt on the diagnosis of PD
- Rapid progression (use of a wheelchair within 5 years of symptom onset)
- Early falls
- Early and severe dysarthria and dysphagia
- Early autonomic failure
- Bilateral, symmetric parkinsonism
- Absence of some of the nonmotor features expected with PD: RBD, hyposmia, constipation, anxiety, depression

Adapted from Postuma RB, Berg D, Stern M, et al. MDS clinical diagnostic criteria for Parkinson's disease. Mov Disord 2015;30(12):1595; with permission.

(note that about one-third of patients with PD do not have tremor). Bradykinesia is characterized by a combination of slowness of movement along with a reduction in the speed or amplitude of sustained repetitive movements (finger, hand, toe, or heel tapping). Tremor is best observed with the hands resting in the lap and sometimes can be brought out by mental distraction such as saying the months of the year backwards. A PD tremor often involves the lower extremity and may begin the foot. The tremor, like other signs of early PD, typically begins unilaterally and this is an important distinction with essential tremor (ET). Rigidity is perceived as a "lead-pipe" resistance to passive movement of the limbs and is best appreciated at the elbow or wrist. Based on these criteria, the abovementioned patient has parkinsonism.

The next step refers to "supportive criteria," that is, features that are typical of PD and usually not seen in other causes of parkinsonism. The most important of these is a "clear and dramatic beneficial response to dopaminergic therapy." Because this patient is not yet on dopaminergic therapy, this criterion cannot be fulfilled at this time, but eventually all patients with PD will require such treatment and until that time, the diagnosis of PD cannot be made with certainty. Additional supportive criteria include a resting tremor (which he has), and olfactory loss, which is also present and will be discussed later as a "prodromal" sign of PD. Although not part of the MDS supportive criteria, PD typically begins unilaterally, unrelated to handedness, and this is considered as an important supportive feature recognizing that no single clinical feature is free of false positives or negatives. Based on this, with the exception of an unknown response to dopaminergic therapy, this patient has other supportive features of PD.

The third criterion is the presence of features that are not expected with PD and point toward an alternative diagnosis. Only several will be discussed here and among them, one of the most important is the lack of exposure to a dopamine blocking or depleting medication in a time frame that could cause parkinsonism, and this typically means within the past year. Dopamine receptor blocking agents include all of the first-generation and many of the second-generation antipsychotics as well as metoclopramide. Because drug-induced parkinsonism may take as long as 1 year to resolve, the patient may no longer be on the offending drug at presentation and therefore it is essential to include this when taking a history. Other "absolute exclusion criteria" include lack of response to dopaminergic therapy, cerebellar signs, cortical sensory loss (agraphesthesia, astereognosis, extinction to double simultaneous stimulation), which suggest corticobasal syndrome, or restriction of vertical gaze, suggesting progressive supranuclear palsy. As will be discussed later, if functional imaging of the pre-synaptic dopamine transporter (DaTScan) is performed as part of the assessment of parkinsonism, and found to be normal, then that is also considered exclusionary for the diagnosis of PD. But, the criteria do not require such imaging and it is usually not necessary.

The final set of criteria are "red flags," which refer to features from the history and examination that do not necessarily reach the level of being an exclusionary feature for PD, yet do cast doubt on the diagnosis particularly when there are several.[7] They generally point toward a parkinsonian syndrome, which will be discussed later. Among several others, these include rapid progression of gait dysfunction, typically necessitating a wheelchair within 5 years of onset of symptoms; severe and early autonomic failure; early bulbar dysfunction such as severe dysarthria or dysphagia, both of which occur in PD, but not early in the course. Similarly, falls are common in PD but only seen in the middle to advanced stages and if present at onset or early in the course, suggest an alternative diagnosis such as MSA or progressive supranuclear palsy (PSP). Earlier it was mentioned that PD typically begins as hemiparkinsonism and as such, bilateral, symmetric parkinsonism should be considered a red flag. Although these criteria accept the presence of dementia at any time in the course of parkinsonism to be in keeping with possible PD, in the authors' opinion and experience, when dementia occurs early in the course of parkinsonism, and especially when it precedes it, this usually suggests an alternative diagnosis such as dementia with Lewy bodies.[8]

In contrast to all other red flags, which refer to the presence of a feature atypical for PD, the absence of certain nonmotor features expected in PD should also make one question the diagnosis. These include the lack of mild dysautonomia (constipation, erectile dysfunction, urinary urgency), the absence of an RBD (dream enactment), normal olfaction, and the lack of psychological features usually seen in PD such as depression and anxiety. The abovementioned patient does not have any exclusionary criteria nor are there any red flags. He has some of the expected nonmotor (premotor) features of PD, including constipation, recent exacerbation of anxiety, and an RBD all pointing to PD as the cause of parkinsonism. Even though the diagnosis of PD seems secure at this time, it is only during long-term follow-up that one is able to be more confident of the diagnosis because red flags may appear later in the course, and it remains to be determined if the patient will respond to levodopa and if so, will he eventually demonstrate fluctuations and dyskinesias that are expected with PD and not with alternative causes of PD. As such, it is important to continually reassess the diagnosis of PD at each visit. Ideally, all patients with parkinsonism should be referred to a neurologist to confirm the diagnosis. **Box 2** lists some additional features that can be helpful in the diagnosis of PD.

Box 2
Some tips for diagnosing Parkinson's disease

- The MDS criteria for PD[6] includes a very useful "completion form" providing a step-by-step checklist through the diagnostic process.

- Be sure to ask about a history of antidopaminergic therapy during the prior year.

- Early PD begins unilaterally, unrelated to handedness.

- Tremor is the most common presenting symptom of PD but one-third of patients do not have tremor and present with unilateral slowness or mild incoordination sometimes sensed as "weakness."

- PD may begin with tremor of the foot.

- The tremor of PD is often present when the patient is walking.

- Whether it begins in the upper or lower extremity, testing rapid repetitive movements will confirm that both limbs on the same side are affected.

- Shoulder shrug is slower on the symptomatic side.

- The resting tremor may "reemerge" while maintaining posture.

- The tremor of PD often involves the chin, tongue, lips, or jaw but typically not the head or voice.

- A handwriting sample is one of the best ways to distinguish PD from ET, assuming that PD involves the dominant hand.

- Refer to the text and the MDS criteria[6] for a list of red flags that cast doubt on the diagnosis of PD.

- Reconsider the diagnosis of PD at each visit because up to 20% of patients will prove to have an alternative cause of parkinsonism, typically a parkinsonian syndrome.

- Be familiar with the nonmotor features of PD because they assist in the diagnosis, are often overlooked, and are important determinants of quality of life.

- Although imbalance is one of the cardinal features of PD, it is not present early in the disease and if so, especially if accompanied by falls, suggests a parkinsonian syndrome.

PARKINSONIAN SYNDROMES

Even though the diagnosis of PD is considered straightforward, often termed a "waiting room diagnosis," autopsy studies have demonstrated that 20% of patients diagnosed with PD during life have an alternative diagnosis at autopsy.[9] The most common mimickers are parkinsonian syndromes—that is, other neurodegenerative disorders that share some features with PD but are distinct in terms of having clinical signs not usually seen with PD (red flags) and demonstrating little or no response to levodopa or the rapid waning of an initially beneficial response. These syndromes are more rapidly progressive and debilitating than PD, with patients usually dying within a decade of onset.

Multiple system atrophy is characterized by the presence of autonomic failure accompanied by either parkinsonism, which is unresponsive to levodopa (MSA-P), or cerebellar ataxia (MSA-C).[10,11] MSA has replaced the prior diagnoses of Shy–Drager syndrome, olivopontocerebellar atrophy (OPCA), and striatonigral degeneration because it was ultimately recognized that they were different presentations of the same disorder. Dementia with Lewy bodies, as MSA, is a synucleinopathy.[12] It is characterized by the presence of dementia either preceding (typically within 2 years) or appearing concurrent with parkinsonism. As mentioned earlier, the authors consider early dementia in the setting of parkinsonism as a red flag pointing away from PD. Other characteristic features of dementia with Lewy bodies include fluctuations in mental status, which are otherwise unexplained; visual hallucinations unrelated to medication; RBD; and sensitivity to dopamine receptor blocking agents.

The other broad category of parkinsonian syndromes is known as tauopathies, in contrast to synucleinopathies, referring to the accumulation of abnormally phosphor-ylated tau in specific brain regions. PSP[13,14] is characterized by early falls, axial parkinsonian signs (stiffness and slowness), frontal-executive dysfunction, and slow vertical saccades (saccades are the eye movements that shift gaze between targets), eventually leading to restricted vertical eye movements (supranuclear vertical ophthal-moplegia). This is the classic form of PSP, also known as Richardson syndrome but it has a heterogeneous clinical picture and may also manifest as freezing of gait, nonflu-ent aphasia, or frontotemporal dementia. Corticobasal degeneration[15] is related to PSP but much less common and typically presents with a combination of cortical signs (agraphesthesia, astereognosis, aphasia, myoclonus) and basal ganglia signs such as dystonia, rigidity, or a "useless" limb. Corticobasal degeneration typically pre-sents unilaterally, as does PD, whereas most of the other parkinsonian syndromes begin symmetrically.

Although not a parkinsonian syndrome, parkinsonism is often attributed to cerebro-vascular disease. This is usually considered in the patient with disproportionate parkinsonian signs from the waist down ("lower half parkinsonism"), lack of benefit from levodopa, and imaging demonstrating evidence of cerebrovascular disease, either discrete strokes or confluent changes in the white matter often attributed to microvascular disease. What is labeled vascular parkinsonism is arguably overdiag-nosed, and it is important to consider other causes such as a parkinsonian syndrome or normal pressure hydrocephalus.[16–18]

IMAGING OF THE PRESYNAPTIC DOPAMINE TRANSPORTER

Single-photon emission computed tomography imaging of the uptake of ioflupane I123 (DaTscan) by the presynaptic dopamine transporter is a marker of integrity of the dopaminergic nigrostriatal pathway and has a high sensitivity to detect its degen-eration.[19–22] It was approved by the Food and Drug Administration in 2011 to distin-guish tremor due to PD from essential tremor. It cannot distinguish between PD and other causes of parkinsonism also associated by nigrostriatal degeneration, which is virtually all of the parkinsonism syndrome (MSA, PSP, etc.) and in most cases the differential boils down to PD versus a related syndrome.

In the authors' view, DaTscan has a limited role in the evaluation of most patients with parkinsonism, particularly if one is familiar with and follows the MDS diagnostic criteria. Circumstances where it can be considered include the following: (1) if there is legitimate uncertainty about the cause of parkinsonism; if everything points toward PD, then imaging is not needed; (2) if the result will change management, and (3) if the diagnosis cannot be obtained in an easier and less expensive way and the first step here should be referral to a specialist in movement disorders.[23] Similarly, for many pa-tients with an unclear cause of parkinsonism, the best test is often the "test of time" along with careful follow-up.

Nonmotor Features of Parkinson's Disease

As discussed earlier, the diagnosis of PD is based on its motor manifestations and these often get the most attention by physicians and patients. Yet, nonmotor symp-toms (NMS) are present in all patients, are often as distressing as motor symptoms, have a significant impact on quality of life, and are generally resistant to PD therapies directed at motor symptoms. Nonmotor symptoms cover a broad range of common PD symptoms and can be broadly classified into neuropsychiatric, sensory, sleep, and autonomic (**Box 3**).[24]

There are several reasons why being familiar with, inquiring about, and treating NMS is important. First, some NMS precede motor signs by years or decades (referred to as prodromal PD) and therefore could potentially be used to predict the onset of disease. These include reduced sense of smell, anxiety, depression, dream enactment (RBD), and constipation.[25] Second, the identification of these symptoms and their link to PD reduces patient and caregiver anxiety about the presence of another disorder. Third, these symptoms require therapies not usually tied to the treatment of motor symptoms

---

Box 3
Nonmotor features of PD

Neuropsychiatric

Mild cognitive impairment

Executive dysfunction

Dementia

Hallucinations

Delusions

Depression

Anxiety

Fatigue

Apathy

Autonomic

Constipation

Neurogenic bladder

Orthostatic hypotension

Erectile dysfunction

Diaphoresis

Drooling

Dysphagia

Sleep

REM behavioral disorder

Insomnia

Excessive daytime sleepiness

Restless legs syndrome and periodic limb movements of sleep

Sensory

Pain

Frozen shoulder

Hyposmia

Diplopia

and the presence of treatment-resistant neuroleptic malignant syndrome heralds increasing overall disability and reduced quality of life. In summary, recognizing and addressing the nonmotor features of PD are crucial to comprehensive care of those with PD.[26,27]

The nonmotor features of PD are reviewed in **Box 3**.

Treatment of Parkinson's Disease

Initiation of therapy

One of the first decisions in treating patients with PD is when to start medical therapy and with which agent. Before considering that, it should be noted that physical therapy intervention and exercise both are likely to be beneficial to patients, although the most useful form of each is uncertain.[28] In the authors' practice they recommend formal "Big and Loud" physical and speech therapies as well as exercise programs geared toward the PD population. Examples include dancing, boxing training, and Tai Chi. Initiating medical therapy is a personalized decision and usually is begun when the signs and symptoms of PD begin to significantly affect a patient's ability to perform their activities related to hobbies, recreational and social activities, and occupation. Less obvious factors such as embarrassment from a tremor, a reduced ability to exercise, and the presence of pain or anxiety should be considered as well.

The mainstay of PD treatment involves medications that deplete dopamine or mimic its effect at the dopamine receptor. The most effective medication is levodopa that is paired with carbidopa, a peripheral inhibitor of its breakdown to reduce side effects and maximize therapeutic efficacy. Alternatives to starting with levodopa include the use of dopamine agonists, monoamine oxidase B (MAO-B) inhibitors and in certain cases anticholinergics.

Medications Used to Treat Parkinson's Disease Motor Symptoms

Levodopa

Levodopa coupled with a DOPA decarboxylase inhibitor (carbidopa in the United States) is the most effective therapy for PD. Carbidopa does not readily pass through the blood-brain barrier, thereby allowing levodopa to be converted to active dopamine preferentially in the central nervous system, because dopamine also does not cross the blood-brain barrier. Initiation of therapy begins with a pill containing 25 mg of carbidopa and 100 mg of levodopa (25/100) titrated up to at least 3 times a day. It should all be given during the waking day (approximately 4–5 hours apart) because most patients do not need medication at night unless symptoms interfere with sleep. Using the 10/100 preparation does not provide adequate carbidopa to prevent the peripheral conversion of levodopa to dopamine and should not be used to initiate therapy. Because levodopa is associated with the onset of wearing off and dyskinesia, its use often had been delayed in favor of other treatments such as MAO-B inhibitors and dopamine agonists in early disease. This idea is now being challenged.[29] The current argument for using levodopa early is that other treatments often have more initial side effects and are less effective than levodopa and that the onset of motor complications is tied to disease duration and levodopa dose magnitude rather than duration of levodopa exposure.[29,30] This is not universally accepted, but initiating levodopa therapy early in the disease course is an acceptable option. Treatment of early PD with levodopa, however, should be limited to the lowest effective dose and some consideration should be given to "levodopa sparing" therapies such as dopamine agonists as the dose requirements of levodopa increase.

Other considerations with the initiation of levodopa therapy include side effects such as dizziness and gastrointestinal (GI) upset. Despite a reduction in therapeutic efficacy, patients may dose with meals to reduce side effects. Protein intake reduces levodopa efficacy by competing with its transport ultimately into the brain, and patients should be aware of this when eating meals containing high-protein loads. Some patients will delay high-protein meals to the evening when optimal symptom control is not required or take extra medication around the time of a high-protein meal. In refractory patients, levodopa-induced nausea can be managed through the use of extra carbidopa, ondansetron, domperidone (not available In the United States), or trimethobenzamide, because more common antiemetics such as promethazine, metoclopramide, and prochlorperazine may worsen Parkinson's symptoms through their antidopaminergic effect.[31]

With advancing disease, levodopa dosing is increased in both dose strength and frequency. As these doses increase other side effects such as hallucinations, delusions, motor complications, and orthostatic hypotension become more common. As dosing increases there is at least the theoretic possibility that carbidopa may cross into the brain and limit levodopa effectiveness. Doses of 450 mg of carbidopa a day do not impair levodopa efficacy,[32] but higher doses should prompt consideration of using preparations such as 10/100 or 25/250 to limit the risk. In addition, the possibility of other side effects from higher dose carbidopa has been suggested, and some recommend reducing daily carbidopa dose to less than 200 to 300 mg/d in susceptible patients.[33]

An increase in the number of daily levodopa doses also increases the number of peaks and troughs in medication concentration and is more burdensome for the patient. In response to this, 2 approved longer-acting formulations of levodopa have been engineered. The controlled release formulation provides minimal extension of the levodopa effect, whereas extended release (C/L-ER, aka Rytary) seems to offer longer-lasting effect with less variation in levodopa concentration.[34,35] Carbidopa/levodopa extended-release capsules (Rytary) are available in 4 dose strengths, each containing 3 formulations of levodopa and carbidopa that generate peak plasma concentration at different times after ingestion. Therapy with this drug is hampered by high cost and difficulties in determining the optimal dose. Tables are available for conversion of standard therapies to C/L-ER; however, more than half of patients require higher doses.[36]

Dopamine agonists

Dopamine agonists mimic the effect of dopamine at the dopamine receptor. They have the benefit of less frequent dosing with pramipexole and ropinirole dosed 3 times a day or once a day if the long-acting preparation is used. Rotigotine comes in a patch formulation for continuous release transdermally. Their use early on delays the need for levodopa and thereby delays the onset of levodopa-induced dyskinesia.[35] Unfortunately, these medications do not offer the same degree of symptom relief as levodopa. In addition, side effects such as peripheral edema, orthostasis, impulse control disorders, skin irritation (seen with rotigotine), psychosis, sleepiness, and a troublesome withdrawal syndrome limit their utility, especially in older patients.[31] They can be used successfully for initial therapy in those patients especially fearful of dyskinesia, in those desiring less frequent medication dosing, and in those who are able to tolerate side effects. They have a role as add-on therapy to levodopa to reduce the length and severity of off time. Given their longer duration effect, dopamine agonists may be better at addressing overnight off time and morning akinesia, when oral dosing of levodopa is inconvenient. Adding a dopamine agonist to levodopa also serves as a levodopa-sparing agent, reducing the need for higher or more frequent levodopa doses and therefore may reduce levodopa-induced side effects.[37] The use of dopamine agonist may worsen dyskinesia necessitating a reduction in levodopa dose or reduction/discontinuation of the dopamine agonist. Apomorphine, another dopamine agonist, is used as an acute rescue therapy for patients with wearing-off symptoms that are troublesome. It is administered as a subcutaneous injection with an onset of action between 7 and 20 minutes and a duration of action of about 90 minutes.[38] Initiation requires the use of trimethobenzamide to avoid nausea and a careful titration to find the optimal, tolerable dose.

Catechol-O-methyl transferase inhibitors
This class of medication inhibits the metabolism of both levodopa and dopamine, therefore prolonging the action of each.[39] In doing so, it also increases the likelihood of levodopa-induced side effects. For practical purposes, entacapone is the only member of this medication class in common use in the United States because tolcapone use is limited by the requirement of monitoring for liver toxicity. Patients should be advised about the propensity of entacapone to cause benign discoloration of urine. It may cause diarrhea, which is typically mild and self-limited and rarely severe, and this side effect can be delayed by weeks to several months after initiation. Entacapone is available in a combination pill along with carbidopa and levodopa. This is a more convenient option and has the added benefit of being available in multiple levodopa dose strengths. A third member of this class opicapone has been found to be clinically useful as a once-a-day medication but is not yet available in the United States.[28]

Monoamine oxidase B inhibitors
These medications impair the metabolism of dopamine and include selegiline, rasagiline, and safinamide. As a class they reduce wearing-off when added to L-DOPA and likely delay the initiation of levodopa when used as monotherapy.

Amantadine
Amantadine has a mild anti-parkinsonian effect but is more often used to reduce levodopa-induced dyskinesia (LID), although duration of the effect and appropriate dosing have been the subjects of debate.[40,41] Nonetheless, amantadine is often used chronically to treat LID usually dosed 2 or 3 times a day. Side effects include psychosis, edema, constipation, and livedo reticularis. More recently, ADS-5102 or Gocovri has been approved for LID. It is an extended release formulation of amantadine that is dosed at bedtime that seems to be more marginally more efficacious than the immediate release form in reducing "off" time and reducing dyskinesia.[42]

Trihexyphenidyl
Anticholinergic medications including trihexyphenidyl are most often used to treat PD tremor and their use is limited by side effects.[43] Older patients may be intolerant of this class due to memory impairment, confusion, and hallucinations. Other side effects include dry mouth, constipation, urinary retention, sedation, tachycardia, reduced perspiration, blurred vision, and GI upset. Despite these drawbacks, trihexyphenidyl can offer tremor relief in patients whose tremor is resistant to levodopa and who demonstrate an ability to tolerate the side effects. They can be used as monotherapy or with other agents, and may have a levodopa sparing effect, reducing the need for higher doses of levodopa that often are required to treat refractory tremor.

Interventional Therapies

Carbidopa/levodopa enteral suspension (Duopa)

Patients with advanced PD whose motor complications, including on-off fluctuation and dyskinesia, are refractory to standard therapies may benefit from a constant infusion of carbidopa and levodopa in the form of an enteral suspension. This therapy involves a surgically implanted jejunostomy connected to a pump that infuses medication directly into the proximal jejunum where levodopa absorption is maximal. Benefits of this therapy include a more constant delivery of drug that bypasses potentially problematic delayed gastric emptying. Patients typically receive a morning bolus dose of medication followed by a continuous maintenance dose. During the course of the day patients have the ability to self-administer extra doses to deal with off periods. The pump is typically disconnected at the end of the waking day. Studies have shown a reduction in daily off time by nearly 2 hours versus the use of standard levodopa oral formulation as well as a reduction in troublesome dyskinesia.[44,45] Drawbacks include surgical and device complications such as abdominal pain, infection, tube occlusion and dislocation, buried bumper syndrome, bezoars, leakage, and polyneuropathy. Also there is the inconvenience of jejunostomy maintenance, pump management, and carrying around the device all day. In selected patients, usually those with a dedicated caregiver to assist with device maintenance and who are reluctant to pursue or are poor candidates for DBS, significant benefit can be seen.

DEEP BRAIN STIMULATION

In a patient whose motor fluctuations are refractory and in those with poorly controlled disabling tremor, stimulation of deep structures of the brain offers significant relief. This therapy consists of placing thin wires containing distal electrodes stereotactically into the brain with the more proximal ends connected to extension cables that tunnel subcutaneously to an impulse generator (IPG). The IPG is placed beneath a patient's skin in the infraclavicular or intraabdominal region and stimulation parameters and location of stimulation among a series of distal contact sites are programmed using a remote device. Programming is done in the clinic and patients may adjust their device using a similar device within parameters set by the clinician programmer. DBS effectively reduces motor signs of the disease and improves off time, dyskinesia, and quality of life.[46] Before surgery, potential side effects of DBS including speech and cognition impairment, gait changes, and neuropsychiatric sequelae need to be considered as do surgical risks.[47] Careful selection of candidates for surgery involves psychiatric and cognitive screening, medical clearance, and involvement of experienced surgeons and device programmers. Patients with significant cognitive, medical, and psychiatric comorbidities are not ideal candidates. Management of expectations is important, and except for potentially better treatment of tremor and dyskinesia, patients should not expect benefit beyond their best preoperative symptom control on optimal medical therapy. Target selection among the 2 most common targets, the subthalamic nucleus and globus pallidus interna, considers the relative benefits of greater medication dose reduction and better tremor control seen in the former, with better dyskinesia control and potentially fewer side effects in the latter.[47] In patients with a tremor dominant presentation, targeting the ventral intermediate nucleus of the thalamus provides significant and sustained tremor relief and is considered in those whose overwhelming complaint is tremor.[48] In addition to site selection, other variables including the type of procedure (awake vs asleep), type of impulse generator (rechargeable or not, current steering or not), and brand of device (Medtronic, Abbott, or Boston Scientific each approved in the United States) and whether to implant unilaterally or bilaterally are decisions made by an experienced clinical team.

REFERENCES

1. Parkinson J. An essay on the shaking palsy. London: Sherwood, Neely, and Jones; 1817. Available at: https://archive.org/details/essayonshakingpa00parkuoft.
2. Obeso JA, Stamelou M, Goetz CG, et al. Past, present, and future of Parkinson's disease: a special essay on the 200th Anniversary of the Shaking Palsy. Mov Disord 2017;32:1264–310.
3. Kalia LV, Lang AE. Parkinson disease in 2015: evolving basic, pathological and clinical concepts in PD. Nat Rev Neurol 2016;12:65–6.
4. Goedert M, Jakes R, Spillantini MG. The synucleinopathies: twenty years on. J Parkinsons Dis 2017;7:S51–69.
5. Deng H, Wang P, Jankovic J. The genetics of Parkinson disease. Ageing Res Rev 2018;42:72–85.
6. Postuma RB, Berg D, Stern M, et al. MDS clinical diagnostic criteria for Parkinson's disease. Mov Disord 2015;30:1591–601.
7. Köllensperger M, Geser F, Seppi K, et al. Red flags for multiple system atrophy. Mov Disord 2008;23:1093–9.
8. Boeve BF, Dickson DW, Duda JE, et al. Arguing against the proposed definition changes of PD. Mov Disord 2016;31:1619–22.
9. Rizzo G, Copetti M, Arcuti S, et al. Accuracy of clinical diagnosis of Parkinson disease: a systematic review and meta-analysis. Neurology 2016;86:566–76.
10. Gilman S, Wenning GK, Low PA, et al. Second consensus statement on the diagnosis of multiple system atrophy. Neurology 2008;71:670–6.
11. Quinn N. Multiple system atrophy-the nature of the beast. J Neurol Neurosurg Psychiatry 1989;(suppl):78–89.
12. McKeith IG, Boeve BF, Dickson DW, et al. Diagnosis and management of dementia with Lewy bodies: fourth consensus report of the DLB Consortium. Neurology 2017;89:88–100.
13. Höglinger GU, Respondek G, Stamelou M, et al, Movement Disorder Society-endorsed PSP Study Group. Clinical diagnosis of progressive supranuclear palsy: The movement disorder society criteria. Mov Disord 2017;32:853–64.
14. Williams DR, Lees AJ. Progressive supranuclear palsy: clinicopathological concepts and diagnostic challenges. Lancet Neurol 2009;8:270–9.
15. Armstrong MJ, Litvan I, Lang AE, et al. Criteria for the diagnosis of corticobasal degeneration. Neurology 2013;80:496–503.
16. Vizcarra JA, Lang AE, Sethi KD, et al. Vascular parkinsonism: deconstructing a syndrome. Mov Disord 2015;30:886–94.
17. Glass PG, Lees AJ, Bacellar A, et al. The clinical features of pathologically confirmed vascular parkinsonism. J Neurol Neurosurg Psychiatry 2012;83:1027–9.
18. Kalra S, Grosset DG, Benamer HT. Differentiating vascular parkinsonism from idiopathic Parkinson's disease: a systematic review. Mov Disord 2010;25:149–56.
19. Ba F, Martin WR. Dopamine transporter imaging as a diagnostic tool for parkinsonism and related disorders in clinical practice. Parkinsonism Relat Disord 2015;21:87–94.

20. Isaacson SH, Fisher S, Gupta F, et al. Clinical utility of DaTscan™ imaging in the evaluation of patients with parkinsonism: a US perspective. Expert Rev Neurother 2017;17:219–25.
21. Brooks DJ. Molecular imaging of dopamine transporters. Ageing Res Rev 2016; 30:114–21.
22. Rodriguez-Porcel F, Jamali S, Duker AP, et al. Dopamine transporter scanning in the evaluation of patients with suspected Parkinsonism: a case-based user's guide. Expert Rev Neurother 2016;16:23–9.
23. Zimmerman S. All my husband needed was a good physical examination. JAMA Intern Med 2015;175:340.
24. Barone P, Antonini A, Colosimo C, et al. The PRIAMO study: a multicenter assessment of nonmotor symptoms and their impact on quality of life in Parkinson's disease. Mov Disord 2009;24:1641–9.
25. Shrestha S, Kamel F, Umbach DM, et al. Nonmotor symptoms and Parkinson disease in United States farmers and spouses. PLoS One 2017;12:e0185510.
26. Titova N, Qamar MA, Chaudhuri KR. The nonmotor features of Parkinson's disease. Int Rev Neurobiol 2017;132:33–54.
27. Santos-Garcia D, de la Fuente-Fernandez R. Impact of non-motor symptoms on health-related and perceived quality of life in Parkinson's disease. J Neurol Sci 2013;332:136–40.
28. Fox SH, Katzenschlager R, Lim SY, et al. International Parkinson and movement disorder society evidence-based medicine review: update on treatments for the motor symptoms of Parkinson's disease. Mov Disord 2018;33(8):1248–66.
29. Matarazzo M, Perez-Soriano A, Stoessl AJ. Dyskinesias and levodopa therapy: why wait? J Neural Transm (Vienna) 2018;125:1119–30.
30. Cilia R, Akpalu A, Sarfo FS, et al. The modern pre-levodopa era of Parkinson's disease: insights into motor complications from sub-Saharan Africa. Brain 2014;137(Pt 10):2731–42.
31. Julius A, Longfellow K. Movement disorders: a brief guide in medication management. Med Clin North Am 2016;100:733–61.
32. Brod LS, Aldred JL, Nutt JG. Are high doses of carbidopa a concern? A randomized, clinical trial in Parkinson's disease. Mov Disord 2012;27:750–3.
33. Lau ACW, Diggle JL, Bring PP. Improvement in severe orthostatic hypotension following carbidopa dose eeduction. Can J Neurol Sci 2018;45:252–3.
34. Margolesky J, Singer C. Extended-release oral capsule of carbidopa-levodopa in Parkinson disease. Ther Adv Neurol Disord 2018;11. 1756285617737728.
35. Connolly BS, Lang AE. Pharmacological treatment of Parkinson disease: a review. JAMA 2014;311:1670–83.
36. Hauser RA, Hsu A, Kell S, et al. Extended-release carbidopa-levodopa (IPX066) compared with immediate-release carbidopa-levodopa in patients with Parkinson's disease and motor fluctuations: a phase 3 randomised, double-blind trial. Lancet Neurol 2013;12:346–56.
37. Talati R, Baker WL, Patel AA, et al. Adding a dopamine agonist to preexisting levodopa therapy vs. levodopa therapy alone in advanced Parkinson's disease: a meta analysis. Int J Clin Pract 2009;63:613–23.
38. Stacy M. Apomorphine: North American clinical experience. Neurology 2004; 62(6 Suppl 4):S18–21.
39. Nutt JG, Woodward WR, Beckner RM, et al. Effect of peripheral catechol-O-methyltransferase inhibition on the pharmacokinetics and pharmacodynamics of levodopa in parkinsonian patients. Neurology 1994;44:913–9.

40. Thomas A, Iacono D, Luciano AL, et al. Duration of amantadine benefit on dyskinesia of severe Parkinson's disease. J Neurol Neurosurg Psychiatry 2004;75: 141–3.

41. Isaacson SH, Fahn S, Pahwa R, et al. Parkinson's Patients with dyskinesia switched from Immediate Release Amantadine to Open-label ADS-5102. Mov Disord Clin Pract 2018;5:183–90.

42. Paik J, Keam SJ. Amantadine extended-release (GOCOVRI™): a review in levodopa-Induced dyskinesia in Parkinson's disease. CNS Drugs 2018;32: 797–806.

43. Olanow CW, Koller WC. An algorithm (decision tree) for the management of Parkinson's disease: treatment guidelines. American Academy of Neurology. Neurology 1998;50(3 Suppl 3):S1–57.

44. Olanow CW, Kieburtz K, Odin P, et al. Continuous intrajejunal infusion of levodopa-carbidopa intestinal gel for patients with advanced Parkinson's disease: a randomised, controlled, double-blind, double-dummy study. Lancet Neurol 2014;13:141–9.

45. Seeberger LC, Hauser RA. Carbidopa levodopa enteral suspension. Expert Opin Pharmacother 2015;16:2807–17.

46. Perestelo-Perez L, Rivero-Santana A, Perez-Ramos J, et al. Deep brain stimulation in Parkinson's disease: meta-analysis of randomized controlled trials. J Neurol 2014;261:2051–60.

47. Almeida L, Deeb W, Spears C, et al. Current practice and the future of deep brain stimulation therapy in Parkinson's disease. Semin Neurol 2017;37:205–14.

48. Cury RG, Fraix V, Castrioto A, et al. Thalamic deep brain stimulation for tremor in Parkinson disease, essential tremor, and dystonia. Neurology 2017;89:1416–23.

Essential Tremor

Stephen G. Reich, MD

KEYWORDS

- Tremor • Essential tremor • Parkinson's disease • Parkinsonism
- Deep brain stimulation • Focused ultrasound

KEY POINTS

- Essential tremor is the most common movement disorder affecting 1% of the population. The prevalence increases by more than five-fold with advancing age.
- Essential tremor is a bilateral postural and action tremor of the upper limbs.
- Essential tremor may also affect the head or voice but must be distinguished from cervical and spasmodic dysphonia, respectively, both of which may be tremulous.
- The two first-line drugs for treatment of ET include propranolol and primidone and they are synergistic.
- Patients with medically refractory disabling ET are candidates for either deep brain stimulation or focused ultrasound of the ventral intermediate nucleus thalamus.

WHAT IS YOUR DIAGNOSIS?

A 66-year-old right-handed woman reports tremor of both hands for at least a decade. It was never much of a problem until the last few years but now interferes with many dexterous tasks, such as writing, pouring, using eating utensils, applying makeup, and fastening jewelry. She finds the tremor embarrassing and tries to avoid writing in front of others. Others have told her that her head shakes but she has not noticed this. Her father and paternal uncle had tremor of the hands as does her brother and she has noticed a mild tremor in her daughter. She has noticed that one glass of wine improves the tremor for about 1 hour. On examination, there is no tremor at rest. While maintaining posture there is a tremor of both hands and this is more pronounced when she holds her hands in front of her nose, "like making wings." The tremor is also present when performing finger-to-nose but does not increase in amplitude as she approaches the target. There is a slight horizontal tremor of the head and a slight tremor of the voice. Her handwriting is of normal size but tremulous as is a spiral (**Fig. 1**A, C). The remainder of the neurologic examination is normal and specifically, no bradykinesia.

Does this patient have essential tremor (ET) or Parkinson's disease (PD)? For most adults with tremor, the differential diagnosis usually boils down to this question. Other causes to consider include drug-induced tremor, which is a side effect of commonly

Disclosure: None.
Department of Neurology, University of Maryland School of Medicine, 110 South Paca Street, 3rd Floor, Baltimore, MD 21201, USA
E-mail address: sreich@som.umaryland.edu

Med Clin N Am 103 (2019) 351–356
https://doi.org/10.1016/j.mcna.2018.10.016
0025-7125/19/© 2018 Elsevier Inc. All rights reserved.

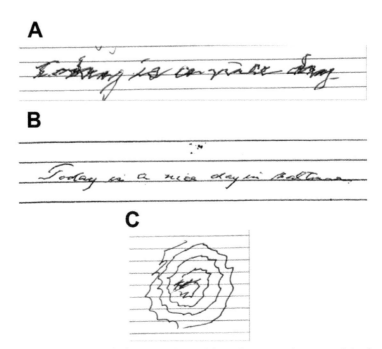

Fig. 1. (*A*) Handwriting sample from a patient with ET demonstrating normal size but tremulousness. (*B*) Handwriting sample from a patient with Parkinson's disease (PD) demonstrating progressive micrographia. (*C*) The spiral in a patient with ET demonstrates tremor, which is typically absent in Parkinson's disease.

used medications including selective serotonin reuptake inhibitors, lithium, tricyclic antidepressants, steroids, and valproate.[1] Medication-induced enhanced physiologic tremor is often asymptomatic; on examination, it, like ET, is present while maintaining posture and with action but it is typically more rapid and of lower amplitude than ET. Hyperthyroidism can cause tremor but is rarely the presenting symptom and takes place in the setting of other clinical clues. In young patients with tremor it is important to keep Wilson disease in mind[2] but this is only rarely a consideration after age 50. A much more common cause of tremor in children and young adults is ET[3] and this is underappreciated because for many years ET was referred to as "senile" tremor. Although ET increases in incidence with advancing age, it is seen across the age spectrum.

The International Parkinson's and Movement Disorder Society recently published an updated consensus statement on the classification of tremors.[4] Tremor is defined as an "involuntary, rhythmic, oscillatory movement of a body part."[4] It is rhythmicity that distinguishes tremor from other hyperkinetic movement disorders. According to the consensus statement, tremor is now classified into two axes. Axis 1 focuses on historical features of the tremor including age of onset, temporal pattern of evolution, family history, and responsiveness to alcohol, and findings on examination, such as body parts affected, position of activation, and frequency. On examination, aside from characteristics of the tremor, it is important to look for other neurologic and systemic findings that may lead to a diagnosis, such as signs of parkinsonism or evidence of systemic illness (eg, liver disease). The second axis is the cause of the tremor. There is a wide spectrum of tremor syndromes and a long list of tremor etiologies but most of them are uncommon, particularly compared with ET and PD, which are the focus of this article.

ET is the most common movement disorder with a prevalence of almost 1%, which increases at least five-fold with advancing age.[5,6] The International Parkinson's and Movement Disorder Society has defined ET as an isolated action tremor of bilateral upper limbs of at least 3 years duration.[4] The term "action" includes maintenance of posture and movement. ET may be accompanied by tremor of the head, voice, or lower limbs, but is otherwise "isolated" meaning that there are no other neurologic signs, such as ataxia or parkinsonism. ET is not just a postural tremor, but also a kinetic tremor apparent when performing finger-to-nose, but unlike an intention tremor (generally synonymous with a cerebellar tremor), which increases in amplitude as the target is approached, the amplitude of ET remains constant between targets. Historically, tremor of the head or voice was considered to be ET but under the new classification, ET of the head or voice can only be diagnosed when there is also ET of upper limbs. This more restrictive definition reflects that tremor of the head or voice (when they exist in isolation) are more likely the result of cervical and laryngeal dystonia, respectively, which are often tremulous.[7]

Distinguishing ET from PD relies on some specific features from the history and examination (Table 1). ET is usually present for several years and often decades before presenting, emphasizing its insidious progression. In contrast, patients with PD who have tremor (recall about one-third do not have tremor) typically present within 1 year of onset. So, a long duration of symptoms favors ET. ET is autosomal dominant in at least 60% of patients,[6] whereas only about 15% of patient with PD have an affected first-degree

Table 1
Clinical features of essential tremor and Parkinson's disease

Feature	PD	ET
Usual duration of symptoms before medical contact	6–12 mo	Usually several years or more
Family history	Generally negative (5%–15% with an affected first-degree relative)	Often positive (>60%), autosomal dominant
Response to small amount of alcohol	Little or none	Often improves
Position of maximal activation	Rest	Maintenance of posture or with movement
Frequency	3–6 Hz	6–12 Hz
Morphology	Pill-rolling	Flexion-extension
Onset	Unilateral	Bilateral
Body parts affected	Upper limb, lower limb, chin, lips, or tongue	Upper limb, head, voice
Handwriting	Micrographic, atremulous	Normal size, tremulous
Associated signs (eg, bradykinesia, hypomimia)	Present	Absent
Is the tremor present when walking?	Yes	No

From Reich SG, Factor S. Therapy of movement disorders: a case-based approach. New York: Springer International Publishing; 2019; with permission.

relative.[8] At least half of patients with ET notice a transient, beneficial effect from alcohol, which usually does not improve the tremor of PD.

On examination, by definition ET is bilateral, whereas PD begins unilaterally, and this is one of the most helpful distinguishing features. A unilateral upper or lower limb tremor in an adult is usually PD. Some patients with ET may report tremor in just one hand, but when examined it is bilateral. The tremor of PD is maximally activated at rest, whereas ET is present with maintenance of posture and movement. A caveat is that the rest tremor of PD may "reemerge" while maintaining posture, usually after a latency of 5 to 10 seconds, and this postural PD tremor has the same frequency and morphology as rest tremor.[9] Aside from the upper limbs, PD tremor may also affect the jaw, lips, tongue, or lower limb but not the head or voice as may be affected with ET. Although PD tremor is of lower frequency than ET, there is overlap between the two so at the bedside frequency is not a particularly helpful feature to make a distinction. Furthermore, it is difficult to estimate frequency. Having the patient walk is another useful way to distinguish ET from PD. It is common for the rest tremor of PD to be present while walking, whereas ET is typically absent while walking.

A handwriting sample is one of the best ways to distinguish ET from PD (**Fig. 1**). Handwriting in PD is small but does not tremor (see **Fig. 1**B). When testing this, it is best to have the patient write a long sentence because it may start out normal sized with the micrographia only appearing toward the end of the sentence or the end of a long word. Having the patient write their name may not demonstrate micrographia. The size of handwriting is not affected by ET but there is tremulousness and this is also seen when drawing a spiral (see **Fig. 1**A, C).

Returning to the patient in the previous example, the long duration of tremor suggests ET. That it affects many daily activities and is embarrassing are key features indicating the need for treatment (discussed next). Note that many patients who are embarrassed by ET are too embarrassed to report it, so it is important to inquire. The strong family history of autosomal-dominant inheritance also suggests ET. On examination, the tremor is bilateral and present with action, typical of ET. The involvement of the head and voice points toward ET and not PD. Her tremulous writing and spiral also indicate ET. Finally, there are no other associated signs, confirming that the upper limb action tremor is "isolated," another criterion for ET.

TREATMENT OF ESSENTIAL TREMOR

The first question is whether treatment is needed. For patients with mild ET, not significantly interfering with daily functioning or causing psychological distress, education and reassurance is the only treatment needed. For patients in whom ET is presenting a problem, and this is either by affecting activities of daily living or causing significant psychological distress in the form of embarrassment, the two first-line medications are propranolol and primidone.[6,10,11] Other β-blockers, including atenolol, sotalol, nadolol, and metoprolol, may be used but are less effective or at least have less evidence for effectiveness according to the practice parameters by the American Academy of Neurology.[10,11] Only propranolol and primidone have level A evidence. Before starting treatment of ET, it is important to review realistic expectations with the patient. Neither of the level A medical therapies cure ET and the goal is to reduce it to a level that allows for better functioning or less embarrassment. It is helpful to follow a few specific tasks to determine the effectiveness of therapy, such as handwriting and ability to use utensils.

Assuming no contraindications, propranolol is a good choice for the patient who also has hypertension because it can serve a dual purpose. In the elderly, I start at a low dose of 10 or 20 mg twice per day and escalate gradually based on the degree of benefit and tolerability. Younger patients can be started on propranolol Long-Acting (LA) 60 mg and escalated gradually. Most patients notice improvement between 60 and 180 mg per day. Equally effective is primidone, which should be started at a low dose of 25 mg at night. Some patients can get by with taking only one dose per day but I typically give it twice per day escalating gradually. Although primidone is increased to 750 mg per day, if there is no improvement at 300 to 400 mg, taking more is usually not beneficial and in the elderly often associated with more side effects, such as drowsiness or imbalance. These are the most effective medications for ET, and it is important to encourage patients to stick with them because initial side effects, particularly from primidone, tend to improve with time. If the maximally tolerated dose of either agent is not sufficiently effective, then they should be combined because the effect is synergistic.

Although there are second-line drugs that are considered for ET, if there is no response to an adequate dose of propranolol and primidone, the chances of another agent offering significant benefit is low. Level B recommendations were given for gabapentin, topiramate, and alprazolam (used with caution). Level C recommendations include clonazepam, nimodipine, and limb injections of botulinum toxin.[10,11]

Patients with disabling tremor refractory to medical therapy are candidates for either deep brain stimulation of the ventral intermediate nucleus of the thalamus, or the recently approved focused ultrasound, which makes a noninvasive thermal lesion of the same area.[12–17] Both have a high rate of success, to the extent of potentially abolishing tremor, and a low risk of side effects. At this stage in the management of tremor, patients should be under the care of a movement disorders specialist.

REFERENCES

1. Morgan JC, Sethi KD. Drug-induced tremors. Lancet Neurol 2005;4:866–76.
2. Bandmann O, Weiss KH, Kaler SG. Wilson's disease and other neurological copper disorders. Lancet Neurol 2015;14:103–13.
3. Jankovic J, Madisetty J, Vuong KD. Essential tremor among children. Pediatrics 2004;114:1203–5.
4. Bhatia KP, Bain P, Bajaj N, et al. Consensus statement on the classification of tremors. From the task force on tremor of the International Parkinson's and Movement Disorder Society. Mov Disord 2018;33:75–87.
5. Louis ED, Ferreira JJ. How common is the most common adult movement disorder? Update on the worldwide prevalence of essential tremor. Mov Disord 2010;25:534–41.
6. Haubenberger D, Hallett M. Essential tremor. N Engl J Med 2018;378:1802–10.
7. Quinn NP, Schneider SA, Schwingenschuh P, et al. Tremor: some controversial aspects. Mov Disord 2011;26:18–23.
8. Deng H, Wang P, Jankovic J. The genetics of Parkinson disease. Ageing Res Rev 2018;42:72–85.
9. Jankovic J, Schwartz KS, Ondo W. Re-emergent tremor of Parkinson's disease. J Neurol Neurosurg Psychiatry 1999;67:646–50.
10. Zesiewicz TA, Elble RJ, Louis ED, et al. Practice parameter: therapies for essential tremor. Neurology 2005;64:2008–20.
11. Zesiewicz TA, Elble RJ, Louis ED, et al. Evidence-based guideline update: treatment of essential tremor. Neurology 2011;77:1752–5.
12. Nazzaro JM, Lyons KE, Pahwa R. Deep brain stimulation for essential tremor. Handb Clin Neurol 2013;116:155–66.

13. Elias WJ, Lipsman N, Ondo WG, et al. A randomized trial of focused ultrasound thalamotomy for essential tremor. N Engl J Med 2016;375:730–9.
14. Fishman PS, Frenkel V. Treatment of movement disorders with focused ultrasound. J Cent Nerv Syst Dis 2017;9. 1179573517705670.
15. Fishman PS, Elias WJ, Ghanouni P, et al. Neurological adverse event profile of magnetic resonance imaging-guided focused ultrasound thalamotomy for essential tremor. Mov Disord 2018;33:843–7.
16. Rohani M, Fasano A. Focused ultrasound for essential tremor: review of the evidence and discussion of current hurdles. Tremor Other Hyperkinet Mov (N Y) 2017;7:462.
17. Chang JW, Park CK, Lipsman N, et al. A meta-analysis of outcomes and complications of magnetic resonance-guided focused ultrasound in the treatment of essential tremor. Ann Neurol 2018;83:107–14.

Entrapment Neuropathies of the Upper Extremity

Christopher T. Doughty, MD[a], Michael P. Bowley, MD, PhD[b],*

KEYWORDS

- Compressive neuropathy • Median neuropathy • Carpal tunnel syndrome
- Ulnar neuropathy • Radial neuropathy

KEY POINTS

- An efficient neurologic examination can diagnose most upper extremity compressive neuropathies and differentiate between other common mimics, including cervical radiculopathy and orthopedic disorders.
- Electrodiagnostic studies assist in the localization of compressive neuropathies when the neurologic examination leaves doubt. By offering insight into the pathophysiology of nerve injury, prognostic information can also be gained.
- Some compressive neuropathies will improve without specific intervention; others will respond to conservative options including splinting or activity modification, while some cases will require surgical intervention.

INTRODUCTION

Focal compression of a nerve is common and may occur under the most ordinary of activities, such as ulnar nerve injury when maintaining a flexed arm position while sleeping. Symptoms and signs of nerve entrapment may be encountered in any medical setting and may lead to significant functional disability. Some entrapment neuropathies improve with observation or conservative measures such as splinting, whereas others require surgical intervention. Therefore, it benefits the internist, specialist, and surgeon alike to be familiar with nerve entrapment syndromes. This article offers a focused review of the pathophysiology of nerve compression and discusses common compressive mononeuropathies affecting the upper extremity.

PATHOPHYSIOLOGY OF NERVE COMPRESSION

Understanding the effects of compression on nerve physiology offers insight into diagnosis and prognosis. Compressive forces are thought to result in microvascular

Disclosure Statement: No disclosures.
a Department of Neurology, Brigham and Women's Hospital, 75 Francis Street, Boston, MA 02115, USA; b Department of Neurology, Massachusetts General Hospital, 55 Fruit Street, WACC 739B, Boston, MA 02114, USA
* Corresponding author.
E-mail address: mpbowley@partners.org

Med Clin N Am 103 (2019) 357–370
https://doi.org/10.1016/j.mcna.2018.10.012
0025-7125/19/© 2018 Elsevier Inc. All rights reserved.

medical.theclinics.com

damage to nerves and their myelin sheaths. Mild degrees of compression may obstruct venous flow, causing congestion and edema, while more severe and consistent compression results in arterial ischemia. Prolonged or repetitive compression results in inflammation, fibrosis, and demyelination.[1] Fibrosis can compound the effects of mechanical compression, as it prevents appropriate gliding or stretching of the nerve. Loss of myelination leads to disruptions in the speed of axonal signaling, and at its most severe can lead to a partial or complete block of action potentials through the affected nerve segment. With persistent compression, the combination of these factors may lead to axonal degeneration. This portends a poorer prognosis and more prolonged recovery; remyelination may take a matter of weeks, while axonal regrowth is glacially slow, approximately 1 mm per day.[2]

Electrodiagnostic studies (EDXs), nerve conduction studies (NCS), and electromyography (EMG) allow for precise localization of nerve injury and may demonstrate the nature (demyelination, axonal degeneration, or both), timing, and severity of injury. Localization can be accomplished by demonstrating focal slowing of conduction across a nerve segment, or by inference using the pattern of muscles that are affected or spared. Certain findings, such as axon loss, have important prognostic relevance and may help guide treatment decisions.

MEDIAN NEUROPATHY AT THE WRIST – CARPAL TUNNEL SYNDROME

The median nerve is formed from the C6-T1 nerve roots. The median nerve innervates the forearm pronators as well as most of the wrist and finger flexors in the forearm. The median nerve enters the hand by passing through the carpal tunnel, an anatomically restricted space that is bounded by carpal bones and the transverse carpal ligament (**Fig. 1**). The distal wrist crease approximates the proximal boundary of the carpal tunnel. After exiting the carpal tunnel, the median nerve provides innervation to the muscles of the thenar eminence (abductor pollicis brevis, opponens pollicis, and flexor

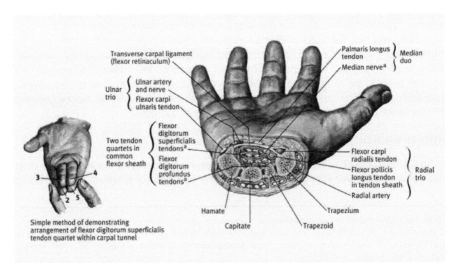

Fig. 1. The carpal tunnel. The anatomic boundaries of the carpal tunnel include a floor formed by the carpal bones of the hand and a roof formed from the thick transverse carpal ligament. The contents of the carpal tunnel include the median nerve and 9 finger flexor tendons. [a] Contents of carpal tunnel. (*From* Ellis H. The carpal tunnel. Surgery 2008;26(10):e6; with permission.)

pollicis brevis), as well as the first and second lumbricals. The sensory territory of the median nerve is exclusively distal to the wrist (**Fig. 2**). A palmar branch, providing sensory innervation from the thenar eminence, originates proximal to the wrist and is spared in carpal tunnel syndrome (CTS).

CTS is the most common compressive neuropathy, with an estimated lifetime risk of 10%.[3] The incidence of CTS increases with age, and women are more likely to be affected than men. Conditions that decrease the size of the carpal tunnel or increase the size of its contents can lead to median nerve compression. Pregnancy, obesity, rheumatoid arthritis, diabetes, hypothyroidism, tenosynovitis, and acromegaly are associated with increased incidence of CTS.[4–7] Activities and occupations that involve high rates of repetitive tasks of hand/wrist flexion while placing the hand under high force (eg, forceful gripping) are also associated with CTS.[8] CTS can occur secondary to trauma or space-occupying lesions within the carpal tunnel such as a ganglion cyst.

Patients first complain of intermittent numbness and paresthesias of the fingers. Patients frequently report symptoms that extend beyond the sensory distribution of the median nerve—tingling in all 5 fingers, or pain that extends into the forearm. Symptoms may be more frequent at night, waking patients from sleep, or brought on by activities that narrow the carpal tunnel such as holding the steering wheel while driving. Shaking out the wrists can relieve discomfort.[9] As CTS worsens, symptoms become more constant and fixed sensory deficits on examination accumulate. Weakness of thenar muscles usually occurs late in the course.[10]

The most useful and accurate diagnostic tests are pinprick sensation in the hand, thumb abduction strength (**Fig. 3**), and use of the Katz diagram.[11] Thenar atrophy

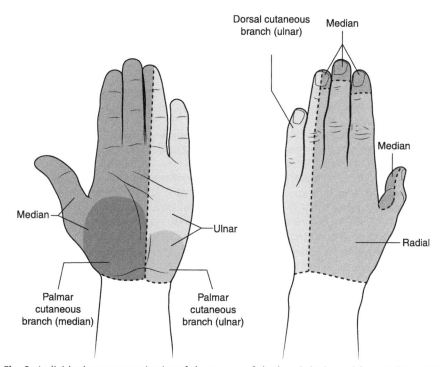

Fig. 2. Individual sensory territories of the nerves of the hand. (*Adapted from* Sullivan EM. Emergency medicine. In: Ballweg R, Sullivan EM, Brown D, et al, editors. Physician assistant: a guide to clinical practice. 5th edition. Philadelphia: Saunders; 2013; with permission.)

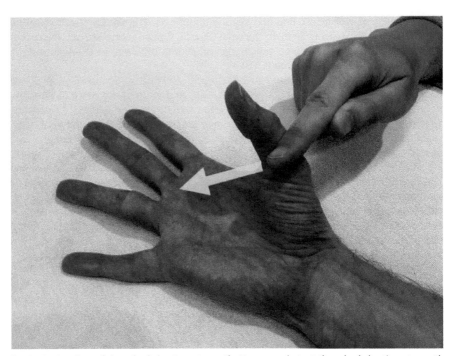

Fig. 3. Evaluation of thumb abduction strength. To properly test thumb abduction strength, ensure the thumb is perpendicular, not parallel, to the palm. Apply force to the metacarpophalangeal joint, attempting to press the thumb straight down toward the second digit, asking the patient to resist.

occurs in severe cases and suggests axonal loss, an important prognostic indicator. In mild cases, the neurologic examination may be normal, so the Katz diagram can be helpful; patients pictorially represent any pain, numbness, and tingling on pictures of the hand.[12] Classic maneuvers including the Tinel or Phalen sign, or pressure applied over the carpal tunnel, may in fact be more sensitive and specific for flexor muscle tenosynovitis rather than CTS.[13]

The neurologic examination can also help differentiate between CTS and important alternative diagnoses, including cervical radiculopathy and proximal median neuropathy (**Table 1**). Tenosynovitis or carpometacarpal joint arthritis may produce pain similar to CTS, but neither leads to sensory loss or weakness. Finally, when there are thenar weakness and atrophy without significant sensory symptoms; look for concurrent atrophy of the first dorsal interosseous (FDI) and hyperreflexia in the arm. This may unfortunately be an early presentation of amyotrophic lateral sclerosis.

EDXs are routinely performed as part of the evaluation of CTS and have been shown to be highly valid, reproducible, and specific.[14] However, CTS remains largely a clinical diagnosis based on characteristic symptoms and signs. EDXs may assist in detecting the mimics discussed previously or concurrent pathologies such as a generalized polyneuropathy that may contribute to symptoms. There is little to no relationship between the severity of clinical symptoms and the severity of findings on EDXs.[15] Studies suggest that 15% to 25% of patients with clinically definite CTS will have normal EDXs.[14,16] In 1 study utilizing sensitive methods of EDXs, however, patients with clinically diagnosed CTS but normal EDXs had lower success rates with surgical

Table 1
Clinical signs and symptoms differentiating carpal tunnel syndrome from common mimics

Site of Lesion	Motor Weakness				Sensory Loss			
	Thumb Abduction	Forearm Pronation	Finger Abduction	Finger Extension	1st and 2nd Digit, Palmar Surface	Thenar Eminence	5th Digit	Brachioradialis and/or Biceps Reflexes
Median neuropathy at the wrist (CTS)	Yes	No	No	No	Yes	No	No	No effect
Proximal median neuropathy	Yes	Yes	No	No	Yes	Yes	No	No effect
C6 radiculopathy	No	Yes	No	No	Yes	Yes	No	May be reduced or absent
C8-T1 radiculopathy	Yes	No	Yes	Yes	No	No	Yes	No effect

carpal tunnel release (CTR) compared to those with mild-to-moderate CTS by electro-physiologic criteria; only 51% had a successful outcome.[17] A pragmatic interpretation is that negative NCS should prompt careful reconsideration of the clinical diagnosis before surgery is contemplated. When patients cannot tolerate EDX, or if confirmation is desired when EDXs are normal, high-resolution ultrasound can support a clinical diagnosis of CTS by demonstration of enlargement of the median nerve at the carpal tunnel.[18]

Multiple effective treatment options exist for CTS. In mild cases without significant motor symptoms, it is reasonable to begin with a trial of conservative therapies including activity modification (avoiding activities that promote excessive flexion/extension at the wrist), physical therapy, and splinting.[19] Corticosteroid injection into the carpal tunnel may be beneficial in up to 70% of patients, with short-term outcomes equivalent to surgery.[20,21] Adverse effects include skin depigmentation, cutaneous atrophy, tendon rupture, or nerve injury, but are less common than with surgery.[22] Up to 50% of patients will have relapse of symptoms after initial improvement; by contrast, relapse after 1 year is quite rare after surgery. The long-term safety of repeated steroid injections is not well studied.

If patients fail to respond to conservative measures after several weeks, surgical referral is suggested. Approximately 75% of patients will have complete or near-complete resolution of symptoms after surgical CTR; an estimated 8% will report worse symptoms after surgery.[20] Other potential complications include postoperative pain, hematoma, scarring, and development of complex regional pain syndrome; severe complications including damage to arteries, tendons, or nerves occur in less than 1% of patients.[23] Immediate surgical referral should be considered in patients with clinical signs of severe CTS—significant APB weakness or thenar muscle atrophy—or signs of median nerve axonal damage on EDXs.[8] The aim is to limit further axon loss. Such patients have been shown to have lower rates of complete response to surgery; pain and paresthesias may improve, but improvement in numbness and weakness is often incomplete.[17,24]

ULNAR NEUROPATHY AT THE ELBOW

The ulnar nerve arises from C8-T1 nerve root fibers. At the elbow, the nerve passes in between the medial epicondyle of the humerus and the ulnar olecranon, a space called the retrocondylar or ulnar groove (**Fig. 4**). Just distal to the medial epicondyle, the ulnar nerve passes below the humeroulnar arcade (HUA), a tendinous arch connecting the humeral and ulnar heads of the flexor carpi ulnaris muscle (FCU). This is the entrance to the cubital tunnel. Near the elbow, the ulnar nerve innervates the FCU and the flexor digitorum profundus (FDP) to digits 4 and 5. The ulnar nerve enters the hand via Guyon canal, formed in part by the pisiform bone and the hook of the hamate. Its sensory territory is solely in the hand (see **Fig. 2**); the dorsal hand and the proximal medial palm are supplied by branches arising proximal to Guyon canal. Motor innervation is provided to the hypothenar muscles including abductor digiti minimi (ADM), the third and fourth lumbricals, the interosseous muscles, and adductor pollicis.

Ulnar neuropathy at the elbow (UNE) is the second most common entrapment neuropathy after CTS.[25] The incidence of UNE is higher in men than women. Ulnar nerve compression at the elbow typically occurs within the ulnar groove or the cubital tunnel. It is difficult to make this distinction either clinically or using EDXs. The nerve lies superficially in the ulnar groove, so it is prone to external compression (eg, resting the elbows on an armchair). Elbow flexion narrows the space within the cubital tunnel, promoting compression, and lengthens the course of the nerve. Activities and

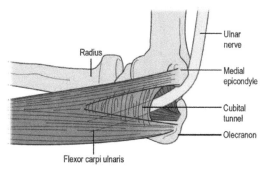

Fig. 4. The ulnar nerve at the elbow. After passing through the ulnar groove in between the medial epicondyle of the humerus and the ulnar olecranon, the ulnar nerve passes through the cubital tunnel. The floor of the cubital tunnel is formed by the medial collateral ligament of the elbow. Its roof is formed by the tendinous arch of the 2 heads of the flexor carpi ulnaris. The nerve can be compressed both at the ulnar groove and within the cubital tunnel. (*From* Kincaid JC. AAEE minimonograph no. 31: The electrodiagnosis of ulnar neuropathy at the elbow. Muscle Nerve 1988;11(10):1005–15; with permission.)

occupations requiring repetitive elbow flexion and extension have been associated with UNE.[26] Elbow trauma can also cause UNE, sometimes in a delayed fashion after fracture. Although less common than UNE, compression of the ulnar nerve can also occur at Guyon canal (eg, with prolonged cycling or propelling a manual wheelchair).

Patients typically complain of numbness and/or paresthesias affecting the medial hand and fourth and fifth digits. In mild cases, these symptoms will be intermittent and may be provoked by prolonged flexion at the elbow. Patients with UNE often present with more advanced disease (ie, weakness and atrophy) compared to patients with CTS.[27] Patients may describe a weak grip or difficulty with fine motor tasks such as buttoning. Crossing the fingers may be difficult because of interosseous weakness; patients may describe the fifth digit getting caught when placing the hand in a pocket. Like CTS, traditional provocative maneuvers for UNE are not sensitive or specific. Thirty-four percent of normal volunteers endorse paresthesia induced by tapping over the ulnar nerve at the elbow, and 20% report symptoms after 3 minutes of elbow flexion.[28]

Findings on the neurologic examination are more reliable, can suggest localization at the elbow, and may also have prognostic relevance. Sensory testing should ensure no deficits are found in the median or radial (dorsal lateral hand) sensory territories. Sensory deficits in the territory of the dorsal ulnar cutaneous or palmar cutaneous support localization to the elbow rather than the wrist. Weakness is most common in FDI and ADM, so testing abduction of the second and fifth digits is of highest yield.[29] Although FDP weakness (flexion at the DIP joint) is less frequent, finding it rules out ulnar neuropathy at the wrist. The presence of severe weakness or muscle atrophy suggests axonal damage. Atrophy is most easily appreciated in the FDI, which lies in the webspace between the thumb and second digit. The major considerations for differential diagnosis include C8/T1 radiculopathy or pathologies affecting the lower brachial plexus (**Table 2**). Medial epicondylitis (golfer's elbow) can cause elbow pain that radiates into the forearm and wrist, but without neurologic deficits.

Because it is difficult to localize ulnar neuropathy to the elbow based on clinical examination alone, EDXs are routinely obtained. Demonstration of focal slowing of motor nerve conduction or conduction block across the elbow allows for localization.[30] The presence of conduction block is also a useful prognostic finding in a patient with

Table 2
Clinical signs and symptoms differentiating ulnar neuropathy at the elbow from common mimics

Site of Lesion	Motor Weakness				Sensory Loss			
	Finger Abduction	Flexion at DIP, 5th Digit (FDP)	Thumb Abduction	Finger Extension	5th Digit, Palmar Surface	Dorsal Medial Hand	Medial Forearm	Brachioradialis, Biceps, Triceps Reflexes
Ulnar neuropathy at the elbow	Yes	Yes	No	No	Yes	Yes	No	No effect
Ulnar neuropathy at the wrist	Yes	No	No	No	Yes	No	No	No effect
C8-T1 radiculopathy	Yes	Yes	Yes	Yes	Yes	Yes	Yes	No effect
Brachial plexopathy, medial cord	Yes	Yes	Yes	No	Yes	Yes	Yes	No effect

Abbreviations: DIP, distal interphalangeal joint; FDP, flexor digitorum profundus.

weakness, as it implies demyelination rather than axon loss and has been associated with greater improvement with treatment.[31] Ultrasound may be useful for patients for whom EDXs are either normal or fail to localize the ulnar neuropathy.[32]

There are no randomized trials comparing surgery with conservative treatment options for UNE. For mild-to-moderate UNE (only mild sensory deficits and/or weakness without atrophy, no signs of axon loss on EDXs), a trial of conservative management is reasonable.[33] Up to 50% of patients may improve with activity modification alone— avoiding prolonged flexion at the elbow (eg, cell phone use), crossing the arms, or resting the elbows when seated or driving.[34] Splints limiting elbow flexion to 45° to 90° can be worn at night. Patients who do not tolerate splinting can be told to wrap a towel around the elbow. In 1 cohort, 88% of patients with mild-to-moderate UNE improved with activity modification and nocturnal splinting.[35] In the only randomized prospective trial of conservative management, however, splinting had no added benefit above and beyond activity modification.[36] Corticosteroid injection at the elbow has been shown to have no benefit in a randomized, double-blind, placebo-controlled trial.[37] Surgery may be offered to patients who fail to improve with conservative therapy, or those with severe disease at onset (severe weakness or sensory loss, atrophy, signs of axon loss on EDXs). Sixty-five percent to 75% of patients will improve with surgery.[38] Patients with axon loss may have poor recovery of motor function, but often have improvement in pain or paresthesias.[39]

RADIAL NEUROPATHY AT THE SPIRAL GROOVE

Fibers originating from the C5-C8 and sometimes T1 nerve roots contribute to the radial nerve. The radial nerve courses through the medial upper arm before traveling laterally across the posterior surface of the humerus through the spiral groove, where it is susceptible to compression (**Fig. 5**). Innervation to the triceps and a sensory branch supplying the posterior upper arm originate proximal to the spiral groove. Distal to the spiral groove, innervation to the brachioradialis and radial wrist extensors are provided. A sensory branch to the posterior forearm originates above the elbow. At the elbow, the radial nerve divides into a deep motor branch (the posterior interosseus nerve) and a superficial sensory branch. The posterior interosseous nerve passes under the Arcade of Fröhse, a fibrous arch along the superficial head of the supinator muscle, and innervates muscles controlling forearm supination, ulnar wrist extension, finger extension, and thumb extension. The superficial sensory branch travels superficially along the lateral distal radius to supply sensory innervation to the dorsal lateral hand (see **Fig. 2**).

The most common etiology of radial neuropathy is trauma, usually related to fractures of the humerus. Compressive neuropathy occurs most frequently at the spiral groove of the humerus, resulting from sustained pressure against the posterior upper arm.[40] The resulting syndrome is typically referred to as Saturday night palsy. Classically, affected patients wake up with acute weakness of wrist and finger extensors (wrist drop and finger drop) after falling asleep inebriated from alcohol or another substance, with the arm outstretched on the arm of a chair. Patients are not always inebriated, however; a sleep partner may similarly compress the arm, resulting in honeymooner's palsy. Weakness is often severe, with up to one-third having complete paralysis. Sensory symptoms are less common than weakness. One-third to one-half of patients will have no sensory symptoms and no demonstrable sensory loss on examination, even in some cases of complete paralysis.[2,41,42]

With Saturday night palsy, brachioradialis is usually weak, but triceps strength and the triceps reflex will be spared. Weakness of the triceps implies a lesion above the spiral groove (**Table 3**), as with compression of the radial nerve in the axilla caused

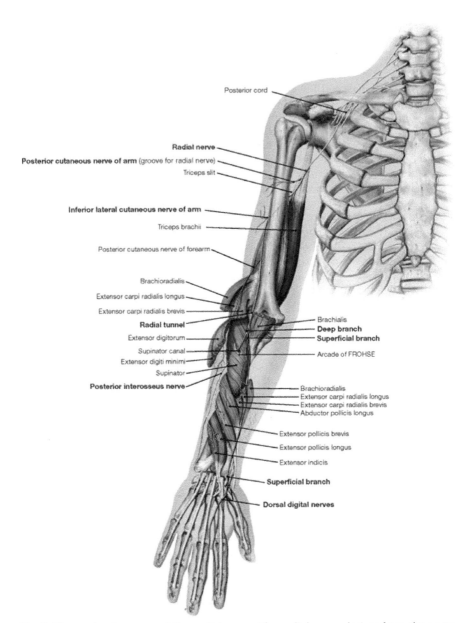

Fig. 5. The anatomic course of the radial nerve. The radial nerve derives from the posterior cord of the brachial plexus. It begins in the medial upper arm but travels laterally to pass along the posterior surface of the humerus in the spiral groove. Due to its direct proximity to the bone, the radial nerve is prone to compression here. At the elbow, the nerve divides into a superficial sensory branch and a deep motor branch (the posterior interosseous nerve). (*From* Paulsen F. Upper extremity. In: Paulsen F, editor. Sobotta atlas of human anatomy. vol. 1. 15th edition. Munich (Germany): Elsevier GmbH; 2013; with permission.)

Table 3
Clinical signs and symptoms differentiating radial neuropathy at different compressive sites

Site of Compression	Motor Weakness				Sensory Loss			Reflexes
	Finger Extension	Wrist Extension	Brachioradialis	Triceps	Dorsal Lateral Hand	Posterior Forearm	Posterior Upper Arm	
Axilla	Yes	Yes	Yes	Yes	Yes	Yes	Yes	Brachioradialis and triceps decreased
Spiral Groove	Yes	Yes	Yes	No	Yes	Yes	No	Brachioradialis decreased, triceps normal
Arcade of Fröhse (posterior interosseous nerve)	Yes	Partially weak, with radial deviation[a]	No	No	Yes	No	No	Brachioradialis and triceps normal
Wrist (superficial radial sensory nerve)	No	No	No	No	Yes	No	No	Brachioradialis and triceps normal

[a] The extensor carpi radialis longus and brevis are spared in posterior interosseous lesions, but the extensor carpi ulnaris is weak.

by improper use of crutches (crutch palsy). The superficial radial sensory nerve can be compressed at the lateral wrist by a tight wristwatch or handcuffs.[43] Affected patients will have no motor deficits. C7 radiculopathy and stroke are also important differential considerations. Upper motor neuron weakness from a stroke preferentially affects elbow, wrist, and finger extensors; sparing of brachioradialis and hyperreflexia are important clues to look for. EDXs aid in the precise localization of radial neuropathy. Demonstration of conduction block or slowed conduction velocity across the spiral groove is helpful confirmatory findings. Conduction block has also been associated with a favorable prognosis.[44]

Saturday night palsy should be treated conservatively, as most patients have complete recovery after an average of 2 to 3 months.[41,42] Patients with more severe weakness may take longer to recover, up to 6 months, but even those with complete paralysis at onset can have a full recovery. Supportive care includes physical therapy to maintain range of motion and avoid disuse. A dorsal cock-up splint should be used to maintain the wrist in a position to allow the normal hand muscles to function appropriately.

FUTURE DIRECTIONS/SUMMARY

Compressive neuropathies are a common cause of peripheral sensory loss, and weakness and may be encountered in any clinical setting. Careful examination of a patient is often sufficient to establish the diagnosis; when uncertainty exists, EDXs and neuromuscular ultrasound can confirm the diagnosis. For patients with transient or pure sensory symptoms, conservative treatment including avoidance of inciting factors and bracing is often sufficient for treatment. When motor weakness and atrophy are evident, referral for consideration of surgical decompression may be indicated.

REFERENCES

1. Rempel DM, Diao E. Entrapment neuropathies: pathophysiology and pathogenesis. J Electromyogr Kinesiol 2004;14(1):71–5.
2. Trojaborg W. Rate of recovery in motor and sensory fibres of the radial nerve: clinical and electrophysiological aspects. J Neurol Neurosurg Psychiatry 1970;33(5):625–38.
3. Stevens JC, Sun S, Beard CM, et al. Carpal tunnel syndrome in Rochester, Minnesota, 1961 to 1980. Neurology 1988;38(1):134–8.
4. Stevens JC, Beard CM, O'Fallon WM, et al. Conditions associated with carpal tunnel syndrome. Mayo Clin Proc 1992;67(6):541–8.
5. Shiri R, Pourmemari MH, Falah-Hassani K, et al. The effect of excess body mass on the risk of carpal tunnel syndrome: a meta-analysis of 58 studies. Obes Rev 2015;16(12):1094–104.
6. Shiri R. Hypothyroidism and carpal tunnel syndrome: a meta-analysis. Muscle Nerve 2014;50(6):879–83.
7. O'Duffy JD, Randall RV, MacCarty CS. Median neuropathy (carpal-tunnel syndrome) in acromegaly. A sign of endocrine overactivity. Ann Intern Med 1973;78(3):379–83.
8. Graham B, Peljovich A, Afra R, et al. The American Academy of Orthopaedic Surgeons evidence-based clinical practice guideline on: management of carpal tunnel syndrome. J Bone Joint Surg Am 2016;98(20):1750–4.
9. Pryse-Phillips WE. Validation of a diagnostic sign in carpal tunnel syndrome. J Neurol Neurosurg Psychiatry 1984;47(8):870–2.

10. Padua L, Padua R, Lo Monaco M, et al. Multiperspective assessment of carpal tunnel syndrome. Neurology 1999;53(10):1654–9.
11. D'Arcy CA, McGee S. The rational clinical examination. Does this patient have carpal tunnel syndrome? JAMA 2000;283(23):3110–7.
12. Katz JN, Stirrat CR. A self-administered hand diagram for the diagnosis of carpal tunnel syndrome. J Hand Surg Am 1990;15(2):360–3.
13. El Miedany Y, Ashour S, Youssef S, et al. Clinical diagnosis of carpal tunnel syndrome: old tests-new concepts. Joint Bone Spine 2008;75(4):451–7.
14. Jablecki CK, Andary MT, Floeter MK, et al. Practice parameter: electrodiagnostic studies in carpal tunnel syndrome: report of the American Association of Electrodiagnostic Medicine, American Academy of Neurology, and the American Academy of Physical Medicine and Rehabilitation. Neurology 2002;58(11):1589–92.
15. Chan L, Turner JA, Comstock BA, et al. The relationship between electrodiagnostic findings and patient symptoms and function in carpal tunnel syndrome. Arch Phys Med Rehabil 2007;88(1):19–24.
16. Witt JC, Hentz JG, Stevens JC. Carpal tunnel syndrome with normal nerve conduction studies. Muscle Nerve 2004;29(4):515–22.
17. Bland JD. Do nerve conduction studies predict the outcome of carpal tunnel decompression? Muscle Nerve 2001;24(7):935–40.
18. Cartwright MS, Hobson-Webb LD, Boon AJ, et al. Evidence-based guideline: neuromuscular ultrasound for the diagnosis of carpal tunnel syndrome. Muscle Nerve 2012;46(2):287–93.
19. Page MJ, Massy-Westropp N, O'Connor D, et al. Splinting for carpal tunnel syndrome. Cochrane Database Syst Rev 2012;(7):CD010003.
20. Bland JD. Treatment of carpal tunnel syndrome. Muscle Nerve 2007;36(2):167–71.
21. Ly-Pen D, Andréu J-L, de Blas G, et al. Surgical decompression versus local steroid injection in carpal tunnel syndrome: a one-year, prospective, randomized, open, controlled clinical trial. Arthritis Rheum 2005;52(2):612–9.
22. Verdugo R, Salinas R, Castillo J, et al. Surgical versus non-surgical treatment for carpal tunnel syndrome. Cochrane Database Syst Rev 2008;(4):CD001552.
23. Benson LS, Bare AA, Nagle DJ, et al. Complications of endoscopic and open carpal tunnel release. Arthroscopy 2006;22(9):919–24, 924-2.
24. Kronlage SC, Menendez ME. The benefit of carpal tunnel release in patients with electrophysiologically moderate and severe disease. J Hand Surg Am 2015;40(3):438–44.
25. Mondelli M, Giannini F, Ballerini M, et al. Incidence of ulnar neuropathy at the elbow in the province of Siena (Italy). J Neurol Sci 2005;234(1–2):5–10.
26. Carter GT, Weiss MD, Friedman AS, et al. Diagnosis and treatment of work-related ulnar neuropathy at the elbow. Phys Med Rehabil Clin N Am 2015;26(3):513–22.
27. Mallette P, Zhao M, Zurakowski D, et al. Muscle atrophy at diagnosis of carpal and cubital tunnel syndrome. J Hand Surg Am 2007;32(6):855–8.
28. Kuschner SH, Ebramzadeh E, Mitchell S. Evaluation of elbow flexion and tinel tests for cubital tunnel syndrome in asymptomatic individuals. Orthopedics 2006;29(4):305–9.
29. Stewart JD. The variable clinical manifestations of ulnar neuropathies at the elbow. J Neurol Neurosurg Psychiatry 1987;50(3):252–8.
30. Campbell E, Greenberg M, Krendel D, et al. The electrodiagnostic evaluation of patients with ulnar neuropathy at the elbow: literature review of the usefulness of

nerve conduction studies and needle electromyography. Muscle Nerve 1999; 22(8):175–205.

31. Friedrich JM, Robinson LR. Prognostic indicators from electrodiagnostic studies for ulnar neuropathy at the elbow. Muscle Nerve 2011;43(4):596–600.
32. Beekman R, Schoemaker MC, Van Der Plas JPL, et al. Diagnostic value of high-resolution sonography in ulnar neuropathy at the elbow. Neurology 2004;62(5):767–73.
33. Dellon AL, Hament W, Gittelshon A. Nonoperative management of cubital tunnel syndrome: an 8-year prospective study. Neurology 1993;43(9):1673–7.
34. Padua L, Aprile I, Caliandro P, et al. Natural history of ulnar entrapment at elbow. Clin Neurophysiol 2002;113(12):1980–4.
35. Shah CM, Calfee RP, Gelberman RH, et al. Outcomes of rigid night splinting and activity modification in the treatment of cubital tunnel syndrome. J Hand Surg Am 2013;38(6):1125–30.e1.
36. Svernlov B, Larsson M, Rehn K, et al. Conservative treatment of the cubital tunnel syndrome. J Hand Surg Eur Vol 2009;43E(2):201–7.
37. vanVeen KEB, Alblas KCL, Alons IME, et al. Corticosteroid injection in patients with ulnar neuropathy at the elbow: a randomized, double-blind, placebo-controlled trial. Muscle Nerve 2015;52(3):380–5.
38. Caliandro P, La Torre G, Padua R, et al. Treatment for ulnar neuropathy at the elbow. Cochrane Database Syst Rev 2016;2016(11):CD006839.
39. Taha A, Galarza M, Zuccarello M, et al. Outcomes of cubital tunnel surgery among patients with absent sensory nerve conduction. Neurosurgery 2004;54(4):891–6.
40. Mondelli M, Morana P, Ballerini M, et al. Mononeuropathies of the radial nerve: clinical and neurographic findings in 91 consecutive cases. J Electromyogr Kinesiol 2005;15(4):377–83.
41. Arnold WD, Krishna VR, Freimer M, et al. Prognosis of acute compressive radial neuropathy. Muscle Nerve 2012;45(6):893–4.
42. Kim KH, Park KD, Chung PW, et al. The usefulness of proximal radial motor conduction in acute compressive radial neuropathy. J Clin Neurol 2015;11(2):178–82.
43. Grant AC, Cook AA. A prospective study of handcuff neuropathies. Muscle Nerve 2000;23(6):933–8.
44. Bsteh G, Wanschitz JV, Gruber H, et al. Prognosis and prognostic factors in non-traumatic acute-onset compressive mononeuropathies - radial and peroneal mononeuropathies. Eur J Neurol 2013;20(6):981–5.

Entrapment Neuropathies of the Lower Extremity

Michael P. Bowley, MD, PhD[a],*, Christopher T. Doughty, MD[b]

KEYWORDS

- Compressive neuropathy • Meralgia paresthetica • Common peroneal neuropathy
- Femoral neuropathy • Tarsal tunnel syndrome • Foot drop

KEY POINTS

- Lower-extremity compressive neuropathies are commonly encountered in the primary care setting and in hospitalized patients. Timely diagnosis may help limit significant pain and functional disability.
- A focused neurologic examination can reliably diagnose most lower-extremity compressive neuropathies and differentiate between other possible conditions, including lumbosacral radiculopathy and orthopedic issues.
- In select cases, electrodiagnostic studies and neuromuscular ultrasound are valuable complements to the neurologic history and examination and may offer additional insight into localization, pathophysiology, and prognosis following nerve entrapment.
- Most compressive neuropathies in the lower extremity will improve with conservative measures, including activity modification, bracing, and pain control. Rarely, surgical intervention is indicated.

INTRODUCTION

Entrapment neuropathies in the lower extremities may occur both during benign activities, such as when the common peroneal nerve is stretched with prolonged kneeling, or in the setting of extreme medical issues, such as when the femoral nerve is compressed following retroperitoneal hemorrhage. As such, symptoms and signs of nerve entrapment may be encountered in any medical setting. Given the significant pain, sensory loss, incoordination, weakness, and functional disability that may result, it benefits the internist, medical specialist, and surgeon alike to be familiar with nerve compression and entrapment syndromes to offer effective intervention. Here, the

Disclosure Statement: The authors have no disclosures.
[a] Department of Neurology, Massachusetts General Hospital, 55 Fruit Street, WACC 739B, Boston, MA 02114, USA; [b] Department of Neurology, Brigham and Women's Hospital, 75 Francis Street, Boston, MA 02115, USA
* Corresponding author.
E-mail address: mpbowley@partners.org

Med Clin N Am 103 (2019) 371–382
https://doi.org/10.1016/j.mcna.2018.10.013

authors offer a focused review of select compressive mononeuropathies affecting the lower extremity.

LOWER EXTREMITY ENTRAPMENT NEUROPATHIES
Femoral Neuropathy

Femoral neuropathy is a rare condition resulting in weakness of hip flexion and knee extension with sensory loss involving the anterior and medial thigh and medial lower leg.

The femoral nerve is formed within the psoas muscle from portions of the L2, L3, and L4 nerve roots and then runs on an inferior course between the psoas and iliacus muscles, beneath the iliacus fascia in the retroperitoneal space. Motor innervation to the psoas and iliacus muscles is provided by the femoral nerve in its course through the abdomen. The nerve then emerges onto the thigh by passing deep to the inguinal ligament, lateral to the femoral artery (**Fig. 1**A). Here it divides into an anterior division, providing motor innervation to the sartorius and pectineus muscles, and sensory information from the skin of the anterior and medial thigh, and into a lateral division that supplies motor innervation to the quadriceps muscles and then continues as the

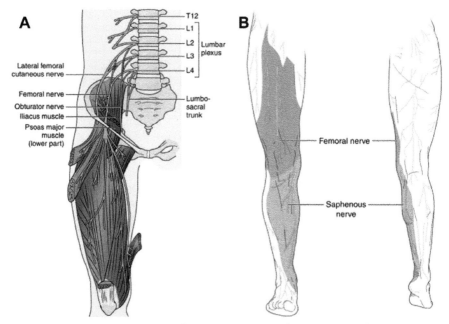

Fig. 1. (*A*) The femoral nerve. The femoral nerve arises from portions of the L2-L4 nerve roots and emerges from the psoas muscle and descends through the pelvis deep to the iliacus fascia to exit deep to the inguinal ligament, lateral to the femoral artery. Common sites of compression include the retroperitoneal space and as the nerve passes deep to the inguinal ligament. (*B*) The femoral nerve supplies sensation from the medial and anterior thigh, and from the medial lower leg (via the saphenous nerve). (*From [A]* Craig EJ, Clinchot DM. Femoral neuropathy. In: Frontera WR, Silver JK, Rizzo TD, editors. Essentials of physical medicine and rehabilitation. 3rd edition. Philadelphia: Saunders; 2015, with permission; and [*B*] Kim DH, Hudson AR, Kline DG. Femoral nerve. In: Kim DH, Hudson AR, Kline DG, editors. Atlas of peripheral nerve surgery. 2nd edition. Philadelphia: Saunders; 2013, with permission.)

pure sensory saphenous nerve, supplying sensation from the skin of the medial lower leg (**Fig. 1**B).

Injury to the femoral nerve can occur in the retroperitoneal space or as it crosses deep to the inguinal ligament. Sustained lithotomy positioning in select urologic or gynecologic procedures or during childbirth can result in excessive stretch or compression of the femoral nerve across the inguinal ligament.[1] Retroperitoneal hemorrhage can compress the nerve under the poorly compliant iliacus fascia and is an especially important consideration if the patient reports concomitant abdominal pain or is on anticoagulation.[2] Femoral injury may also occur following surgery or procedures at the femoral triangle, such as vascular catheterization.

Diagnosis of a femoral neuropathy is largely based on the clinical examination, showing sensory and motor deficits limited to this nerve. Weakness of hip flexion is a key examination finding for localization; lesions above the inguinal ligament in the retroperitoneal space can impair hip flexion, whereas those at or below the inguinal ligament do not. It is important to consider disorders of the lumbar plexus or lumbar radiculopathy (L2-L4) in the differential diagnosis; the neurologic examination can help differentiate between these (**Table 1**). Sensory deficits in the proximal medial thigh (innervated by the obturator nerve) or lateral thigh (via the lateral femoral cutaneous nerve) should suggest an alternative diagnosis. Similarly, weakness of hip adductors (innervated by the obturator nerve) or ankle dorsiflexion (innervated by the peroneal nerve) would be inconsistent with a femoral neuropathy.

Nerve conduction studies offer a limited role in confirming femoral nerve entrapment. Evaluation of the nerve is restricted to its segment distal to the inguinal ligament; therefore, direct demonstration of nerve compression in the abdomen or at the inguinal ligament is not possible. Nerve conduction studies can assist with prognostication after unilateral femoral injury. Patients with a greater than 50% reduction in motor response amplitude on the affected side compared with the unaffected side (which correlates with axon loss) are more likely to have an incomplete or delayed recovery.[3]

In cases of diagnostic or etiologic uncertainty, neuromuscular ultrasound may be helpful.[4] The femoral nerve can be visualized on ultrasound from 10 cm above to 5 cm below the inguinal ligament and thus can visualize the nerve across a site of known entrapment. Abnormalities in the nerve's shape, cross-sectional area, or echotexture may help support a clinical suspicion of nerve entrapment and injury. Additional imaging modalities, such as computed tomography or MRI, are essential when there is suspicion for an intra-abdominal mass or hematoma causing femoral nerve compression. Identification of a hematoma is important, because early intervention via reversal of anticoagulation and possible surgical decompression may be critical to a patient's recovery and degree of lifelong disability. Although surgical decompression in all cases is controversial, evidence of hemodynamic instability and worsening neurologic dysfunction are both thought to be appropriate indications for pursuing surgical intervention.[5]

Treatment of femoral mononeuropathy involves removing or limiting inciting factors that lead to nerve compression. Care is otherwise symptomatic and may include physical therapy, bracing, and orthoses. Prognosis is overall favorable, with two-thirds of patients showing evidence of functional improvement within 2 years of symptom onset.[3]

Lateral Femoral Cutaneous Neuropathy (Meralgia Paresthetica)

Injury to the lateral femoral cutaneous nerve results in the classic syndrome of burning pain, paresthesias, numbness, and tactile hypersensitivity isolated to the skin of the anterolateral thigh (known as meralgia paresthetica; **Fig. 2**). It is considered the

Table 1
Clinical signs and symptoms differentiating femoral neuropathy from common mimics

Site of Lesion	Motor Weakness				Sensory Loss				Reflexes
	Hip Flexion	Hip Adduction	Knee Extension	Ankle Dorsiflexion	Anterior Thigh	Lateral Thigh	Medial Thigh	Medial Calf	Patellar
Femoral nerve (above inguinal ligament)	Yes	No	Yes	No	Yes	No	Yes (distal only)	Yes	Reduced
Femoral nerve (below inguinal ligament)	No	No	Yes	No	Yes	No	Yes (distal only)	Yes	Reduced
Lumbar plexopathy	Yes	Yes	Yes	Yes	Yes	Yes	Yes (proximal & distal)	Yes	Reduced
L2-L4 lumbosacral radiculopathy	Yes	Yes	Yes	Yes	Yes	Yes	Yes (proximal & distal)	Yes	Reduced (L4)

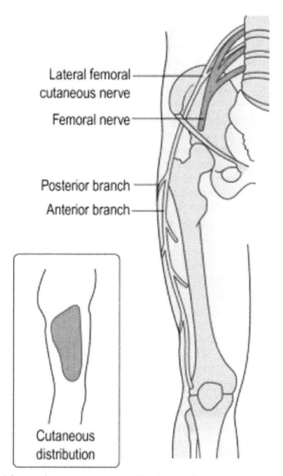

Fig. 2. The lateral femoral cutaneous nerve. The lateral femoral cutaneous nerve is formed from portions of the L2 and L3 nerve roots, crosses the abdomen, and emerges into the subcutaneous tissues of the thigh in close approximation to the anterior superior iliac spine, inguinal ligament, and tendinous insertion of the sartorius muscle. This pure sensory nerve supplies sensation from the lateral thigh, from the greater trochanter to the patella. (*From* Preston DC, Shapiro BE. Lumbosacral plexopathy. In: Preston DC, Shapiro BE, editors. Electromyography and neuromuscular disorders. 3rd edition. Philadelphia: Saunders; 2013; with permission.)

second most common mononeuropathy in the lower extremities (after common peroneal neuropathy) and has an incidence estimated at 33 in 100,000. Diabetes and obesity are known risk factors.[6]

The lateral femoral cutaneous nerve is derived from the L2 and L3 nerve roots and takes an oblique course through the abdomen, exiting near the inguinal ligament and anterior superior spine of the ilium (ASIS) (see **Fig. 2**). Its proximity to these structures at the pelvic brim places the nerve at risk for entrapment. Detailed anatomic studies demonstrate significant variation in the course of the nerve, with some trajectories more associated with risk for compression, specifically courses that take the nerve over the iliac crest, exiting within the inguinal ligament, or within the tendinous insertion of the sartorius muscle.[7]

The reported causes of lateral femoral cutaneous neuropathy are numerous and include compression or excessive stretch injury from outerwear such as tight fitting pants and belts,[8] from a Smart phone carried on the belt or tablet rested too frequently in a patient's lap,[9] from the weight of a large abdomen in obesity,[10] pregnancy, or ascites in liver failure,[11] or in acute compression from a seatbelt during a motor vehicle accident.[12] Damage to the nerve may also be iatrogenic during anterior surgical approaches to the hip or pelvis, in pin insertion into the ASIS for external fixation of the pelvis, or in bone graft harvesting.[13]

The diagnosis of meralgia paresthetica is largely clinical and depends on a detailed history and examination demonstrating pain, paresthesias, numbness, and/or hypersensitivity of the skin strictly limited to the sensory distribution of this singular nerve. Examination of a patient with meralgia paresthetica will demonstrate a sharply demarcated area of sensory loss or sensitivity restricted to the anterolateral thigh, extending from the trochanter of the femur to the superior margin of the patella, or a more restricted area within these boundaries (see **Fig. 2**). As the lateral femoral cutaneous nerve is a pure sensory nerve, there should be no motor deficits. The presence of motor deficits can differentiate meralgia paresthetica from a radiculopathy at L2, which exhibits similar sensory abnormalities but may present with hip flexion difficulties due to psoas muscle weakness. Sensory abnormalities in L2 radiculopathy are often less sharply demarcated than in a lateral femoral cutaneous mononeuropathy (due to the overlap of sensory dermatomes between L2 and its adjacent nerve roots), and the medial thigh may also be involved.

Electrodiagnostic evaluation of the lateral femoral cutaneous nerve can be performed to aid in diagnosis, although this is not routinely pursued. Examination of this nerve is technically challenging given variability in the path of the nerve as it exits the abdomen and its course through the subcutaneous tissues of the thigh.

Treatment is largely supportive with most cases improving spontaneously.[6] Care should generally focus on reassurance, avoiding potential exacerbating factors, and promoting weight loss when obesity is thought to be a factor. Antiseizure and antidepressant medications can help reduce neuropathic pain. Interventional therapies such as corticosteroid or anesthetic injections and surgical decompression are rarely used.

Peroneal Neuropathy

Peroneal neuropathy is the most common compressive neuropathy in the lower extremities. Injury to this nerve classically causes foot drop with weakness of ankle and toe dorsiflexion and foot eversion, numbness over the lateral lower leg and dorsum of the foot, and a characteristic steppage gait.

Nerve fibers destined for the peroneal nerve are derived from the L4, L5, and S1 nerve roots. They travel through the lumbosacral plexus before forming the sciatic nerve in combination with nerve fibers destined for the tibial nerve. The sciatic nerve courses through the posterior thigh before branching into the common peroneal and tibial nerves above the popliteal fossa. The common peroneal nerve wraps around the head of the fibula in the proximal lateral lower leg. The nerve is prone to compression or excessive stretch injury here against this bony protuberance (**Fig. 3**). Below the fibular head, the nerve divides into superficial and deep branches. The superficial branch supplies sensation from the dorsum of the foot and lateral aspect of the distal lower leg (see **Fig. 3**) as well as motor innervation to the peroneus longus muscle, which everts the foot. The deep branch of the peroneal nerve supplies sensation from the first digital webspace of the foot and motor innervation to ankle dorsiflexors (tibialis anterior muscle) and toe dorsiflexors (extensor hallucis longus and extensor hallucis brevis muscles).

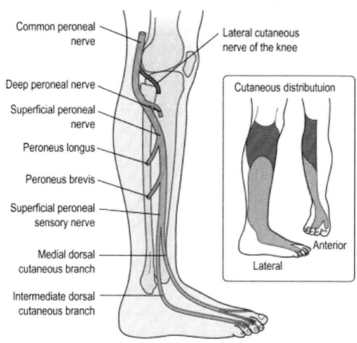

Cutaneous distributuion

Anterior

Lateral

Fig. 3. The anatomic course of the peroneal nerve. The sciatic nerve divides into the common peroneal and tibial nerve in the posterior thigh, proximal to the popliteal fossa. In its lateral course, the common peroneal nerve wraps around the head of the fibula, where it is prone to compression from external forces and excessive stretch injury. In addition to supplying motor innervation to muscles for foot eversion and ankle and toe dorsiflexion, the peroneal nerve also supplies sensation from the lateral aspect of the lower leg and dorsum of the foot. (*From* Haymaker W, Woodhall B. Peripheral nerve injuries. 2nd edition. Philadelphia: WB Saunders; 1953; with permission.)

Compression of the peroneal nerve most commonly occurs at the fibular head. Compression may occur from trauma or from more chronic external compression from a mass lesion (eg, ganglion cyst[14]), from pressure during prolonged immobilization (eg, during anesthesia,[15] or when wearing a cast or orthosis[16]), or with habitual leg crossing. Thin body habitus or rapid weight loss are risk factors for peroneal neuropathy, presumably because loss of subcutaneous soft tissues puts the nerve at greater risk of compression.[17] Excessive stretch from prolonged squatting[18] can also lead to nerve damage.

Foot drop from peroneal neuropathy must be differentiated from more proximal lesions of the sciatic nerve, lumbosacral plexus, or L4-S1 nerve roots (**Table 2**), which can all cause weakness of ankle and toe dorsiflexion and foot eversion. Foot inversion, mediated by the tibial-innervated tibialis posterior muscle, will not be present in a peroneal mononeuropathy but could be present in sciatic mononeuropathy, in lumbosacral plexus lesions, or with a lumbosacral radiculopathy (principally with L5 root involvement). When evaluating inversion in the setting of foot drop, the affected foot should be passively dorsiflexed to a neutral position before testing foot inversion, because testing in the "dropped" or plantarflexed position may result in a false sense of weakness. Ankle plantarflexion weakness (mediated by tibial innervated gastrocnemius muscles; L5-S2) or hip abduction weakness (mediated by the superior gluteal

Table 2
Clinical signs and symptoms differentiating peroneal neuropathy at the fibular head from common mimics

| Site of Lesion | Motor Weakness | | | | | | Sensory Loss | | Reflexes |
	Ankle Dorsiflexion	Ankle Plantarflexion	Foot Eversion	Foot Inversion	Hip Abduction	Dorsum of Foot	Medial, Lateral, or Sole of Foot		Achilles
Peroneal neuropathy (at fibular head)	Yes	No	Yes	No	No	Yes	No		Normal
Sciatic nerve	Yes	Yes	Yes	Yes	No	Yes	Yes		Reduced
Lumbosacral plexopathy	Yes	Yes	Yes	Yes	No	Yes	Yes		Reduced
L4-S1 radiculopathy	Yes	Yes	Yes	Yes	Yes	Yes	Yes		Reduced (S1)

innervated gluteus medius muscle; L5-S1) should also prompt consideration of alternative causes. Last, an isolated peroneal mononeuropathy does not affect the deep tendon reflexes, whereas the patellar reflex (L4) or gastrocnemius/soleus reflex (S1) may be affected by more proximal lesions.

Electrophysiologic studies are of great utility in the evaluation of peroneal neuropathy at the fibular head. Nerve conductions and needle electromyography can assist in localizing the site of injury solely to the peroneal nerve and show evidence of focal compression across the fibular head causing interruption of nerve conduction. Moreover, the severity of nerve compression and extent of axonal injury can be evaluated to help guide in prognosis. Other diagnostic modalities, such as nerve ultrasound[19] or MRI,[20] are not routinely used, but add value when a mass lesion compressing the nerve is suspected. A reasonable approach would be to consider imaging in any patient with a clinical or electrophysiologic diagnosis of peroneal neuropathy, but who does not have a clear history or risk factors to support compression.

Prognosis following compressive peroneal neuropathy is overall favorable. Care is supportive, focusing on patient education, removing inciting factors when possible, and offering supportive devices, such as an ankle-foot orthosis to assist with foot drop. Predictors of poorer outcome include evidence of denervation injury on electromyography, severe weakness at onset, and age.[21] Surgical decompression is controversial and surgical referral should be limited to patients who do not improve despite months of conservative management, or who have progressive symptoms without a clear underlying cause for entrapment.[22]

Posterior Tibial Neuropathy (Tarsal Tunnel Syndrome)

Compression of the posterior tibial nerve at the tarsal tunnel (tarsal tunnel syndrome) is rare and is characterized by pain, sensory loss, and paresthesias over the medial ankle and heel, sole of the foot, and toes. Patients may also complain of cramping of the foot and in severe cases report weakness of toe flexion and abduction with atrophy of the plantar foot muscles. Symptoms tend to be worse with activities such as standing, walking, and running and correspondingly worsen over the course of the day.

The tarsal tunnel is located at the medial ankle, with a bony floor formed by the distal tibia, talus, and calcaneal bones, and a roof formed by the fibrous flexor retinaculum extending from the medial malleolus to the calcaneal bone (**Fig. 4**). The contents of the tarsal tunnel include the posterior tibial nerve, artery, and vein, as well as the tendons of the tibialis posterior, flexor hallucis longus, and flexor digitorum longus muscles. Compression of the nerve may occur when the volume of the tarsal tunnel is physically restricted. Certain positions of the foot, particularly eversion and plantarflexion at the ankle, are known to restrict its dimensions. Other potential causes include soft tissue inflammation (eg, rheumatoid arthritis, flexor tendonitis), masses (eg, tumor), edema (eg, myxedema in hypothyroidism, pitting edema from volume overload), vascular disorders (eg, varicose veins), or bony lesions (eg, osteophytes or osteochondroma).

The spectrum of symptoms in posterior tibial neuropathy can vary considerably depending on the root cause of nerve compression and the anatomic relationship of the nerve and its branches to the tarsal tunnel. The nerve has 3 terminal branches: the medial calcaneal nerve (providing sensation from the medial heel), and the medial and lateral plantar nerves, which supply sensation from their respective sides of the sole of the foot and motor innervation to the deep muscles of the plantar aspect of the foot. The site where the posterior tibial nerve divides into each of its respective branches varies and can be proximal, within, or distal to the tarsal tunnel. Thus, the

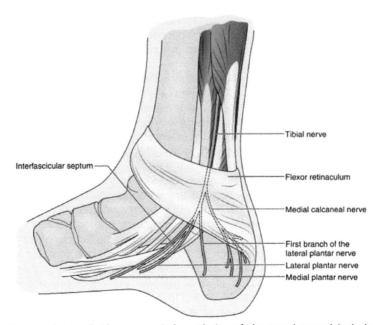

Fig. 4. The tarsal tunnel. The anatomic boundaries of the tarsal tunnel include a floor formed from the tibia, talus, and calcaneus and a roof from the flexor retinaculum which attaches at the medial malleolus and calcaneus. Its contents include the posterior tibial nerve, artery and vein, as well as the tendons of the tibialis posterior, flexor hallucis longus, and flexor digitorum longus muscles. (*From* Del Toro DR. Tibial neuropathy (tarsal tunnel syndrome). In: Frontera WR, Silver JK, Rizzo TD, editors. Essentials of physical medicine and rehabilitation. 3rd edition. Philadelphia: Saunders; 2015; with permission.)

site of origin for the nerve terminal branches in relation to the site of compression can result in heterogeneity in the presenting symptoms between patients.

Tarsal tunnel syndrome is rare, so foot pain and sensory symptoms often have an alternative explanation. Other neurologic disorders to consider include radiculopathy (L4-S1), proximal tibial neuropathy, polyneuropathy, and Morton neuroma. Nonneurologic mimics include calcaneal spurs or bursitis, flexor hallucis longus or flexor digitorum longus tendonitis, or plantar fasciitis.[23]

Examination of a patient with suspected tarsal tunnel syndrome should include a careful sensory examination, confirming abnormalities limited to the heel, sole, and toes, as well as motor examination to assess for toe flexion or abduction weakness. Evidence of frank sensory loss helps to limit the differential to neurologic conditions and would argue against musculoskeletal mimics. Multiple provocative maneuvers have been proposed to assist in the diagnosis. Tinel sign, where the nerve is percussed at the tarsal tunnel and paresthesias are appreciated by the patient in the distribution of the nerve, has poor sensitivity (0.58),[24] and a positive test may be seen in patients with polyneuropathy and in normal subjects.[21] Additional provocative maneuvers include the following:

1. The dorsiflexion-eversion test whereby passive dorsiflexion and eversion at the ankle for 5 to 10 seconds results in pain or numbness at the ankle or sole,[25]
2. The Trepman test whereby passive plantarflexion and inversion results in pain or numbness at the ankle or sole,[26] and
3. The triple-compression test, which combines the Trepman and Tinel tests.

The dorsiflexion-eversion and triple-compression tests have better diagnostic utility with sensitivities and specificities of 0.98 and 1.00 and 0.86 and 1.00, respectively. Nerve conduction studies are of questionable importance because reliable information about their sensitivity and specificity does not exist.[27] MRI and ultrasound of the tarsal tunnel can confirm a clinical suspicion of the disorder and offer further information about the type of compression, whereas ultrasound offers a further option evaluating for compression of the nerve demonstrated under dynamic conditions.[28]

Conservative management of tarsal tunnel syndrome is the rule, especially in the absence of motor weakness or atrophy. This may include custom orthoses, taping, stretching, bracing, massage, and anti-inflammatory and analgesic medications.[29] In the setting of weakness, imaging should be pursued, along with a surgical referral for considerations of microsurgical decompression, although it is important to note that evidence regarding efficacy of tarsal tunnel release is largely equivocal.[23]

FUTURE DIRECTIONS/SUMMARY

Compressive neuropathies are a common cause of weakness and sensory loss in the leg and may lead to significant functional disability. Familiarization with the symptoms, signs, and inciting factors that contribute to nerve compression is important for any physician across any discipline. Careful examination of a patient is often sufficient to establish the diagnosis, and when uncertainty exists, electrophysiologic and imaging studies, including neuromuscular ultrasound, may offer valuable additional information. For patients with transient or pure sensory symptoms, conservative treatment, including avoidance of inciting factors and bracing, is often sufficient for treatment. When progressive motor weakness is evident, consideration for surgical decompression may be considered.

REFERENCES

1. Al-Ajmi A, Rousseff RT, Khuraibet AJ. Iatrogenic femoral neuropathy: Two cases and literature update. J Clin Neuromuscul Dis 2010. https://doi.org/10.1097/CND.0b013e3181f3dbe7.
2. Young MR, Norris JW. Femoral neuropathy during anticoagulant therapy. Neurology 1976;26(12):1173–5.
3. Kuntzer T, Van Melle G, Regli F. Clinical and prognostic features in unilateral femoral neuropathies. Muscle Nerve 1997;20(2):205–11.
4. Gruber H, Peer S, Kovacs P, et al. The ultrasonographic appearance of the femoral nerve and cases of iatrogenic impairment. J Ultrasound Med 2003. https://doi.org/10.7863/jum.2003.22.2.163.
5. Parmer SS, Carpenter JP, Fairman RM, et al. Femoral neuropathy following retroperitoneal hemorrhage: Case series and review of the literature. Ann Vasc Surg 2006. https://doi.org/10.1007/s10016-006-9059-2.
6. Parisi TJ, Mandrekar J, Dyck PJB, et al. Meralgia paresthetica: Relation to obesity, advanced age, and diabetes mellitus. Neurology 2011. https://doi.org/10.1212/WNL.0b013e318233b356.
7. Aszmann OC, Dellon ES, Dellon AL. Anatomical course of the lateral femoral cutaneous nerve and its susceptibility to compression and injury. Plast Reconstr Surg 1997. https://doi.org/10.1097/00006534-199709000-00008.
8. Boyce JR. Meralgia paresthetica and tight trousers. JAMA 1984. https://doi.org/10.1001/jama.1984.03340360021010.
9. Karwa KA, Patel D, Tavee JO. Smart device neuropathy. J Neurol Sci 2016. https://doi.org/10.1016/j.jns.2016.09.040.

10. Deal CL, Canoso JJ. Meralgia paresthetica and large abdomens. Ann Intern Med 1982;96(6 Pt 1):787–8.
11. Radvan GH, Vidikan P. Meralgia paresthetica and liver disease. Ann Intern Med 1982;96(2):252–3.
12. Beresford HR. Meralgia paresthetica after seat-belt trauma. J Trauma 1971. https://doi.org/10.1097/00005373-197107000-00017.
13. Grothaus MC, Holt M, Mekhail AO, et al. Lateral femoral cutaneous nerve: an anatomic study. Clin Orthop Relat Res 2005. https://doi.org/10.1097/01.blo.0000164526.08610.97.
14. Mulligan EP, McCain K. Common fibular (peroneal) neuropathy as the result of a ganglion cyst. J Orthop Sports Phys Ther 2012. https://doi.org/10.2519/jospt.2012.0421.
15. Sawyer RJ, Richmond MN, Hickey JD, et al. Peripheral nerve injuries associated with anaesthesia. Anaesthesia 2000. https://doi.org/10.1046/j.1365-2044.2000.01614.x.
16. Ryan MM, Darras BT, Soul JS. Peroneal neuropathy from ankle-foot orthoses. Pediatr Neurol 2003. https://doi.org/10.1016/S0887-8994(03)00043-2.
17. Cruz-Martinez A, Arpa J, Palau F. Peroneal neuropathy after weight loss. J Peripher Nerv Syst 2000. https://doi.org/10.1046/j.1529-8027.2000.00007.x.
18. Babayev M, Bodack MP, Creatura C. Common peroneal neuropathy secondary to squatting during childbirth. Obstet Gynecol 1998. https://doi.org/10.1016/S0029-7844(97)00717-5.
19. Grant TH, Omar IM, Dumanian GA, et al. Sonographic evaluation of common peroneal neuropathy in patients with foot drop. J Ultrasound Med 2015. https://doi.org/10.7863/ultra.34.4.705.
20. Donovan A, Rosenberg ZS, Cavalcanti CF. MR imaging of entrapment neuropathies of the lower extremity. Radiographics 2010. https://doi.org/10.1148/rg.304095188.
21. Bsteh G, Wanschitz JV, Gruber H, et al. Prognosis and prognostic factors in non-traumatic acute-onset compressive mononeuropathies - radial and peroneal mononeuropathies. Eur J Neurol 2013. https://doi.org/10.1111/ene.12150.
22. Mont M a, Dellon a L, Chen F, et al. The operative treatment of peroneal nerve palsy. J Bone Joint Surg Am 1996;78(6):863–9.
23. McSweeney SC, Cichero M. Tarsal tunnel syndrome-A narrative literature review. Foot (Edinb) 2015. https://doi.org/10.1016/j.foot.2015.08.008.
24. Schwieterman B, Haas D, Columber K, et al. Diagnostic accuracy of physical examination tests of the ankle/foot complex: a systematic review. Int J Sports Phys Ther 2013;8(4):416–26.
25. Kinoshita M, Okuda R, Morikawa J, et al. The dorsiflexion-eversion test for diagnosis of tarsal tunnel syndrome. J Bone Joint Surg Am 2001;83-A(12):1835–9.
26. Trepman E, Kadel NJ, Chisholm K, et al. Effect of foot and ankle position on tarsal tunnel compartment pressure. Foot Ankle Int 1999. https://doi.org/10.1177/107110079902001108.
27. Patel AT, Gaines K, Malamut R, et al. Usefulness of electrodiagnostic techniques in the evaluation of suspected tarsal tunnel syndrome: an evidence-based review. Muscle Nerve 2005. https://doi.org/10.1002/mus.20393.
28. Fantino O. Role of ultrasound in posteromedial tarsal tunnel syndrome: 81 cases. J Ultrasound 2014. https://doi.org/10.1007/s40477-014-0082-9.
29. Hudes K. Conservative management of a case of tarsal tunnel syndrome. J Can Chiropr Assoc 2010;54(2):100–6.

Peripheral Neuropathy

Kelsey Barrell, MD[a],*, A. Gordon Smith, MD[b]

KEYWORDS

- Peripheral neuropathy • Polyneuropathy • Idiopathic peripheral neuropathy
- Diabetic peripheral neuropathy • Neuropathic pain

KEY POINTS

- Peripheral neuropathy is a commonly encountered disorder in clinical practice.
- The most common pattern, a distal sensory polyneuropathy, is linked to diabetes and the metabolic syndrome in many cases.
- Red flag features that suggest a different or more severe neuropathy require a specific diagnostic approach.

INTRODUCTION

Peripheral neuropathies encompass a broad range of disorders affecting the peripheral nervous system in a number of different patterns. The most common pattern is a distal sensory polyneuropathy (DSP), a term used to refer to a group of disorders that share in a common length-dependent peripheral nerve injury resulting in distal predominant sensory loss, pain, and when severe weakness resulting in gait instability, fall risk, and in some instances foot ulceration and amputations.[1] Less common patterns include mononeuritis multiplex where multiple individual nerves are injured causing a patchy pattern of injury, neuronopathy causing non–length-dependent pan-modal sensory loss or weakness and polyradiculopathies causing proximal and distal weakness and numbness. In light of the heterogeneous presentation and the many etiologies, a systematic approach is important for evaluation and management. This article reviews the clinical and diagnostic approach to the most common forms of neuropathy as well a guide to recognizing red flag features that suggest a different or more severe neuropathy requiring a specific diagnostic approach.

EPIDEMIOLOGY

DSP is one of the most common neurologic disorders. The prevalence is increasing owing to an aging population and the increasing prevalence of diabetes and obesity.[2]

Disclosure: The authors declare that they have no relevant or material financial interests that relate to the information covered in this article.
[a] Department of Neurology, University of Utah School of Medicine, 175 North Medical Drive, Salt Lake City, UT 84132, USA; [b] Department of Neurology, Virginia Commonwealth University, 417 North 11th Street, Richmond, VA 23298, USA
* Corresponding author.
E-mail address: Kelsey.barrell@hsc.utah.edu

The most common cause is diabetes, accounting for 50% of cases.[3] DSP affects more than one-half of people with diabetes and is a major cause of morbidity and reduced quality of life owing to pain, gait instability, and associated depression.[3] The second most common cause, accounting for approximately 40% of cases, is idiopathic or cryptogenic polyneuropathy, which is associated with an increased risk of prediabetes and the metabolic syndrome.

SYMPTOMS

Peripheral neuropathies cause a range of symptoms based on the distribution and types of nerve fibers involved. Peripheral nerves are subdivided based on myelination and fiber diameter. Small-diameter, thinly myelinated or unmyelinated fibers convey thermal and mechanical pain information and their injury causes burning, tingling, pins-and-needles, electric shocks, hyperalgesia (increased sensitivity to painful stimuli), or allodynia (painful sensation to an innocuous stimuli).[4] Medium and large myelinated sensory fibers convey vibration and joint position sense and injury results in numbness and imbalance. Injury to large myelinated motor axons causes distal weakness and atrophy. Neuropathic pain, common in diabetic polyneuropathy, is one of the most disabling symptoms, impacting 20% to 30% of patients with diabetic neuropathy.[5]

Autonomic symptoms, most commonly with diabetic and amyloid neuropathies, are frequently underreported because they are nonspecific, thought to be age related, or perceived as embarrassing. They have a significant impact on quality of life unless promptly recognized and treated and, in the setting of diabetes, cardiac autonomic failure portends a poor prognosis.[6] Autonomic symptoms include the cardiovascular (orthostatic hypotension), gastrointestinal (constipation, nausea or diarrhea), urogenital (neurogenic bladder or erectile dysfunction), and secretomotor (abnormalities of sweating) systems.[7]

DIAGNOSIS
Diagnostic Tests

Nerve conduction studies (NCS) and electromyography (EMG), referred to collectively as EMG, provide useful information regarding neuroanatomical localization, severity, chronicity, and physiology (demyelinating vs axonal). NCS are performed by electrically stimulating a nerve and recording the response at a different site along the nerve or a muscle. The amplitude of the response reflects axonal integrity and is decreased or absent in an axonal neuropathy. The speed of conduction reflects the function of large myelinated fibers and is decreased in demyelinating neuropathies. EMG is performed by inserting a small needle electrode into a muscle and recording electrical activity at rest and with activity. EMG differentiates neuropathy from myopathy and provides information regarding chronicity. Autonomic testing evaluates cardiovagal (parasympathetic), sympathetic adrenergic, and sudomotor (sweating) function.[7]

A biopsy of a sensory nerve may be useful in the diagnosis of specific forms of peripheral neuropathy, particularly peripheral nerve vasculitis (**Fig. 1**) and amyloidosis.[8] A biopsy of a nearby muscle increases diagnostic yield.[9] Skin biopsy with assessment of intraepidermal nerve fiber density is a useful means of confirming a suspected diagnosis of small fiber neuropathy in patients with normal NCS.[10] The standard technique consists of performing a 3-mm punch biopsy in the distal leg and distal and proximal thigh. The biopsies are immunostained with an antibody that binds to all axons (PGP 9.5) allowing for measurement of intraepidermal nerve fiber density. Small fiber

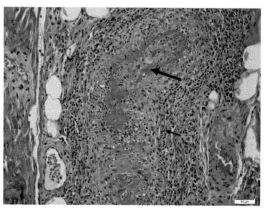

Fig. 1. Sural nerve biopsy (stain: hematoxylin and eosin stain; original magnification ×20) showing typical vasculitic features marked by necrosis and inflammation of the epineurial arteriole with intraluminar thrombosis (*large arrow*) surrounded by mononuclear inflammatory cells (*small arrow*).

neuropathy is diagnosed based on a quantitatively reduced intraepidermal nerve fiber density compared with published age- and sex-matched normative values (**Fig. 2**).

Peripheral nerve and muscle MRI and ultrasound examinations can be useful diagnostic tools in the evaluation of select forms of neuropathy, particularly focal and

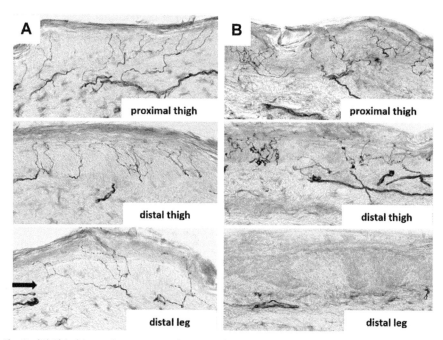

Fig. 2. (*A*) Skin biopsy from a control patient shows normal intraepidermal nerve fiber density (IENFD) at distal and proximal biopsy sites. (*B*) Skin biopsy from a patient with small fiber neuropathy shows reduced IENFD at distal site in a length-dependent pattern. IENFD is measured by counting the darkly staining nerve fibers that cross the dermal–epidermal junction shown by the arrow (Immunostain with anti-PGP 9.5, original magnification ×200).

multifocal patterns including polyradiculopathies and plexopathies. Peripheral nerve ultrasound has the advantage of being noninvasive and inexpensive, and allows for a dynamic examination of a long nerve segment. Ultrasound examination is commonly used to evaluate entrapment neuropathies and other focal nerve lesions.[11]

Diagnostic Approach to Peripheral Neuropathy

The diagnostic approach is based on pattern recognition reflecting neuroanatomic localization. The vast majority of patients present with slowly progressive DSP. Symptoms start in the toes and progress up the leg to the knee and occasionally the hands. DSP diagnosis is based on a suggestive history and a neurologic examination revealing a symmetric stocking–glove pattern sensory loss, diminished or absent Achilles deep tendon reflexes, and absent or mild distal weakness.

NCS and EMG are commonly used to confirm DSP, although their diagnostic value in this setting is questionable because they rarely change treatment and are a major driver of neuropathy-related diagnostic health care costs.[12] In early DSP, which preferentially involves small diameter axons, NCS are normal in 40% of patients.[13] Patients with atypical features (acute onset, asymmetry, proximal involvement, or unexpected severity) require NCS and EMG to define the localization and underlying physiology.

Having recognized DSP, the next step is to identify the underlying etiology and exclude potentially treatable causes. Current guidelines recommend screening every patient with a glucose tolerance test or hemoglobin A1c, serum protein electrophoresis with immunofixation to exclude a monoclonal gammopathy, and vitamin B_{12}.[14] In the absence of toxic exposure history, risk of malnutrition, or clinical evidence of a systemic disorder, additional diagnostic evaluation beyond this basic laboratory evaluation is usually unhelpful.

DIFFERENTIAL DIAGNOSIS

The differential diagnosis depends primarily on neuroanatomic localization based on pattern recognition. The presence of significant asymmetry, proximal involvement, acute/subacute progression, weakness, prominent autonomic features, and young onset are diagnostic red flags suggesting a unique differential diagnosis and diagnostic evaluation (**Table 1**). Specific neuroanatomic patterns and atypical features and their differential diagnosis and treatment are reviewed elsewhere in this article.

Distal Sensory Polyneuropathy

Although a large number of disorders cause DSP, the majority of patients have one of several different underlying etiologies. No cause is identified in up to 40% of patients (idiopathic or cryptogenic sensory peripheral neuropathy). Identifying and managing the underlying risk factors is paramount because, by eliminating offending agents and treating the underlying disease, often one can halt the progression and improve symptoms.

Diabetic peripheral neuropathy

Diabetes is the most common cause for DSP worldwide. DSP occurs in one-half of patients with both type 1 and type 2 diabetes, and in 10% to 25% of those with prediabetes.[5,15] Treatment-induced neuropathy of diabetes, previously termed insulin neuritis is a clinically distinct entity marked by the acute onset of a small fiber–predominant DSP associated with severe neuropathic pain and autonomic involvement in the setting of rapid correction of chronic hyperglycemia.[16] It is most common

Table 1

Atypical "red flag" features and their neuroanatomic localization with differential diagnosis and diagnostic evaluation

Atypical Features	Neuroanatomical Localization	Differential Diagnosis	Evaluation/Laboratory Tests
Asymmetric	Mononeuritis multiplex Mononeuropathies	Vasculitic syndromes Hereditary neuropathy with liability to pressure palsies Infectious Carpal tunnel syndrome Ulnar nerve entrapment at the elbow	ANA, P-ANCA, C-ANCA, HgA1c, ESR, HIV antibodies, cryoglobulins, hepatitis C, ACE level, Lyme titer, CMV PCR, WNV PCR, HTLV 1 Nerve biopsy—suspected vasculitis
Proximal involvement	Polyradiculoneuropathy Plexopathy	AIDP (when acute) CIDP (nadir AFTER 8 wk) DLRPN (diabetic patient) Meningeal based disease (carcinoma, lymphoma, sarcoid, infectious) Idiopathic	CSF analysis (include cell count, culture and stain, protein, glucose IgG index and depending on scenario may add cytology, ACE level and infectious studies) MRI with or without neurography with contrast
Acute/subacute progression	Variable	Toxic Infectious Paraneoplastic Porphyria	Vitamin B₆, heavy metals, paraneoplastic panel, porphyrin titers, rheumatologic screen
Motor predominant (symmetric)	Motor neuropathy Motor neuronopathy	SMA and Kennedy disease POEMS Lead intoxication Acute porphyria CMT AIDP or CIDP some sensory	CSF analysis, ganglioside panel, porphyrin titers, heavy metal panel, may consider genetic testing, SPEP/IFE

(continued on next page)

Table 1
(continued)

Atypical Features	Neuroanatomical Localization	Differential Diagnosis	Evaluation/Laboratory Tests
Motor predominant (asymmetric)	Motor neuropathy Motor neuronopathy	MMN ALS	CSF analysis Ganglioside panel
Prominent autonomic features	Autonomic nervous system	Diabetic neuropathy Amyloidosis Paraneoplastic/autoimmune CIPN (vincristine) Porphyria Hereditary sensory autonomic neuropathy	HbA1c with or without GTT SPEP/IFE, free light chains (serum and urine) Paraneoplastic panel Porphyrins Autonomic lab testing (if severe) Genetic testing (young onset)
Non length dependent	Sensory neuronopathy (dorsal root ganglionopathy)	Sjögren syndrome CIPN (platinums) Paraneoplastic Vitamin B_6 toxicity HIV	ACE level, rheumatologic screen Paraneoplastic panel (anti-Hu) Vitamin B_6 levels HIV antibodies
Young onset	Often polyneuropathy	Inherited neuropathy (CMT) Toxic exposure Vitamin deficiency	Genetic testing Heavy metals and vitamin levels in appropriate context

Abbreviations: ACE, angiotensin-converting enzyme; AIDP, acute inflammatory demyelinating polyneuropathy; ALS, amyotrophic lateral sclerosis; ANA, antinuclear antibody; C-ANCA, cytoplasmic antineutrophil cytoplasmic antibody; CIDP, chronic inflammatory demyelinating polyneuropathy; CIPN, chemotherapy-induced peripheral neuropathy; CMT, Charcot-Marie-Tooth disease; CMV, cytomegalovirus; CSF, cerebrospinal fluid; DLRPN, diabetic lumbosacral radiculoplexus neuropathy; ESR, erythrocyte sedimentation rate; GTT, glucose tolerance test; HgA1c, hemoglobin A1c; HIV, human immunodeficiency virus; HTLV, human T-cell leukemia virus; MMN, multifocal motor neuropathy; P-ANCA, perinuclear antineutrophil cytoplasmic antibody; PCR, polymerase chain reaction; POEMS, polyneuropathy, organomegaly, endocrinopathy, monoclonal gammopathy, and skin changes; SMA, spinal muscular atrophy; SPEP/IFE, serum protein electrophoresis with immunofixation; WNV, West Nile virus.

among patients with type 1 diabetes mellitus treated with insulin. The risk is proportionate to the rate of correction with a 20% risk associated with a 2% to 3% decrease in hemoglobin A1c over 3 months and an 80% risk with a 4% decrease.[16] Aggressive glycemic control decreases the risk and rate of progression of DSP in type 1 diabetes but not in type 2 diabetes.[17] This observation suggests that hyperglycemia is not the only metabolic cause. Growing evidence suggests obesity and dyslipidemia and the metabolic syndrome are important potentially modifiable risk factors.[4]

Cryptogenic sensory peripheral neuropathy

A diagnosis of cryptogenic sensory peripheral neuropathy is based on excluding other DSP etiologies. The metabolic syndrome, obesity, and prediabetes are associated with cryptogenic sensory peripheral neuropathy risk.[4] Several studies suggest that individualized diet and exercise training may slow progression and improve symptoms.[18,19] Despite promising preclinical and early phase clinical data, clinical trials of the antioxidant benfotiamine, glutathione, L-glutamine, N-acetylcysteine, and magnesium failed to show efficacy.[20] Alpha lipoic acid, considered the most successful antioxidant in clinical trials, was approved for the treatment of diabetic peripheral neuropathy in Europe but not in the United States.[21]

Toxic and nutritional neuropathies

Toxic and deficiency-related neuropathies must be considered in at-risk patients. A list of medications and toxic exposures associated with DSP is included in **Table 2**. Chemotherapy-induced peripheral neuropathy is an increasingly frequent problem as cancer survivorship increases. It affects more than 30% of patients receiving potentially neurotoxic agents making it one of the main dose-limiting side effects of chemotherapy with the highest prevalence in platinum-based drugs (oxaliplatin and cisplatin), taxanes (paclitaxel), and vinca alkaloids (vincristine).[22] Chemotherapy-induced peripheral neuropathy develops during chemotherapy and may progress for up to 3 months after discontinuation, a phenomenon called coasting. Chemotherapy-induced peripheral neuropathy resolves in up to two-thirds of patients. Heavy alcohol use is associated with DSP in 25% to 66% of chronic alcoholics in the United States.[23]

Vitamin B_{12} deficiency is the most common vitamin deficiency seen in general practice, especially in patients with severe dietary restriction (ie, vegan diet) or abnormal absorption (ie, pernicious anemia, inflammatory bowel disease, or a history of gastric bypass). Vitamin B_{12} deficiency may also be observed in metformin-treated diabetics.[24] Vitamin B_{12} deficiency causes subacute combined degeneration of the

Table 2	
Medications and toxins associated with the development of peripheral neuropathy	
Type of Neurotoxin	**Selected Toxins**
Chemotherapy drugs	Paclitaxel, cisplatin, oxaliplatin, bortezomib, thalidomide
Antibiotics	Chloroquine, dapsone, isoniazid, metronidazole, nitrofurantoin
Antiarrhythmia drugs	Amiodarone, perhexiline, hydralazine
Other medications	Colchicine, gold salts, phenytoin, disulfiram, pyridoxine
Heavy metals	Lead (wrist drop), arsenic, thallium (alopecia), mercury
Organic solvents	Hexane, acrylamide, vacor

Data from London Z, Albers JW. Toxic neuropathies associated with pharmaceutical and industrial agents. Neurol Clin 2007;25(1):257–76.

corticospinal tracts and posterior columns of the spinal cord in addition to DSP. The clinical presentation in subacute combined degeneration is distinguished from DSP by prominent impairment of position and vibration sense and an ataxic gait disorder related to spinal cord involvement. Acquired copper deficiency (most frequently caused by zinc overload) and vitamin E deficiency are often clinically indistinguishable from vitamin B_{12} deficiency.[25,26] Vitamin B_1 (thiamine) deficiency is an important consideration in alcoholics or malnourished patients. This entity can manifest as progressive axonal sensorimotor neuropathy that may be subacute, as well as heart failure and cognitive problems.[27] Vitamin B_6 (pyridoxine) is noteworthy in that it is associated with peripheral neuropathy with deficiency or overload.[28] Vitamin B_6 toxicity may cause DSP with lower levels but higher levels of exposure cause a non–length-dependent sensory neuronopathy with associated ataxia.[29]

Monoclonal gammopathy

Monoclonal gammopathies encompass a spectrum of clonal plasma cell disorders, the most common of which are monoclonal gammopathy of uncertain significance and multiple myeloma. Monoclonal gammopathies are relatively common, with a prevalence of 3% to 4% in those older than 50 years.[30] Monoclonal gammopathy of uncertain significance has a 1% annual risk of progression to multiple myeloma or a related disorder.[31] DSP is present in 11% to 13% of patients with multiple myeloma at presentation and nearly 75% develop this over the disease course.[32] Light chain amyloidosis is a rare multisystem disorder that causes a progressive form of DSP in 15% to 20% of patients with frequent autonomic dysfunction. The treatment of choice for eligible patients is stem cell transplantation and combination chemotherapy for the remainder of patients.[32] POEMS syndrome is a clonal plasma cell disorder characterized by polyneuropathy, organomegaly, endocrinopathy, monoclonal protein, and skin changes and is usually associated with osteosclerotic myeloma or angiofollicular lymph node hyperplasia (Castleman disease). POEMS syndrome causes a progressive neuropathy characterized by distal weakness and sensory loss, often with evidence of demyelination. It is sometimes mistaken for chronic inflammatory demyelinating polyneuropathy (CIDP).[33] Elevated serum vascular endothelial growth factor levels are usually observed. The treatment of POEMS is targeted at the underlying plasma cell disorder.

Monoclonal gammopathies may also cause antibody specific neuropathy syndromes. The most common are associated with IgM gammopathies reactive to GM1 ganglioside (multifocal motor neuropathy, reviewed elsewhere in this article) and myelin-associated glycoprotein (anti-MAG neuropathy). Anti-MAG neuropathy causes slowly progressive distal weakness with numbness and prominent tremor. NCS reveal a distal demyelinating pattern. Treatment with rituximab may be effective.[34]

Inherited neuropathies

Inherited neuropathies can often be distinguished by an early age of onset and lack of positive sensory symptoms. Charcot-Marie-Tooth (CMT) disease, is the most common form. CMT disease causes distal weakness and is reviewed under motor neuropathies. Hereditary sensory and autonomic neuropathies refer to phenotypes where sensory and autonomic symptoms predominate.

Familial amyloid polyneuropathy, a rare inherited neuropathy, can manifest as a DSP and is important to identify owing to emerging treatment options for this otherwise life-threatening disorder. Familial amyloid polyneuropathy is caused by mutations in 3 genes, namely, transthyretin, the most commonly implicated gene, apolipoprotein A1, and gelsolin. The mutation destabilizes the protein, resulting in the formation of amyloid deposits in the peripheral nerves and other tissues.[35] Diagnostic clues to familial amyloid polyneuropathy include a progressive course, early autonomic features, bilateral carpal tunnel syndrome, unexplained cardiomyopathy, and a family history.

Sensory Neuronopathy

Sensory neuronopathies cause non–length-dependent panmodel sensory loss that is asymmetric and often associated with gait ataxia. The most common causes are paraneoplastic (particularly associated with anti-Hu antibodies in small cell lung carcinoma) and Sjögren syndrome. Idiopathic forms are also observed.[36]

Mononeuritis Multiplex

Mononeuritis multiplex refers to the involvement of multiple individual nerves resulting in a patchy, asymmetric pattern of weakness and numbness caused by multifocal nerve infarctions in the setting of vasculitis. Peripheral nervous system vasculitis can be caused by a systemic disorder, in which case there are often diagnostic clues, including weight loss, constitutional symptoms, rashes, or adult-onset asthma/sinus disease. Common etiologies include polyarteritis nodosa, microscopic polyangiitis, rheumatoid arthritis, systemic lupus erythematosus, Wegner granulomatosis, eosinophilic vasculitis (Churg-Strauss syndrome), cryoglobulinemia (often in the setting of hepatitis C), Sjögren syndrome, sarcoidosis, and infectious vasculopathy.[37] The most common treatment is pulse intravenous cyclophosphamide with corticosteroids, with transition to azathioprine.[37]

Polyradiculoneuropathies

Polyradiculoneuropathies, often owing to inflammatory immune neuropathies, present with proximal and distal weakness and numbness. Guillain-Barré syndrome (GBS), the most common type, typically presents as an acute demyelinating form (acute inflammatory demyelinating polyneuropathy [AIDP]), but rare subtypes include acute motor and sensory axonal neuropathy, acute motor axonal neuropathy, and Miller-Fisher syndrome. AIDP is characterized by rapidly ascending symmetric weakness and sensory symptoms reaching its nadir in less than 4 weeks, which can quickly progress to quadriplegia and respiratory failure. During the course, patients become hyporeflexic or areflexic and the cerebrospinal fluid typically reveals cytoalbuminologic dissociation (elevated protein with low/normal white blood cells). AIDP is preceded by an infectious prodrome in two-thirds of cases, with *Campylobacter jejuni* being the most common pathogen. Miller-Fisher syndrome, comprising 5% to 10% of GBS cases, consists of a triad of ophthalmoparesis, areflexia, and gait ataxia.[38] GBS is treated with intravenous immunoglobulin or plasma exchange starting within 2 weeks of onset. CIDP has a more protracted course, reaching its nadir in more than 8 weeks, with a higher likelihood of incomplete recovery or reoccurrence. Otherwise, CIDP clinically resembles AIDP in most respects. In addition to intravenous immunoglobulin and plasma exchange, CIDP can also it be treated with corticosteroids as well as steroid-sparing immunosuppressants. Diabetic lumbosacral radiculoplexus neuropathy, or diabetic amyotrophy, causes painful asymmetric polyradiculoneuropathy associated with weight loss and type 2 diabetes. It presents with acute/subacute severe proximal leg pain followed by atrophy and weakness and progressive involvement of the contralateral limb and distal muscles. Although diabetic lumbosacral radiculoplexus neuropathy is self-limited and most patients experience recovery over months, many are left with partial disability such as a footdrop.[39] Data regarding the usefulness of immunomodulatory therapy is limited, but there is some evidence suggesting that corticosteroids may be helpful in acute neuropathic pain management.[39]

Motor Neuropathies

Symmetric motor neuropathies

Many inherited neuropathies will have prominent motor symptoms, although few have pure motor symptoms. CMT, one of the most common inherited neurologic disorders, has a population prevalence 1 in 2500 with the demyelinating form CMT1 accounting for 50% of cases followed by the axonal form CMT2 (20%).[40] Most forms of CMT will present with distal weakness and painless sensory loss in the first 2 decades often associated with characteristic high arched feet (pes cavus), hammertoes, and distal leg atrophy. POEMS syndrome, distal acquired demyelinating symmetric neuropathy, and some toxic neuropathies cause a symmetric distal motor neuropathy. Rare but important considerations include genetic forms of motor neuron disease, namely, spinal muscular atrophy, an autosomal-recessive motor neuronopathy of childhood, and spinal bulbar muscular atrophy (Kennedy disease), an adult-onset X-linked motor neuron disease marked by bulbar and proximal predominant weakness and endocrinologic changes. Lead poisoning often presents with abdominal pain and encephalopathy, but characteristically can result in weakness involving wrist and finger extensors.[41]

Asymmetric motor neuropathies

Amyotrophic lateral sclerosis (ALS) is the most common motor neuron disease. The diagnostic hallmark of classic ALS is a combination of upper (spasticity and/or hyperreflexia) and lower motor neuron dysfunction (fasciculations, muscle atrophy, and weakness). Onset typically begins in 1 limb (80% of cases) or with cranial nerve involvement marked by bulbar dysfunction (20% of cases) and progresses to other body segments.[42] Variants of ALS include pure upper motor neuron involvement (primary lateral sclerosis) or lower motor neuron involvement (progressive muscular atrophy). ALS is diagnosed clinically but NCS/EMG is important to confirm the diagnosis and exclude mimics. The 2 US Food and Drug Administration–approved disease-modifying drug treatments for ALS, riluzole and edaravone, are shown to modestly slow disease progression in some patients.

Multifocal motor neuropathy is characterized by progressive distal predominant asymmetric weakness affecting primarily the upper extremities. Multifocal motor neuropathy is associated with monoclonal anti-GM1 antibodies in up to one-half of patients, and partial motor conduction block is common.[43] It is imperative to distinguish multifocal motor neuropathy from motor neuron disease because the former is a treatable disorder with intravenous immunoglobulin as the standard first-line therapy.[44]

Mononeuropathies

Carpal tunnel syndrome, the most common peripheral entrapment neuropathy, is seen in 3.8% of the general population.[45] Compression of the median nerve between the carpal bones, flexor tendons, and the carpal ligament results in episodic wrist pain and paresthesia's involving the first 3 fingers, which is often provoked by repetitive movements or sleep. With progression, persistent numbness, grip weakness, and atrophy of the thenar eminence occur. The dominant hand is typically affected and, when presenting bilaterally, it is important to consider diabetes, hypothyroidism, amyloidosis, and rheumatoid arthritis. Ulnar nerve entrapment at the elbow or cubital tunnel syndrome, the second most common entrapment neuropathy, results in numbness, tingling, and weakness involving the fourth and fifth digits. Carpal tunnel syndrome treatment decisions are based on symptom severity; mild symptoms are treated conservatively with nocturnal wrist splinting, ergonomic positioning, or corticosteroid injections; more severe or resistant cases require a carpal tunnel release, which holds a high-long term success rate in 75% to 90% of patients.[46] Likewise, ulnar entrapment is also amenable to surgical decompression in carefully selected patients.

Acute Neuropathies

Acute or subacute onset suggests toxic, immune-mediated, or infectious etiologies. GBS is the most common acute neuropathy. GBS and its variants usually cause proximal and distal weakness. Therefore, the presence of distal predominant weakness should raise suspicion for an alternative etiology. Porphyric neuropathy can cause acute motor neuropathy mimicking GBS with a prodrome of abdominal pain and psychosis.[47]

SYMPTOMATIC MANAGEMENT
Neuropathic Pain

Neuropathic pain is a common feature in peripheral neuropathies, seen in up to 30% of patients with diabetic DPN.[3] The most commonly used agents for neuropathic pain include tricyclic antidepressants (amitriptyline and nortriptyline), anticonvulsants (gabapentin and pregabalin), and serotonin-norepinephrine reuptake inhibitors (duloxetine and venlafaxine). The European Federation of Neurologic Societies published revised evidence-based guidelines in 2010 concluding that these drugs have similar efficacy in painful polyneuropathy.[48] However, given the paucity of large-scale comparative studies and the short duration of most clinical trials, clinicians rely heavily on clinical judgment based on a patients comorbidities, potential adverse effects, medication interactions, and cost.[49] Despite evidence suggesting comparable effectiveness, only duloxetine and pregabalin are approved by the US Food and Drug Administration to treat neuropathic pain in diabetes.[50] These 2 agents are significantly more expensive than other first-line agents.[50] Both controlled-release oxycodone and tramadol with acetaminophen were recommended with level A evidence by the European Federation of Neurologic Societies; however given their side effect profile and addiction potential, they are generally used as second- or third-line drugs.[48] A rational diagnostic approach starts with either gabapentin, amitriptyline or nortriptyline given similar efficacy and lower cost. If there is an inadequate response after an appropriate trial and dose, pregabalin or duloxetine may be tried next. If there is no response polytherapy may be tried. Rarely there is a role for oral opiate therapy or procedural intervention (eg, spinal cord stimulation). Generally, at this juncture referral to a specialty pain clinic is recommended. It is very important to address relevant comorbidities, particularly mood and sleep.

Given the potential side effects and perceived lack of efficacy among conventional analgesics, complementary and alternative medicine has become increasingly popular despite lack of rigorous evidence supporting their efficacy. Complementary and alternative medicine encompasses a large group of therapies including physical therapy, acupuncture, megavitamins, magnets, herbal remedies, chiropractic manipulation, and meditation, among others.[20] In a prospective prevalence study of 180 outpatients with peripheral neuropathy, 43% of patients used complementary and alternative medicine.[51]

Management of comorbidities and autonomic dysfunction

Previous studies show that peripheral neuropathy markedly increases fall risk, which can lead to injury, emergency room visits, and loss of independence.[52] Primary fall prevention should start with the primary care provider and include a fall risk assessment, education, and referral to physical therapy when appropriate. The burden of illness in patients with peripheral neuropathy extends beyond the peripheral nervous system. In painful neuropathy, the severity of pain has been correlated with increased rates of insomnia, decreased productivity and function, and increased depression.[53] Given this well-described impact on well-being, addressing sleep, pain, and mood are important aspects of care.

The treatment of autonomic neuropathies primarily focuses on symptomatic management. Most cases of orthostatic hypotension can be initially managed with non-pharmacologic treatments including avoidance of triggers, a 30° head-up tilt of the bed at night, adequate hydration, physical countermaneuvers (crossing legs, squatting), and compression stockings. Gastroparesis can be more difficult to manage and, if supportive measures are inadequate (small regular meals 4–5 times a day; low-fat and low residue meals; avoidance of carbonation, alcohol, and tobacco; and optimization of liquid nutrition), referral to a specialist is recommended.[54–56]

SUMMARY

Peripheral neuropathy is commonly seen in the primary care office setting given its high population prevalence. Most patients present with the prototypic presentation of a symmetric distal polyneuropathy and can be accurately diagnosed and managed expeditiously. However, recognizing red flags for a more serious process is fundamental for early identification, appropriate referral and management.

REFERENCES

1. Tesfaye S, Selvarajah D. Advances in the epidemiology, pathogenesis and management of diabetic peripheral neuropathy. Diabetes Metab Res Rev 2012;28: 8–14.
2. Gregg EW, Sorlie P, Paulose-Ram R, et al. Prevalence of lower-extremity disease in the U.S. adult population ≥40 years of age with and without diabetes: 1999–2000 national health and nutrition examination survey. Diabetes Care 2004;27: 1591–7.
3. Tesfaye S, Vileikyte L, Rayman G, et al. Painful diabetic peripheral neuropathy: consensus recommendations on diagnosis, assessment and management: painful diabetic peripheral neuropathy. Diabetes Metab Res Rev 2011;27: 629–38.
4. Stino AM, Smith AG. Peripheral neuropathy in prediabetes and the metabolic syndrome. J Diabetes Investig 2017;8:646–55.
5. Zilliox L, Russell JW. Treatment of diabetic sensory polyneuropathy. Curr Treat Options Neurol 2011;13:143–59.
6. Spallone V, Ziegler D, Freeman R, et al. Cardiovascular autonomic neuropathy in diabetes: clinical impact, assessment, diagnosis, and management: diabetic cardiovascular autonomic neuropathy in clinical practice. Diabetes Metab Res Rev 2011;27:639–53.
7. Freeman R. Autonomic peripheral neuropathy. Lancet 2005;365:1259–70.
8. Lacomis D. Clinical utility of peripheral nerve biopsy. Curr Neurol Neurosci Rep 2005;5:41–7.

9. Vital C, Vital A, Canron MH, et al. Combined nerve and muscle biopsy in the diagnosis of vasculitic neuropathy. A 16-year retrospective study of 202 cases. J Peripher Nerv Syst 2006;11:20–9.
10. Lauria G, Hsieh ST, Johansson O, et al. European Federation of Neurological Societies/peripheral nerve society guideline on the use of skin biopsy in the diagnosis of small fiber neuropathy. Report of a joint task force of the European Federation of Neurological Societies and the Peripheral Nerve Society. Eur J Neurol 2010;17:e44–9.
11. Bianchi S. Ultrasound of the peripheral nerves. Joint Bone Spine 2008;75:643–9.
12. Callaghan BC, Kerber KA, Lisabeth LL, et al. Role of neurologists and diagnostic tests on the management of distal symmetric polyneuropathy. JAMA Neurol 2014; 71:1143–9.
13. Smith AG. Do all neuropathy patients need an EMG at least once? Continuum (Minneap Minn) 2014;20:1430–4.
14. England JD, Gronseth GS, Franklin G, et al. Practice parameter: evaluation of distal symmetric polyneuropathy: role of laboratory and genetic testing (an evidence-based review): report of the American Academy of Neurology, American Association of Neuromuscular and Electrodiagnostic Medicine, and American Academy of Physical Medicine and Rehabilitation. Neurology 2009;72: 185–92.
15. Papanas N, Vinik AI, Ziegler D. Neuropathy in prediabetes: does the clock start ticking early? Nat Rev Endocrinol 2011;7:682–90.
16. Gibbons CH, Freeman R. Treatment-induced neuropathy of diabetes: an acute, iatrogenic complication of diabetes. Brain 2015;138:43–52.
17. Callaghan BC, Little AA, Feldman EL, et al. Enhanced glucose control for preventing and treating diabetic neuropathy. Cochrane Database Syst Rev 2012;(6):CD007543.
18. Smith AG, Russell J, Feldman EL, et al. Lifestyle intervention for pre-diabetic neuropathy. Diabetes Care 2006;29:1294–9.
19. Balducci S, Iacobellis G, Parisi L, et al. Exercise training can modify the natural history of diabetic peripheral neuropathy. J Diabetes Complications 2006;20: 216–23.
20. Peripheral neuropathy: pathogenic mechanisms and alternative therapies. Available at: http://www.biomedsearch.com/article/Peripheral-neuropathy-pathogenic-mechanisms-alternative/157656145.html. Accessed June 15, 2018.
21. Oyenihi AB, Ayeleso AO, Mukwevho E, et al. Antioxidant strategies in the management of diabetic neuropathy. Biomed Res Int 2015;2015:515042.
22. Grisold W, Cavaletti G, Windebank AJ. Peripheral neuropathies from chemotherapeutics and targeted agents: diagnosis, treatment, and prevention. Neuro Oncol 2012;14:iv45–54.
23. Chopra K, Tiwari V. Alcoholic neuropathy: possible mechanisms and future treatment possibilities. Br J Clin Pharmacol 2012;73:348–62.
24. Fogelman Y, Kitai E, Blumberg G, et al. Vitamin B12 screening in metformin-treated diabetics in primary care: were elderly patients less likely to be tested? Aging Clin Exp Res 2017;29:135–9.
25. Kumar N, Gross JB. Copper deficiency myelopathy produces a clinical picture like subacute combined degeneration. Neurology 2004;63(1):33–9.
26. Traber MG, Sokol RJ, Ringel SP, et al. Lack of tocopherol in peripheral nerves of vitamin E-deficient patients with peripheral Ne27uropathy. N Engl J Med 1987; 317:262–5.

27. Abdou E, Hazell AS. Thiamine deficiency: an update of pathophysiologic mechanisms and future therapeutic considerations. Neurochem Res 2015;40:353–61.
28. Berger AR, Schaumburg HH, Schroeder C, et al. Dose response, coasting, and differential fiber vulnerability in human toxic neuropathy: a prospective study of pyridoxine neurotoxicity. Neurology 1992;42:1367–70.
29. Kulkantrakorn K. Pyridoxine-induced sensory ataxic neuronopathy and neuropathy: revisited. Neurol Sci 2014;35:1827–30.
30. Kelly JJ, Kyle RA, O'Brien PC, et al. Prevalence of monoclonal protein in peripheral neuropathy. Neurology 1981;31:1480–3.
31. Kyle RA, Therneau TM, Rajkumar SV, et al. A long-term study of prognosis in monoclonal gammopathy of undetermined significance. N Engl J Med 2002; 346:564–9.
32. Raheja D, Specht C, Simmons Z. Paraproteinemic neuropathies. Muscle Nerve 2014;51:1–13.
33. Chaudhry HM, Mauermann ML, Rajkumar SV. Monoclonal gammopathy-associated peripheral neuropathy: diagnosis and management. Mayo Clin Proc 2017;92:838–50.
34. Lunn MP, Nobile-Orazio E. Immunotherapy for IgM anti-myelin-associated glycoprotein paraprotein-associated peripheral neuropathies. Cochrane Database Syst Rev 2016;(10):CD002827.
35. Planté-Bordeneuve V, Said G. Familial amyloid polyneuropathy. Lancet Neurol 2011;10:1086–97.
36. Sheikh SI, Amato AA. The dorsal root ganglion under attack: the acquired sensory ganglionopathies. Pract Neurol 2010;10:326–34.
37. Younger DS. Vasculitis of the nervous system. Curr Opin Neurol 2004;17:317–36.
38. Dimachkie MM, Barohn RJ. Guillain-Barré syndrome and variants. Neurol Clin 2013;31:491–510.
39. Dyck PJB, Windebank AJ. Diabetic and nondiabetic lumbosacral radiculoplexus neuropathies: new insights into pathophysiology and treatment. Muscle Nerve 2002;25:477–91.
40. Saporta MA. Charcot-Marie-Tooth disease and other inherited neuropathies. Continuum (Minneap Minn) 2014;20:1208.
41. Thomson RM, Parry GJ. Neuropathies associated with excessive exposure to lead. Muscle Nerve 2006;33:732–41.
42. Tiryaki E, Horak HA. ALS and other motor neuron diseases. Continuum (Minneap Minn) 2014;20:1185.
43. Parry GJG. Antiganglioside antibodies do not necessarily play a role in multifocal motor neuropathy. Muscle Nerve 1994;17:97–9.
44. Nobile-Orazio E, Gallia F. Multifocal motor neuropathy: current therapies and novel strategies. Drugs 2013;73:397–406.
45. Ghasemi-rad M, Nosair E, Vegh A, et al. A handy review of carpal tunnel syndrome: from anatomy to diagnosis and treatment. World J Radiol 2014;6: 284–300.
46. Mintalucci DJ, Leinberry CF. Open versus endoscopic carpal tunnel release. Orthop Clin North Am 2012;43:431–7.
47. Albers JW, Fink JK. Porphyric neuropathy. Muscle Nerve 2013;30:410–22.
48. Attal N, Cruccu G, Baron R, et al. EFNS guidelines on the pharmacological treatment of neuropathic pain: 2010 revision: treatment of neuropathic pain. Eur J Neurol 2010;17:1113-e88.

49. Griebeler ML, Morey-Vargas OL, Brito JP, et al. Pharmacologic interventions for painful diabetic neuropathy: an umbrella systematic review and comparative effectiveness network meta-analysis. Ann Intern Med 2014;161:639.
50. Callaghan BC, Feldman EL. Painful diabetic neuropathy: many similarly effective therapies with widely dissimilar costs. Ann Intern Med 2014;161:674.
51. Brunelli B, Gorson KC. The use of complementary and alternative medicines by patients with peripheral neuropathy. J Neurol Sci 2004;218:59–66.
52. Richardson JK, Hurvitz EA. Peripheral neuropathy: a true risk factor for falls. J Gerontol A Biol Sci Med Sci 1995;50A:M211–5.
53. Taylor-Stokes G, Pike J, Sadosky A, et al. Association of patient-rated severity with other outcomes in patients with painful diabetic peripheral neuropathy. Diabetes Metab Syndr Obes 2011;4:401–8.
54. Freeman R, Miyawaki E. The treatment of autonomic dysfunction. J Clin Neurophysiol 1993;10:61–82.
55. Finnerup NB, Otto M, McQuay HJ, et al. Algorithm for neuropathic pain treatment: an evidence based proposal. Pain 2005;118:289–305.
56. Dworkin RH, O'Connor AB, Backonja M, et al. Pharmacologic management of neuropathic pain: evidence-based recommendations. Pain 2007;132:237–51.

Moving?

Make sure your subscription moves with you!

To notify us of your new address, find your **Clinics Account Number** (located on your mailing label above your name), and contact customer service at:

Email: journalscustomerservice-usa@elsevier.com

800-654-2452 (subscribers in the U.S. & Canada)
314-447-8871 (subscribers outside of the U.S. & Canada)

Fax number: 314-447-8029

Elsevier Health Sciences Division
Subscription Customer Service
3251 Riverport Lane
Maryland Heights, MO 63043

*To ensure uninterrupted delivery of your subscription, please notify us at least 4 weeks in advance of move.